Methods in Molecular Biology

Series Editor
John M. Walker
School of Life and Medical Sciences
University of Hertfordshire
Hatfield, Hertfordshire, AL10 9AB, UK

For further volumes:
http://www.springer.com/series/7651

Targeted Drug Delivery

Methods and Protocols

Edited by

Rachael W. Sirianni

Vivian L. Smith Department of Neurosurgery, University of Texas Health Science Center at Houston, Houston, TX, USA; Barrow Neurological Institute, Phoenix, AZ, USA

Bahareh Behkam

Department of Mechanical Engineering, Virginia Tech, Blacksburg, VA, USA; School of Biomedical Engineering and Sciences, Virginia Tech, Blacksburg, VA, USA; Macromolecules Innovation Institute, Virginia Tech, Blacksburg, VA, USA

Humana Press

Editors
Rachael W. Sirianni
Vivian L. Smith Department of Neurosurgery
University of Texas Health Science
Center at Houston
Houston, TX, USA

Barrow Neurological Institute
Phoenix, AZ, USA

Bahareh Behkam
Department of Mechanical Engineering
Virginia Tech
Blacksburg, VA, USA

School of Biomedical Engineering and Sciences
Virginia Tech
Blacksburg, VA, USA

Macromolecules Innovation Institute
Virginia Tech
Blacksburg, VA, USA

ISSN 1064-3745 ISSN 1940-6029 (electronic)
Methods in Molecular Biology
ISBN 978-1-4939-8659-0 ISBN 978-1-4939-8661-3 (eBook)
https://doi.org/10.1007/978-1-4939-8661-3

Library of Congress Control Number: 2018948358

Printed on acid-free paper

This Humana Press imprint is published by the registered company Springer Science+Business Media, LLC part of Springer Nature.
The registered company address is: 233 Spring Street, New York, NY 10013, U.S.A.

Preface

Our species has long recognized that *where* and *how* a drug is applied to the body will alter its biological potency. Inhalation of nicotine produces mild and transient euphoria; ingestion of the same substance is lethal. An antibiotic washed over the surface of the skin may become ineffective quickly; the same substance administered as a systemic therapy, or released slowly from a carefully prepared topical bandage, can halt a life-threatening infection.

Modern approaches to drug delivery originated in a happenstance experiment performed by the great angiogenesis researcher Judah Folkman. While utilizing Silastic® (silicone rubber) tubing as an arterio-venous shunt in rabbits, Folkman and colleagues noticed that exposing the external surface of the tubing to anesthetic gases produced sedation [1]. Perhaps most significantly, the silastic tubing could be implanted, and altering the thickness of the tubing changed the rate at which molecules were transported through the material. Several years later, a scientist by the name of Robert Langer would conduct postdoctoral research in Folkman's laboratory. In 1976, Folkman and Langer published the first report utilizing polymeric biomaterials to deliver and control the action of macromolecules [2]. Thus the field of drug delivery was born.

From these basic beginnings, drug delivery has become an essential consideration in fields ranging from oncology to infectious disease, endocrinology, and reproductive medicine. Drug-loaded biomaterials are integrated into many kinds of medical practice, with the greatest clinical successes observed for implants and coatings that locally release their active agents. More recent innovations highlight the potential of miniaturizing these biomaterials to serve as circulating or mobile carriers for active agents. Our challenge as scientists invested in the field of nanocarrier drug delivery has become even greater and focused across an even smaller length scale: can we design therapeutic approaches that will redirect drug distribution to target tissue and cellular compartments? Such targeting will enhance drug potency to treat disease while reducing systemic exposure and toxicity.

In this volume on *Targeted Drug Delivery*, we will address important methods that enable therapeutic molecules to be targeted for site-specific delivery. In Part I, we will describe approaches to formulate biologically derived and synthetic nanocarriers. Part II will overview diverse strategies to facilitate nanocarrier targeting to specific cells and tissues. In Part III, we will cover select methods for evaluating delivery and efficacy of these new classes of agents.

As is often observed in the field of bioengineering, these methods will integrate chemistry, physics, and biology to solve important medical problems. It is our hope that this volume will serve as a valuable resource to understand the diversity of scientific methods available to achieve targeted drug delivery.

Houston, TX, USA *Rachael W. Sirianni*
Blacksburg, VA, USA *Bahareh Behkam*

References

1. Folkman J, Long DM (1964) The use of silicone rubber as a carrier for prolonged drug therapy. J Surg Res 4(3):139–142
2. Langer R, Folkman J (1976) Polymers for the sustained release of proteins and other macromolecules. Nature 263:797–800

Contents

Part III Measuring Delivery and Efficacy

Contributors

IRVING C. ALLEN • *Department of Biomedical Sciences and Pathobiology, Virginia-Maryland College of Veterinary Medicine, Virginia Tech, Blacksburg, VA, USA; Graduate Program in Translational Biology, Medicine, and Health, Virginia Tech, Blacksburg, VA, USA; Department of Biomedical Sciences, Carilion School of Medicine, Virginia Tech, Roanoke, VA, USA*

JULI R. BAGÓ • *Division of Molecular Pharmaceutics, UNC Eshelman School of Pharmacy, The University of North Carolina at Chapel Hill, Chapel Hill, NC, USA*

BAHAREH BEHKAM • *Department of Mechanical Engineering, Virginia Tech, Blacksburg, VA, USA; School of Biomedical Engineering and Sciences, Virginia Tech, Blacksburg, VA, USA; Macromolecules Innovation Institute, Virginia Tech, Blacksburg, VA, USA*

MICHAEL R. CAPLAN • *School of Biological and Health Systems Engineering, Fulton Schools of Engineering, Arizona State University, Tempe, AZ, USA*

EUGENE P. CHUNG • *Barrow Brain Tumor Research Center, Barrow Neurological Institute, St. Joseph's Hospital and Medical Center, Phoenix, AZ, USA*

SHERYL L. COUTERMARSH-OTT • *Department of Biomedical Sciences and Pathobiology, Virginia-Maryland College of Veterinary Medicine, Virginia Tech, Blacksburg, VA, USA*

EMILY S. DAY • *University of Delaware Biomedical Engineering, Newark, DE, USA*

MATTHEW R. DEWITT • *Virginia Tech- Wake Forest School of Biomedical Engineering and Sciences, Blacksburg, VA, USA*

DANIELLE M. DIPERNA • *Barrow Brain Tumor Research Center, Barrow Neurological Institute, St. Joseph's Hospital and Medical Center, Phoenix, AZ, USA*

JACOB ELMER • *Department of Chemical Engineering, Villanova University, Villanova, PA, USA*

STEPHEN L. HAYWARD • *Department of Chemical and Biomolecular Engineering, University of Nebraska-Lincoln, Lincoln, NE, USA; Division of Hematology/Oncology, Department of Internal Medicine, University of Michigan Medical School, Ann Arbor, MI, USA*

XIAOMING HE • *Fischell Department of Bioengineering, University of Maryland, College Park, MD, USA*

SHAWN D. HINGTGEN • *Division of Molecular Pharmaceutics, UNC Eshelman School of Pharmacy, The University of North Carolina at Chapel Hill, Chapel Hill, NC, USA; Biomedical Research Imaging Center, The University of North Carolina at Chapel Hill, Chapel Hill, NC, USA; Lineberger Comprehensive Cancer Center, The University of North Carolina at Chapel Hill, Chapel Hill, NC, USA*

KULLERVO HYNYNEN • *Physical Sciences Platform, Sunnybrook Research Institute, Toronto, ON, Canada; Department of Medical Biophysics, University of Toronto, Toronto, ON, Canada; Institute of Biomaterials and Biomedical Engineering, University of Toronto, Toronto, ON, Canada*

STEVEN M. JAY • *Fischell Department of Bioengineering, University of Maryland, College Park, MD, USA; Program in Oncology, Marlene and Stewart Greenebaum Cancer Center, University of Maryland, College Park, MD, USA; Program in Molecular and Cell Biology, University of Maryland, College Park, MD, USA*

JOHN R. KAGEL • *Translational Oncology and Nanoparticle Drug Development Initiative (TOND2I) Lab, UNC Eshelman School of Pharmacy, UNC Lineberger Comprehensive Cancer Center, Carolina Center for Cancer Nanotechnology Excellence, The University of North Carolina at Chapel Hill, Chapel Hill, NC, USA*

SRIVATSAN KIDAMBI • *Department of Chemical and Biomolecular Engineering, University of Nebraska-Lincoln, Lincoln, NE, USA; Fred & Pamela Buffett Cancer Center, University of Nebraska Medical Center, Omaha, NE, USA; Nebraska Center for Integrated Biomolecular Communication, University of Nebraska, Lincoln, NE, USA; Nebraska Center for the Prevention of Obesity Diseases, University of Nebraska, Lincoln, NE, USA; Nebraska Center for Materials and Nanoscience, University of Nebraska, Lincoln, NE, USA; Mary and Dick Holland Regenerative Medicine Program, University of Nebraska Medical Center, Omaha, NE, USA*

TEK N. LAMICHHANE • *Fischell Department of Bioengineering, University of Maryland, College Park, MD, USA*

ANDREW T. LUCAS • *Translational Oncology and Nanoparticle Drug Development Initiative (TOND2I) Lab, UNC Eshelman School of Pharmacy, UNC Lineberger Comprehensive Cancer Center, Carolina Center for Cancer Nanotechnology Excellence, The University of North Carolina at Chapel Hill, Chapel Hill, NC, USA*

WILLIAM MARSH • *School of Biological and Health Systems Engineering, Ira A. Fulton Schools of Engineering, Arizona State University, Tempe, AZ, USA*

DYLAN K. MCDANIEL • *Department of Biomedical Sciences and Pathobiology, Virginia-Maryland College of Veterinary Medicine, Virginia Tech, Blacksburg, VA, USA*

JILIAN R. MELAMED • *University of Delaware Biomedical Engineering, Newark, DE, USA*

MEAGHAN A. O'REILLY • *Physical Sciences Platform, Sunnybrook Research Institute, Toronto, ON, Canada; Department of Medical Biophysics, University of Toronto, Toronto, ON, Canada*

TORAL R. PATEL • *Department of Neurological Surgery, UT Southwestern Medical Center, Dallas, TX, USA*

THRIMOORTHY POTTA • *Chemical Engineering, School for Engineering of Matter, Transport and Energy, Arizona State University, Tempe, AZ, USA*

ALESIA V. PRAKAPENKA • *Barrow Brain Tumor Research Center, Barrow Neurological Institute, St. Joseph's Hospital and Medical Center, Phoenix, AZ, USA; Department of Psychology, Arizona State University, Tempe, AZ, USA*

KAUSHAL REGE • *Chemical Engineering, School for Engineering of Matter, Transport and Energy, Arizona State University, Tempe, AZ, USA*

RACHEL S. RILEY • *University of Delaware Biomedical Engineering, Newark, DE, USA*

VERONICA M. RINGEL-SCAIA • *Graduate Program in Translational Biology, Medicine, and Health, Virginia Tech, Blacksburg, VA, USA*

M. NICHOLE RYLANDER • *Department of Mechanical Engineering, University of Texas at Austin, Austin, TX, USA; Department of Biomedical Engineering, University of Texas at Austin, Austin, TX, USA*

ALI SAHARI • *School of Biomedical Engineering and Sciences, Virginia Tech, Blacksburg, VA, USA*

ALLISON N. SCHORZMAN • *Translational Oncology and Nanoparticle Drug Development Initiative (TOND2I) Lab, UNC Eshelman School of Pharmacy, UNC Lineberger Comprehensive Cancer Center, Carolina Center for Cancer Nanotechnology Excellence, The University of North Carolina at Chapel Hill, Chapel Hill, NC, USA*
KEVIN T. SHEETS • *Division of Molecular Pharmaceutics, UNC Eshelman School of Pharmacy, The University of North Carolina at Chapel Hill, Chapel Hill, NC, USA*
RACHAEL W. SIRIANNI • *Vivian L. Smith Department of Neurosurgery, University of Texas Health Science Center at Houston, Houston, TX, USA; Barrow Neurological Institute, Phoenix, AZ, USA*
SARAH E. STABENFELDT • *School of Biological and Health Systems Engineering, Ira A. Fulton Schools of Engineering, Arizona State University, Tempe, AZ, USA*
JILL M. STEINBACH-RANKINS • *Department of Bioengineering and Center for Predictive Medicine, University of Louisville, Louisville, KY, USA*
MAHAMA A. TRAORE • *Department of Mechanical Engineering, Virginia Tech, Blacksburg, VA, USA; School of Biomedical Engineering and Sciences, Virginia Tech, Blacksburg, VA, USA*
HAI WANG • *Fischell Department of Bioengineering, University of Maryland, College Park, MD, USA*
AMANDA WITTEN • *School of Biological and Health Systems Engineering, Ira A. Fulton Schools of Engineering, Arizona State University, Tempe, AZ, USA*
XINGWANG WU • *Department of Neurosurgery, Yale University, New Haven, CT, USA; Department of Radiology, The First Affiliated Hospital of Anhui Medical University, Hefei, Anhui, China*
WILLIAM C. ZAMBONI • *Translational Oncology and Nanoparticle Drug Development Initiative (TOND2I) Lab, UNC Eshelman School of Pharmacy, UNC Lineberger Comprehensive Cancer Center, Carolina Center for Cancer Nanotechnology Excellence, The University of North Carolina at Chapel Hill, Chapel Hill, NC, USA*
JIANGBING ZHOU • *Department of Neurosurgery, Yale University, New Haven, CT, USA*

Part I

Drug Carrier Design

Chapter 1

Synthesis of Cationic Polymer Libraries for Gene Delivery Using Diglycidyl Ethers

Jacob Elmer, Thrimoorthy Potta, and Kaushal Rege

Abstract

Gene therapy has the potential to cure many different genetic diseases, if safe and effective gene delivery vectors can be developed. This chapter describes protocols for the synthesis of novel polymers using diglycidyl ether and diamine or polyamine monomers for transgene delivery and expression. The resulting poly (amino ethers) are able to transfect a higher number of cells, with lower cytotoxicity than other commercially available polymers (e.g., Polyethyleneimine, PEI).

Key words Polymers, Gene therapy, Gene delivery, Polyplex, Aminoglycosides, Diglycidyl ethers

1 Introduction

Point mutations in the genome can cause hundreds of different genetic disorders (e.g., hemophilia [1] and cancer [2]). Gene therapy could potentially treat many of these diseases by replacing or supplementing these mutated genes. Indeed, one form of blindness (e.g., Leber's Congenital Amaurosis, LCA) has been cured by using an adenovirus to deliver a functional RPE65 gene that replaces the mutated RPE65 gene in patients with LCA [3]. Viral gene therapy has also shown promise in treating other genetic diseases like immunodeficiency, but ~20% of the patients receiving the therapy also developed leukemia when the virus inserted its gene near oncogenes [4].

In addition to carcinogenesis, some viral gene therapy strategies are also induce inflammation [5] and are limited by low payload capacity (i.e., gene size [6]), high production costs, and other issues [7]. These issues have motivated researchers to develop alternative "non-viral" gene delivery vectors that do not have the same safety concerns as viral vectors. For example, several cationic lipids [8], polymers [9], and dendrimers [10] have been designed to bind anionic DNA to form polyplexes that are endocytosed by cells. Unfortunately, while these non-viral vectors

Rachael W. Sirianni and Bahareh Behkam (eds.), *Targeted Drug Delivery: Methods and Protocols*, Methods in Molecular Biology, vol. 1831, https://doi.org/10.1007/978-1-4939-8661-3_1, © Springer Science+Business Media, LLC, part of Springer Nature 2018

have shown some promise, they are typically limited by low transfection efficiency (i.e., percent of cells expressing the transgene) and high toxicity [11, 12].

In this chapter, we describe methods to synthesize cationic polymers for gene delivery. These polymers, described in our previous reports [13, 14], are formed by a ring-opening polymerization reaction between epoxides on diglycidyl ether monomers and primary/secondary amines on polyamine or aminoglycoside monomers. Several of the resulting Poly(polyamino ether) (PPAE) or Poly(amino glycoside ether) (PAGE) polymers demonstrate significantly higher transgene expression efficacies and lower cytotoxicities than other cationic polymers (e.g., 25 kDa polyethyleneimine, PEI) [13, 14].

2 Materials

All solutions should be prepared using ultra pure water, unless otherwise mentioned. Cell culture materials and recombinant plasmid DNA should be disposed by following proper biosafety procedures.

2.1 Synthesis of Poly(Polyamino Ether) Polymers

Any combination of diglycidyl ether and polyamine monomers can be used to prepare cationic poly(polyamino ether) (PPAE) polymers, but for the purposes of this discussion we will focus on the reaction of 1,4-cyclohexanedimethanol diglycidyl ether (1,4C) and 1,4-bis(3-aminopropyl) piperazine (1,4Bis) to form a 1,4C-1,4Bis polymer.

1. 20 mL glass scintillation vials and 50 mL tubes.
2. 10× PBS: 40.9 g NaCl, 1.0 g KCl, 7.1 g Na_2HPO_4, 1.2 g KH_2PO_4, 500 mL water, pH 7.4.
3. Diglycidyl Ether (DE) monomers (Sigma Aldrich, St. Louis, MO; partial list):
   (a) 1,4-butanmediol diglycidyl ether (1,4B).
   (b) 1,4-cyclohexanedimethanol diglycidyl ether (1,4C).
   (c) 4-vinylcyclohexene diepoxide (4VCD).
   (d) Ethylene glycol diglycidyl ether (EDGE).
   (e) Glycerol diglycidyl ether (GDE).
   (f) Neopentylglycol diglycidyl ether (NPDGE).
   (g) Poly(ethylene glycol) diglycidyl ether (PEGDE).
   (h) Poly(propylene glycol) diglycidyl ether (PPGDE).
   (i) Resorcinol diglycidyl ether (RDE).

4. Mono, di, and polyamino monomers (Sigma Aldrich, St. Louis, MO; partial list):
   (a) 1-(2-aminoethyl) piperidine.
   (b) 1,4-bis(3-aminopropyl) piperazine (1,4Bis).
   (c) 3,3′-diamino-N-methyl dipropylamine.
   (d) 4,7,10-trioxa-1,13-tridecanediamine.
   (e) Aniline.
   (f) Butylamine.
   (g) Diethylenetriamine.
   (h) Ethylenediamine.
   (i) N-(2-aminoethyl)-1,3-propanediamine.
   (j) Pentaethylenehexamine.
5. Dialysis tubing (3.5 kDa MWCO) (Spectrum Labs, Rancho Dominguez, CA).
6. Hydrochloric Acid (HCl) for titration.
7. Nitrogen gas (N_2).

2.2 Synthesis of Poly(Amino Glycoside Ether) Polymers

The same diglycidyl ethers listed in Subheading 2.1 may be used in this section.

1. 0.01× PBS (*see* Subheading 2.1).
2. 20 mL glass vials.
3. Diglycidyl Ethers (*see* Subheading 2.1).
4. Aminoglycoside monomers (Sigma Aldrich, St. Louis, MO):
   (a) Apramycin sulfate.
   (b) Paramomycin sulfate.
   (c) Sisomicin sulfate.
   (d) Amikacin hydrate.
   (e) Neomycin sulfate.
   (f) Kanamycin A sulfate.
   (g) Streptomycin sulfate.
5. Amberlite anion exchange resin (Sigma Aldrich, St. Louis, MO).
6. Acetone.
7. Dimethylformamide (DMF).
8. Dialysis Tubing (3.5 kDa MWCO) (Spectrum Labs, Rancho Dominguez, CA).
9. Hydrochloric Acid (HCl) for titration.
10. Nitrogen gas (N_2).

2.3 Quantification of Polymer Toxicity (MTT Assay)

For the purposes of this discussion, we will use the MTT assay kit and human prostate cancer cells (PC3) from the American Type Culture Collection (ATCC, Manassas, VA). However, many other cell lines and cell viability assays are available from other manufacturers.

1. PC3 human prostate cancer cells (ATCC, Manassas, VA).
2. MTT Cell Proliferation Assay Kit (ATCC, Manassas, VA). This kit contains the MTT dye and a detergent solution for cell lysis.
3. Tissue-culture treated 24-well plates.
4. Fetal bovine Serum (FBS).
5. Cell Culture Media, with (SCM) and without (SFM) serum (FBS).
6. Aluminum Foil.

2.4 Cell Transfection and Luciferase Assay

For the purposes of this discussion, we will use the pGL4.50 luciferase expression plasmid and luciferase assay kit from Promega (Madison, WI) to test the transfection efficacy of the polymers from Subheadings 3.1 and 3.2 with PC3 human prostate cancer cells (ATCC).

1. PC3 human prostate cancer cells (ATCC, Manassas, VA).
2. Tissue-culture treated 24-well plates.
3. Clear 96-well plates.
4. Half-area white 96-well plates.
5. Fetal bovine Serum (FBS).
6. Cell Culture Media, with (SCM) and without (SFM) serum (FBS).
7. 1×PBS (*see* Subheading 2.1).
8. Cationic polymers from Subheading 3.1 or 3.2.
9. Luciferase expression plasmid pGL4.50 (Promega, Madison, WI).
10. Cell Culture Lysis Reagent (CCLR) (Promega, Madison, WI).
11. Luciferase Assay Kit (Promega, Madison, WI). This kit contains Luciferase Assay Buffer and Luciferin powder.
12. Bicinchoninic Acid (BCA) Assay Kit (Thermo-Fisher Scientific, Rockford, IL). This kit contains Reagents A and B and a bovine serum albumin (BSA) standard.

3 Methods

The following protocols (Subheadings 3.1–3.4) describe methods for synthesizing cationic polymers, determining their effects on cell viability, and evaluating the efficacy of their transgene delivery to mammalian cells. Cell culture steps are performed at 37 °C with 5% CO_2, but all other experiments are performed at room temperature in aqueous solution, unless otherwise noted.

3.1 Synthesis of Poly(Polyamino Ether) (PPAE) Polymers

The following protocol describes the general synthesis of cationic polymers with alternating diglycidyl ether and amino monomers (e.g., 1,4 Cyclohexanedimethanol diglycidyl ether (1,4C) and 1,4-Bis(3-aminopropyl) piperazine (1,4Bis), respectively. *See* Figs. 1 and 2 for monomer structures). The monomers polymerize in a chain reaction in which primary and secondary amines react with the epoxide rings in the diglycidyl ethers to form hydroxyls in the growing polyamino ether polymer (*see* Fig. 3). [13, 15].

1. Add the amine and diglycidyl ether monomers in a 1:1 molar ratio in a glass vial (*see* **Note 1**). For example, mix 238.2 μL 1,4C with 269.5 μL 1,4Bis.
2. Briefly vortex the vial to completely mix the monomers.
3. Incubate the vial at room temperature (25 °C) for approximately 16 h (*see* **Note 2**).
4. Weigh the polymer mixture and add enough 1× PBS to prepare a 10 mg/mL solution (*see* **Note 3**).
5. Vortex the vial to resuspend the polymer solution and transfer it to a 50 mL tube (*see* **Note 4**).

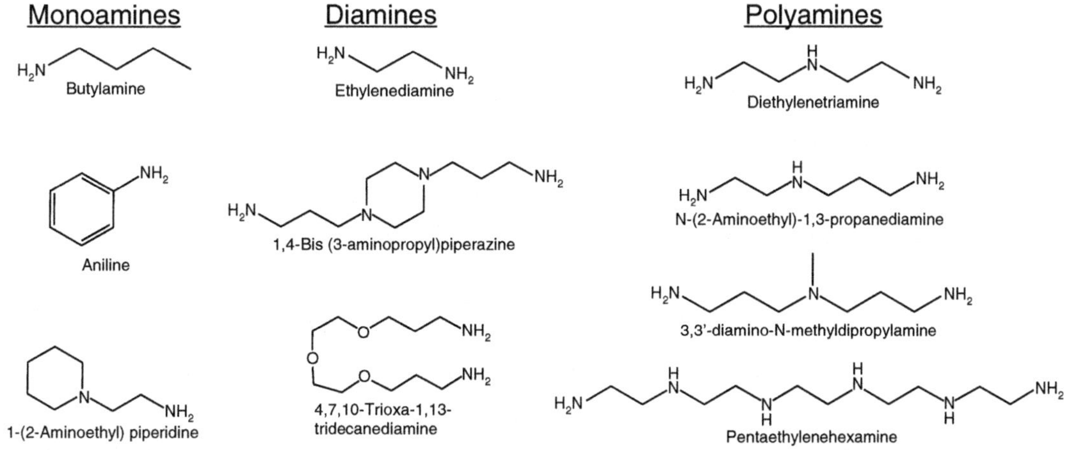

Fig. 1 Mono, di, and poly-amine monomers

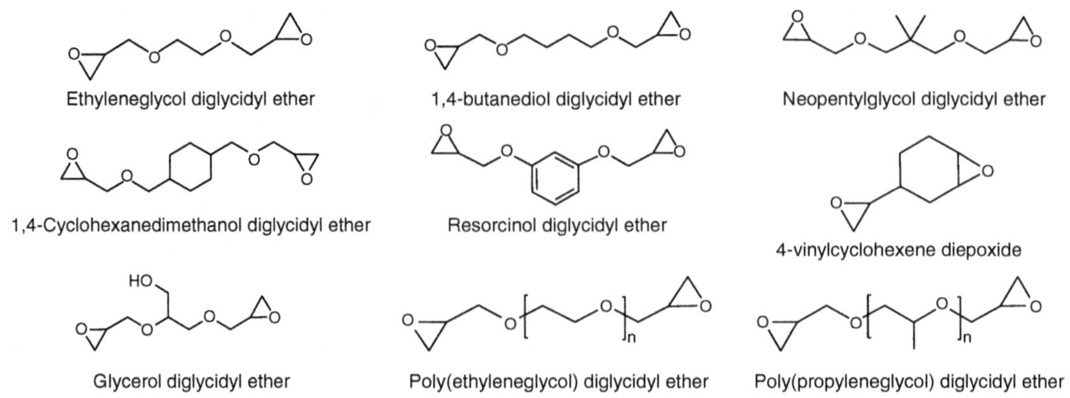

Fig. 2 Diglycidyl ether monomers

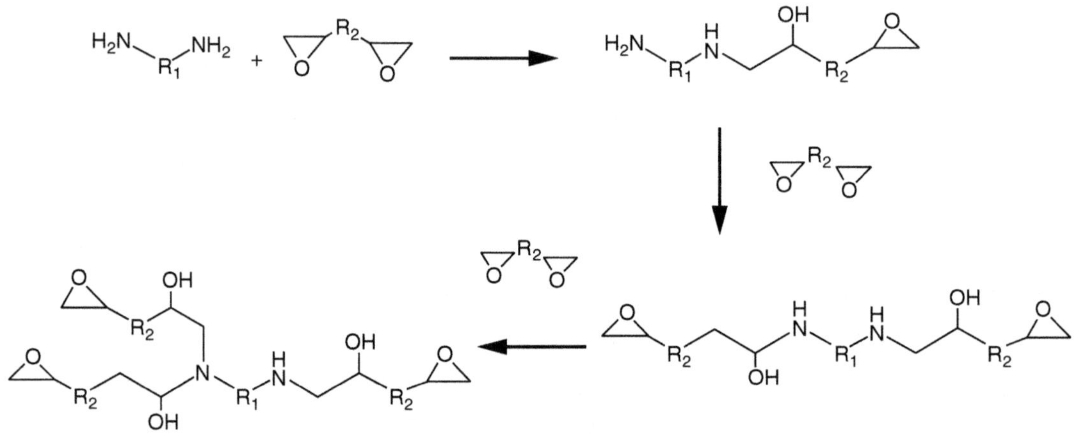

Fig. 3 Polymerization of diglycidyl ethers (e.g., 1,4C) and polyamino monomers (e.g., 1,4Bis). Reprinted with permission from (Sutapa Barua, Amit Joshi, Akhilesh Banerjee, Dana Matthews, Susan T. Sharfstein, Steven M. Cramer, Ravi S. Kane, and Kaushal Rege. Parallel synthesis and screening of polymers for nonviral gene delivery. *Mol Pharm* 6:86–97.). Copyright (2009) American Chemical Society

6. Adjust the pH of the polymer solution to 7.4 using HCl.
7. Incubate the polymer solution with shaking (100 rpm) at room temperature (25 °C) for an additional 12 h to completely dissolve any remaining polymer. Check the pH of the polymer solution as often as possible to maintain a pH of 7.4.
8. Remove unreacted monomers and small polymers from the polymer solution by transferring it to dialysis membrane tubing with a molecular weight cutoff of 3.5 kDa. Submerge the dialysis tubing in 2–4 L of distilled water and change the water twice a day for 2 days.
9. Transfer the dialyzed polymer solution to a new 50 mL tube and freeze at −80 °C for ≥3 h.

10. Freeze dry the frozen polymer solution to obtain dry polymer powder (*see* **Note 5**).
11. Store the solid polymer at −20 °C in nitrogen gas (N_2) (*see* **Note 6**).

3.2 Synthesis of Poly(Amino Glycoside Ether) (PAGE) Polymers

PAGE polymer synthesis [14] is highly similar to the PPAE polymer synthesis described in Subheading 3.1, but with aminoglycoside monomers (*see* Fig. 4) and a few other key differences, as shown in the protocol below. Since this protocol requires DMF and acetone, caution must be taken when working with these solvents. Use appropriate personal protective equipment and only use these solvents in a chemical fume hood.

1. The sulfates associated with the aminoglycoside monomers must be replaced with chlorides via anion exchange with Amberlite resin to increase reactivity (*see* **Note 7**)
2. Mix the aminoglycoside and diglycidyl ether monomers in a 1:1–1:3 molar ratio. Specifically, amikacin:diglycidyl ether(1:1), kanamycin:diglycidyl ether (1:2), steptomycin:diglycidyl ether(1:2) apramycin:diglycidyl ether (1:2.1), paramomycin:diglycidyl ether (1:2.2), sisomycin:diglycidyl ether (1:2), neomycin:diglycidyl ether(1:3) (*see* **Note 8**).
3. Transfer the required amount of aminoglycoside monomer (in the chloride form) into a 20 mL glass vial and add 1.5 mL of water. Vortex for 5 min to dissolve the monomer, then add 1 mL of DMF and stir the monomer mixture at 60 °C for 5 h.
4. Cool the polymer mixture to room temperature.

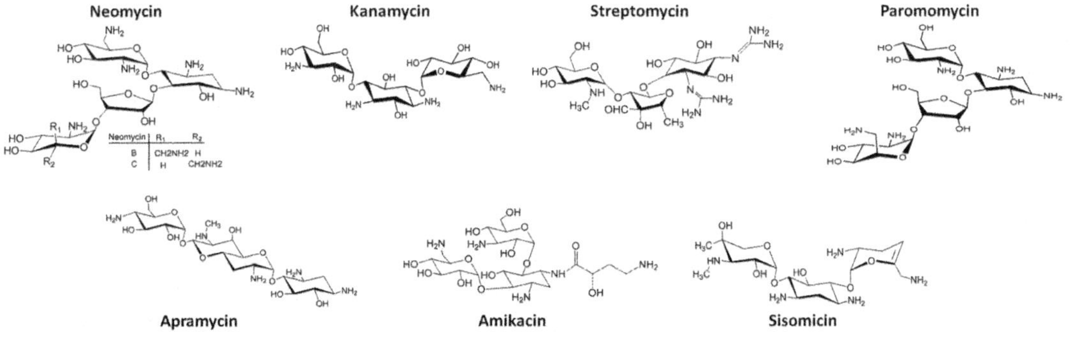

Fig. 4 Aminoglycoside monomers used for polymerization. All of these monomers formed polymers that were able to successfully transfect human prostate (PC3) and pancreatic (Mia PaCa-2) cancer cell lines with the following transfection efficiencies: Apramycin-RDE > Paromomycin-RDE > Paromomycin-GDE > Sisomicin-RDE > Sisomicin-GDE > Amikacin-EGDE > Neomycin-GDE

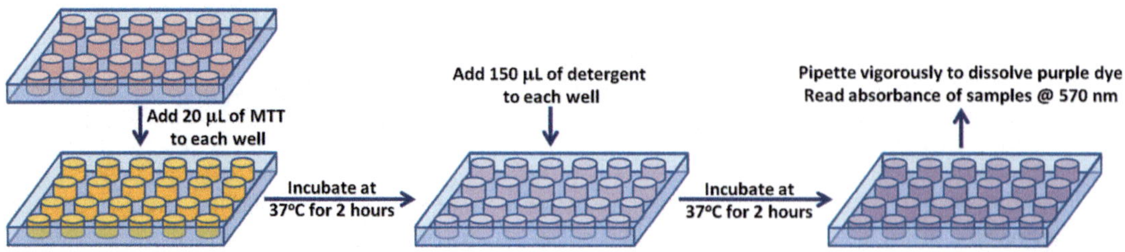

Fig. 5 Overview of MTT Assay procedure. Start by adding 20 μL of MTT reagent to each well and incubate at 37 °C for 2 h. Then add 150 μL of detergent solution to each well and incubate for an additional 2 h at 37 °C. Finally, resuspend the purple dye by vigorously pipetting each well and read the absorbance of the solution at 570 nm

5. Transfer the reaction mixture into 50 mL falcon tube, add 40 mL of acetone and keep aside overnight to precipitate the polymer.
6. Remove the supernatant. Wash the precipitate twice with 40 mL of acetone.
7. Air dry the precipitate for 1 h to remove acetone.
8. Dissolve the dried precipitate in 10 mL nanopure water.
9. Remove unreacted aminoglycosides and small polymers from the polymer solution by transferring it to dialysis membrane tubing with a molecular weight cutoff of 3.5 kDa.
   (a) Submerge the dialysis tubing in 2–4 L of distilled water.
   (b) Change the water twice a day for 2 days.
10. Transfer the dialyzed polymer solution to a new 50 mL tube and freeze at −80 °C for ≥3 h.
11. Freeze-dry the frozen polymer solution to obtain dry polymer powder (*see* **Note 5**).
12. Store the solid polymer at −20 °C in nitrogen gas (N_2) (*see* **Notes 6** and **9**).

3.3 Measuring the Effects of PPAE and PAGE Polymers on Cell Viability

The cytotoxicity of cationic polymers may be quantified using the MTT Assay [16] (Fig. 5). In this assay, a yellow tetrazolium dye (3-(4,5-dimethylthiazol-2-yl)-2,3-diphenyltetrazolium bromide) is reduced to an insoluble purple formazan dye by NADPH-dependent oxidoreductase enzymes inside living cells. Since these enzymes are not found in the cell culture media or inside dead cells, the amount of yellow tetrazolium converted to purple formazan may be measured and used to estimate the number of metabolically active cells in a sample [16]. Therefore, this assay may be used as an indirect indicator of living cell concentrations. Since MTT is light sensitive, protect it from light whenever possible.

1. Passage 50,000 cells into each well of a 24-well plate and incubate at 37 °C and 5% CO_2 for at least 16 h with 500 μL of media per well.
2. Perform a transfection with the polymer(s) as described in Subheading 3.4. Be sure to leave at least three wells on each plate for a live (untreated) control that is not exposed to any polymer or DNA.
3. Add 20 μL of MTT reagent (yellow dye) directly to the media in each well.
4. The MTT dye is light sensitive, so wrap the plate(s) in aluminum foil and incubate them at 37 °C for 2–4 h (*see* **Note 10**).
5. Add 150 μL of detergent to each well and incubate at 37 °C for another 2–4 h (*see* **Note 11**).
6. Vigorously pipette the liquid in each well until the formazan dye is completely dissolved.
7. Transfer 150 μL from each well to a clear 96-well plate (*see* **Note 12**).
8. Read the absorbance of each well at 570 nm (A_{570}).
9. Transfer the remaining liquid from each well of the 24-well plate to a weigh dish on an analytical balance and record the masses (m).
10. Correct the absorbance values obtained in **step 8** for any volume lost to evaporation (*see* **Note 13**) during the 37 °C incubation steps with Eq. 1 (*see* **Note 14**):

$$A_{570,\mathrm{corrected}} = A_{570}\frac{m + 150\ \mathrm{mg}}{570\ \mathrm{mg}} \quad (1)$$

11. Use the corrected absorbance values ($A_{C,570}$) and Eq. 2 to calculate the cell viability relative to the live control ($A_{C,570\ \mathrm{Live}}$) for each well (*see* **Note 15**).

$$\%\mathrm{Viability} = \frac{A_{C,570}}{A_{C,570\ \mathrm{Live}}} \cdot 100\% \quad (2)$$

3.4 Cell Transfection and Luciferase Assay

The transfection efficiency of polymers may be determined by using them to transfect mammalian cells with a plasmid containing a gene for a luciferase enzyme (Fig. 6). This protocol will describe the transfection of cells with the plasmid pGL4.50 from Promega, which carries a gene for the luciferase from the common firefly *Photinus pyralis* [17]. However, it is important to mention that plasmids carrying genes for other luciferases (e.g., from the sea pansy *Renilla reniformis* [18] or the shrimp

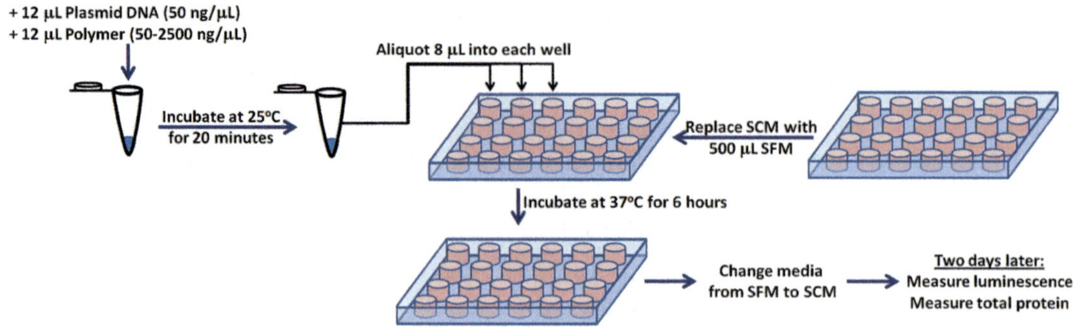

Fig. 6 Overview of Transfection procedure. DNA (50 ng/μL) and polymer (at desired concentration) are mixed in a separate tube and incubated at room temperature for 20 min for polyplex formation. Meanwhile, the SCM media in the 24-well plates is exchanged for SFM media. Eight microliters of polyplex is dispensed into each well and the plate is incubated at 37 °C for 6 h, after which time the media is changed back to SCM and the plates are incubated for an additional 2 days to allow luciferase to be expressed

Oplophorus gracilirostris [19]) are also available and may provide higher luminescence signals, if needed. Regardless of which enzyme is used, the amount of luciferase expressed can be measured by adding its substrate luciferin and measuring the light produced (i.e., luminescence). The amount of luminescence can then be used to determine the transfection efficiency (i.e., amount of reporter protein expressed) of each polymer.

1. Passage 50,000 cells into each well of a 24-well plate and incubate at 37 °C and 5% CO_2 for at least 16 h with 500 μL of serum-containing media per well.
2. Immediately before the transfection, dissolve the required amount of polymer in 0.01× PBS buffer (*see* **Note 16**).
3. Titrate the pH of the polymer solution to 7.4, if necessary.
4. Mix the polymer with plasmid DNA (we recommend pGL4.50 from Promega) in the desired weight ratio (*see* **Note 17**).
5. Incubate the polymer-DNA mixture at room temperature for 20 min to allow polyplexes to form.
6. Meanwhile, remove the serum-containing media (SCM) from each well and replace it with 500 μL of serum-free media (SFM) (*see* **Note 18**).
7. Add the desired amount of polyplex to each well (*see* **Note 19**) and incubate at 37 °C for 6 h (*see* **Note 20**).
8. Replace the SFM with SCM and incubate the cells at 37 °C for 2 days (48 h).
9. Remove the media from each well and rinse with 150 μL of 1× PBS (*see* **Note 21**).
10. Remove the 1× PBS from each well and add 150 μL of 1× Cell Culture Lysis Reagent.

11. Incubate the plate at 37 °C for 10–20 min to ensure complete cell lysis (*see* **Note 22**).
12. Add 500 μL of 1× PBS to each of the cell lysates. These samples will be used for the luciferase assay in **step 14**.
13. Transfer 50 μL of each cell lysate to a new 24-well plate and dilute with 450 μL of 1× PBS (Dilution factor, $D = 10$). These diluted samples will be used to measure for the BCA assay in **step 15**.
14. Perform a luciferase assay to quantify the amount of luciferase enzyme in each sample:
    (a) Immediately prior to the assay, prepare fresh substrate (luciferin) solution by adding the provided Luciferase Assay Buffer to the Luciferin Powder (*see* **Note 23**).
    (b) Transfer 15 μL of cell lysate (V_{lysate}) to a half-area 96-well plate.
    (c) Add 30 μL of luciferin solution to each cell lysate well.
    (d) Immediately record the luminescence (L) in each well (*see* **Note 24**).
15. Perform a BCA Assay to quantify the total protein concentration in each lysate:
    (a) Add 10 μL of the diluted cell lysates from **step 13** to a clear 96-well plate.
    (b) Prepare stocks of Bovine Serum Albumin (BSA) at concentrations of 0.025–2 mg/mL and transfer 10 μL of those solutions to the same 96-well plate.
    (c) If using the Pierce® BCA Protein Assay Kit, mix Reagent A and Reagent B in a 50:1 ratio to make fresh working reagent (*see* **Note 25**).
    (d) Add 190 μL of working reagent to each well and incubate the plate(s) at 37 °C for 30 min (*see* **Note 26**).
    (e) Read the absorbance in each well at 562 nm.
    (f) Use the absorbance values of the BSA samples to prepare a standard curve and estimate the total protein concentration ([P_{total}], mg/mL) of each lysate.
16. Use Eq. 3 (*see* **Note 27**) to calculate the Relative Luminescence Units (RLU) for each sample:

$$\text{RLU} = \frac{L}{D\left[P_{\text{total}}\right]V_{\text{lysate}}} \quad \left(\frac{\text{luminescence units}}{\text{mg of total protein}}\right) \tag{3}$$

17. The RLU values may then be compared to determine the relative transgene expression levels of each polymer.

4 Notes

1. Since most monomers are supplied as viscous liquid solutions, use a pipette to transfer a small amount of each monomer to a glass vial and check their masses using an analytical balance to ensure 1:1 molar ratio of the monomers.
2. Optimum times for polymerization vary depending upon the monomers used (i.e., some monomers may require more or less than the recommended 16 h).
3. The polymer mixture should be a viscous liquid.
4. The pH of the dissolved polymer solution will be highly basic (pH = 10–12) and may appear cloudy. Titration of the polymer solution to pH = 7.4 will reduce the cloudiness of the solution and increase the solubility of any undissolved polymer. Any polymer that refuses to dissolve may be discarded when the solution is transferred to the new 50 mL tube.
5. The freeze-dried polymer may appear white or pale yellow in color.
6. Polymers should always be stored in an anaerobic atmosphere (e.g., nitrogen, N_2). Oxygen (O_2) will likely oxidize the polymers and affect their functionality.
7. A 1:1 ratio must be used for amikacin, since a 1:2 ratio produces an insoluble product.
8. The acetone washes are used to remove excess diglycidyl ethers.
9. Expected yields for PPAE polymers vary between 50 and 60% after dialysis, while PAGE polymers typically have a lower yield (35–45%) after dialysis.
10. Cells will still need oxygen during their incubation with MTT, so be sure to leave enough of an opening in the aluminum foil for gas exchange.
11. Cells should now be visibly purple from formazan dye formation.
12. Bubbles may form in the 96-well plate, and will interfere with absorbance readings. Pop the bubbles before making any measurements.
13. Wells near the outer edge of the plate are especially prone to volume loss by evaporation and may lose as much as 10% of their original volume while wells near the center of the plate experience almost no change in volume. Therefore, it is important to determine actual liquid volumes in each well.
14. In Eq. 1, m is the measured mass of the solution in each well, 150 mg reflects the mass/volume transferred to the 96-well

plate, and 570 mg is the expected mass in each well (500 μL media + 20 μL MTT + 150 μL detergent).

15. In Eq. 2, $A_{C,570}$ is the corrected absorbance value from one of the wells treated with polymer and $A_{C,570\ Live}$ is the average absorbance value of the live cell wells.
16. Do not resuspend polymers in 1× PBS buffer—the large amount of negatively charged phosphates (i.e., high salt concentration) may interfere with polyplex formation, which is driven by electrostatic interactions.
17. Different polymers will have different optimum weight ratios. For example, Polyethyleneimine (PEI) provides the highest transgene expression levels at a 1:1 m:m PEI:pDNA ratio. Values for PPAE and PAGE polymers range from 1:1 to 50:1. All polymers were initially screened at a polymer:DNA w:w ratio of 50:1, but this ratio was lowered for some polymers based on dose response data.
18. The serum in SCM contains albumin and other proteins which are known to bind and sequester charged molecules, including cationic polymers. Therefore, serum is typically removed to prevent it from interfering with the transfection. If SCM is used during the transfection, luminescence values will likely be lower than those obtained when transfections performed with SFM.
19. 100–200 ng of plasmid DNA per well is usually sufficient for transfections. The amount of plasmid DNA may be increased depending on experimental requirements.
20. In some cases, transgene expression can be seen after as little as 3 h incubation with the polyplex.
21. Add PBS to the wells slowly to avoid sloughing off any of the attached cells.
22. Cell lysis can be tracked with a light microscope.
23. Luciferase Assay Buffer contains ATP, which may be damaged by multiple freeze-thaw cycles. Luciferin may also be light sensitive, so protect it from light.
24. Luciferase Assays vary between manufacturers, but most only provide a 1–2 min window in which reliable luminescence data may be recorded after the luciferin solution is mixed with cell lysates. This is a highly non-linear response.
25. Reagent B should be blue, while the working reagent should have a green color.
26. The lysates should change from green to purple, if any protein is present.
27. In Eq. 3, L is the luminescence measured in **step 14d**, D is the dilution factor (e.g., 10) used in **step 13**, $[P_{total}]$ is the total

protein concentration measured in **step 15f**, and V_{lysate} is the volume of the cell lysate used in **step 14b** for the luciferase assay (e.g., 15 μL).

Acknowledgments

We are grateful to the NIH/NIGMS (Grant 1R01GM093229-01A1) for financial support of this study. Chemical structures were drawn using ChemDraw based on those available on the MilliporeSigma website.

References

1. Chen SH, Thompson AR, Zhang M, Scott CR (1989) Three point mutations in the factor IX genes of five hemophilia B patients. Identification strategy using localization by altered epitopes in their hemophilic proteins. J Clin Invest 84:113–118
2. Forbes SA et al (2008) The Catalogue of Somatic Mutations in Cancer (COSMIC). Curr Protoc Hum Genet Chapter 10:Unit 10.11
3. Simonelli F et al (2010) Gene therapy for Leber's congenital amaurosis is safe and effective through 1.5 years after vector administration. Mol Ther 18:643–650
4. Kohn DB, Sadelain M, Glorioso JC (2003) Occurrence of leukaemia following gene therapy of X-linked SCID. Nat Rev Cancer 3:477–488
5. Nayak S, Herzog RW (2010) Progress and prospects: immune responses to viral vectors. Gene Ther 17:295–304
6. Atkinson H, Chalmers R (2010) Delivering the goods: viral and non-viral gene therapy systems and the inherent limits on cargo DNA and internal sequences. Genetica 138:485–498
7. Thomas CE, Ehrhardt A, Kay MA (2003) Progress and problems with the use of viral vectors for gene therapy. Nat Rev Genet 4:346–358
8. Junquera E, Aicart E (2014) Cationic lipids as transfecting agents of DNA in gene therapy. Curr Top Med Chem 14:649–663
9. De Smedt SC, Demeester J, Hennink WE (2000) Cationic polymer based gene delivery systems. Pharm Res 17:113–126
10. Svenson S, Tomalia DA (2012) Dendrimers in biomedical applications—reflections on the field. Adv Drug Deliv Rev 64:102–115
11. Tros de Ilarduya C, Sun Y, Düzgüneş N (2010) Gene delivery by lipoplexes and polyplexes. Eur J Pharm Sci 40:159–170
12. Lv H, Zhang S, Wang B, Cui S, Yan J (2006) Toxicity of cationic lipids and cationic polymers in gene delivery. J Control Release 114:100–109
13. Barua S et al (2009) Parallel synthesis and screening of polymers for nonviral gene delivery. Mol Pharm 6:86–97
14. Potta T et al (2014) Discovery of antibiotics-derived polymers for gene delivery using combinatorial synthesis and cheminformatics modeling. Biomaterials 35:1977–1988
15. Kasman LM, Barua S, Lu P, Rege K, Voelkel-Johnson C (2009) Polymer-enhanced adenoviral transduction of CAR-negative bladder cancer cells. Mol Pharmacol 6:1612–1619
16. Mosmann T (1983) Rapid colorimetric assay for cellular growth and survival: application to proliferation and cytotoxicity assays. J Immunol Methods 65:55–63
17. De Wet JR, Wood KV, DeLuca M, Helinski DR, Subramani S (1987) Firefly luciferase gene: structure and expression in mammalian cells. Mol Cell Biol 7:725–737
18. Hori K, Cormier MJ (1973) Structure and chemical synthesis of a biologically active form of Renilla (sea pansy) luciferin. Proc Natl Acad Sci 70:120–123
19. Hall MP et al (2012) Engineered luciferase reporter from a deep sea shrimp utilizing a novel imidazopyrazinone substrate. ACS Chem Biol 7:1848–1857

Chapter 2

Generation of Ultra-Small PLGA Nanoparticles by Sequential Centrifugation

Xingwang Wu, Jiangbing Zhou, and Toral R. Patel

Abstract

Direct, local delivery of polymer nanoparticles to the brain is a promising strategy to bypass the blood-brain barrier (BBB) and safely deliver a large therapeutic payload. However, even with the aid of convection-enhanced delivery (CED) techniques, this approach has been limited by the inability to fabricate appropriately sized polymer nanoparticles. Here, we outline a versatile and efficient method for producing polymer nanoparticles that are <100 nm in diameter and can be delivered to the brain via CED.

Key words Nanoparticle, Polymer, Convection-enhanced delivery, PLGA, Brain, Blood-brain barrier

1 Introduction

Nanocarriers for drug delivery are typically colloidal systems that range in size from 1 to 500 nm and contain a therapeutic agent. They can be fabricated from a wide variety of biomaterials, including polymers, lipids, and inorganic molecules, based on the desired application. Historically, several polymers have demonstrated excellent safety profiles, and thus, have been utilized for a variety of clinical applications. Of these, the co-polymer poly(lactic-co-glycolic acid) (PLGA), which was approved by the Food and Drug Administration (FDA) in 1969, has been in continuous, safe clinical use for decades [1–3].

Recently, there has been substantial interest in developing polymeric nanoparticles for drug delivery applications. In comparison to free drug, polymer nanoparticles can improve delivery efficiency, reduce off-target effects, improve drug kinetics, and allow delivery of a chemically diverse range of therapeutic agents. These advantages are particularly important when considering drug delivery strategies for central nervous system (CNS) disorders, which are isolated from the systemic circulation by the blood-brain barrier (BBB).

Rachael W. Sirianni and Bahareh Behkam (eds.), *Targeted Drug Delivery: Methods and Protocols*, Methods in Molecular Biology, vol. 1831, https://doi.org/10.1007/978-1-4939-8661-3_2, © Springer Science+Business Media, LLC, part of Springer Nature 2018

Polymer nanoparticles can be designed for either systemic or local delivery [1, 2]. Systemic delivery platforms seek to bypass the BBB by utilizing receptor-mediated and adsorptive-mediated transcytosis pathways, typically by coating the nanoparticles with specific targeting ligands. Local delivery platforms completely bypass the BBB and rely on convection-enhanced delivery (CED) to achieve adequate distribution through the brain interstitium.

One of the biggest challenges to employing polymer nanoparticles for local delivery to the CNS is the production of appropriately sized particles. It has been demonstrated that the pore size of the normal brain extracellular matrix is between 38–64 nm [4]. The pore size is enlarged in brain tumors and can reach up to 100 nm [5]. However, typical fabrication protocols will produce polymer nanoparticles that are approximately 100–200 nm in diameter. To distribute to a large volume in the brain via CED, nanoparticles must be less than 100 nm in diameter. Here, we outline a versatile method for producing ultra-small PLGA nanoparticles, with an average diameter of ~70 nm, using a single-emulsion solvent evaporation technique and sequential centrifugation protocol. These nanoparticles are well suited for local delivery to the CNS [6].

2 Materials

Store all reagents at room temperature, unless otherwise indicated.

1. PLGA (50:50 PLGA; inherent viscosity ~0.67 dL/g; LACTEL Absorbable Polymers, Birmingham, AL). Store at −20 °C.
2. Poly(vinyl alcohol) (PVA; Sigma-Aldrich). Make 2.5% PVA (2.5 g PVA/100 mL PBS) and 0.3% PVA (0.3 g PVA/100 mL PBS) stock solutions. Store at 4 °C.
3. Dichloromethane (DCM; Sigma-Aldrich).
4. Ethyl acetate (EA; Sigma-Aldrich).
5. α-Trehalose (Sigma-Aldrich).
6. Drug/agent (to be encapsulated).

3 Methods

Carry out all procedures at room temperature, unless otherwise indicated (Fig. 1).

1. Dissolve 100 mg of PLGA in 2 mL of DCM or EA (*see* **Notes 1** and **2**).

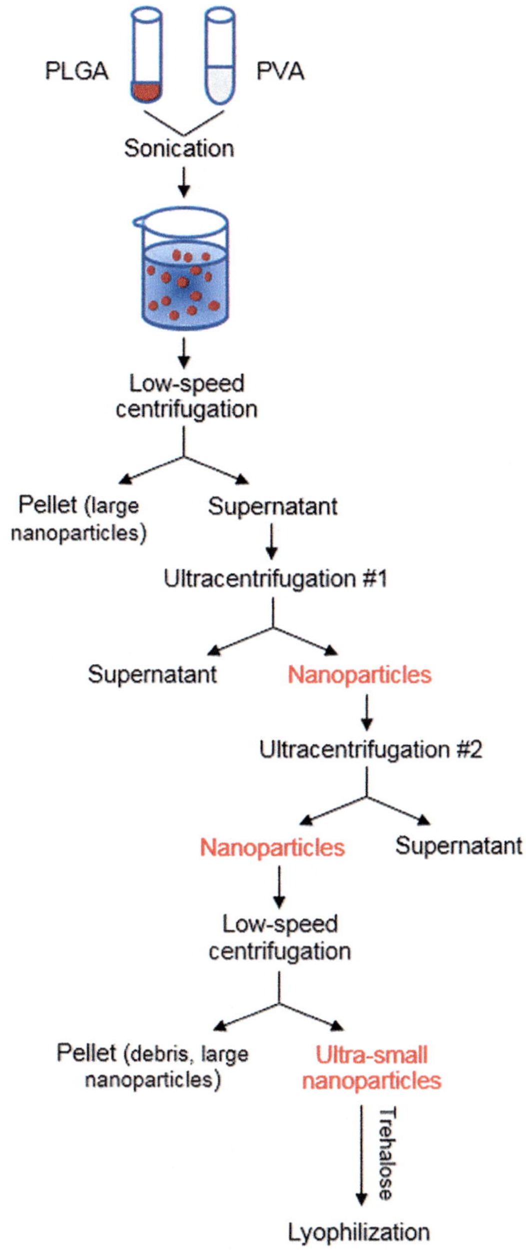

Fig. 1 Schematic diagram outlining the fabrication protocol for ultra-small nanoparticles

2. Add the desired drug/agent (to be encapsulated) to the polymer solution (*see* **Note 3**).
3. Vortex the polymer/drug solution until grossly mixed.
4. Add the polymer/drug solution dropwise to 4 mL of 2.5% PVA under vortex. Continue to vortex the tube for an additional 10 s once all components have been added (*see* **Note 4**).

5. Using a probe sonicator (at 38% amplitude), sonicate the mixture from **step 4** on ice three times for 10 s each to form an emulsion (*see* **Note 5**).
6. Add the sonicated emulsion from **step 5**, dropwise, into a beaker containing 100 mL of aqueous 0.3% PVA and stir at room temperature for 3 h (DCM as solvent) or 5 h (EA as solvent), using a magnetic stir plate. This allows the solvent to evaporate and the particles to harden.
7. Following solvent evaporation, centrifuge the nanoparticle solution at low speed (8000 × *g*) for 10 min. The larger particles will form a pellet at this stage. Collect the supernatant, which contains the ultra-small nanoparticles (*see* **Note 6**).
8. Centrifuge the supernatant from **step 7** using a high-speed ultracentrifuge (100,000 × *g*) for 30 min. Collect the pellet, which contains the ultra-small nanoparticles. Discard the supernatant (*see* **Note 7**).
9. Take the pellet from **step 8**, add 15 mL of deionized water, and resuspend the particles using a water bath sonicator (Branson 2510).
10. Centrifuge the nanoparticle suspension from **step 9** using a high-speed ultracentrifuge (100,000 × *g*) for 30 min. Collect the pellet, which contains the ultra-small nanoparticles. Discard the supernatant (*see* **Note 8**).
11. Take the pellet from **step 10**, add 10 mL of deionized water, and resuspend the particles using a water bath sonicator (Branson 2510).
12. Centrifuge the particle suspension from **step 11** at low speed (1000 × *g*) for 10 min. Any remaining debris and residual large particles will form a pellet. Collect the supernatant, which contains the ultra-small nanoparticles, in a fresh centrifuge tube and discard the pellet.
13. Add trehalose to the final aqueous ultra-small nanoparticle solution (from **step 12**), at a ratio of 0.1–0.5:1 (trehalose:nanoparticles), by mass. Trehalose is an excipient which prevents nanoparticle aggregation, thus improving their ability to distribute to large volumes in the brain. The yield of ultra-small nanoparticles will depend on the solvent that is used. For example, for particles made with EA, 100 mg of PLGA typically yields ~45 mg of ultra-small nanoparticles; thus, 4.5–22.5 mg of trehalose should be added. For particles made with DCM, 100 mg of PLGA typically yields ~28 mg of ultra-small nanoparticles; thus, 2.8–14 mg of trehalose should be added. Prior to adding the trehalose, reserve a small sample (~100 μL) of the nanoparticle solution in an Eppendorf tube for scanning electron microcopy (SEM) (*see* **Note 9**).

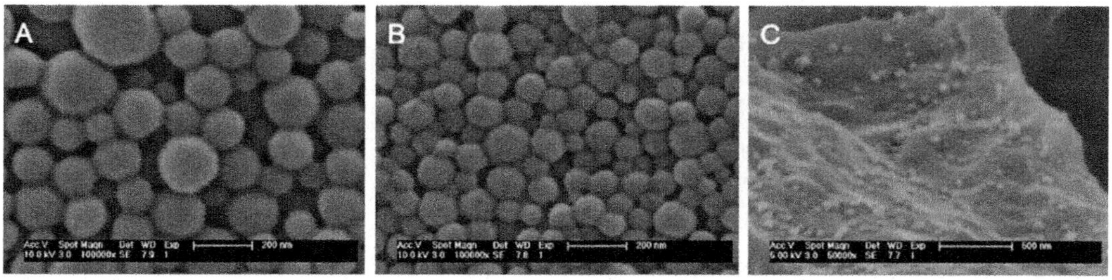

Fig. 2 Scanning electron microscopy images of PLGA nanoparticles. (**a**): nanoparticles fabricated using conventional centrifugation techniques (diameter: 150 ± 30 nm). (**b**): ultra-small nanoparticles fabricated using our sequential centrifugation protocol (diameter: 68 ± 16 nm). (**c**): ultra-small nanoparticles with added trehalose, to prevent aggregation. Scale bars = 200 nm in panels **a** and **b** and 500 nm in panel **c**

14. Cover the opening of the centrifuge and Eppendorf tubes with a Kimwipe or similarly porous paper; secure this in place with a rubber band. Place the tubes in the lyophilizer for 3 days to remove all remaining water.
15. Store the fully dehydrated particles at −20 °C.
16. Characterize the size and morphology of the nanoparticles using SEM (*see* **Note 9**) (Fig. 2).

4 Notes

1. Use glass test tubes and/or containers for this step. The PLGA may be dissolved in the solvent overnight. If this is done, be sure to use a glass container with a screw-top, to prevent solvent evaporation. The solvent choice (EA or DCM) is critical to determining the size and yield of the nanoparticles. In general, compared to DCM, EA produces smaller nanoparticles and greater yields (Fig. 3). The size of particles may also be affected by the drug that is encapsulated.
2. Perform **steps 1–6** of Subheading 3 under a chemical fume hood.
3. Hydrophobic drugs/agents may be added directly to the polymer solution. For hydrophilic drugs/agents, a water to oil (organic solvent) emulsion is performed during this step. If no drug/agent is added to the polymer solution, then "blank" (control) particles will be fabricated.
4. Use a glass pipette to dispense organic solutions.
5. The power (energy input) of the probe sonicator is important for forming ultra-small nanoparticles. We used the Tekmar Ultrasonic Processor (600 W) (Fig. 4).
6. The size and yield of the ultra-small nanoparticles depends on the speed used in the initial low-speed centrifugation (**step 7**).

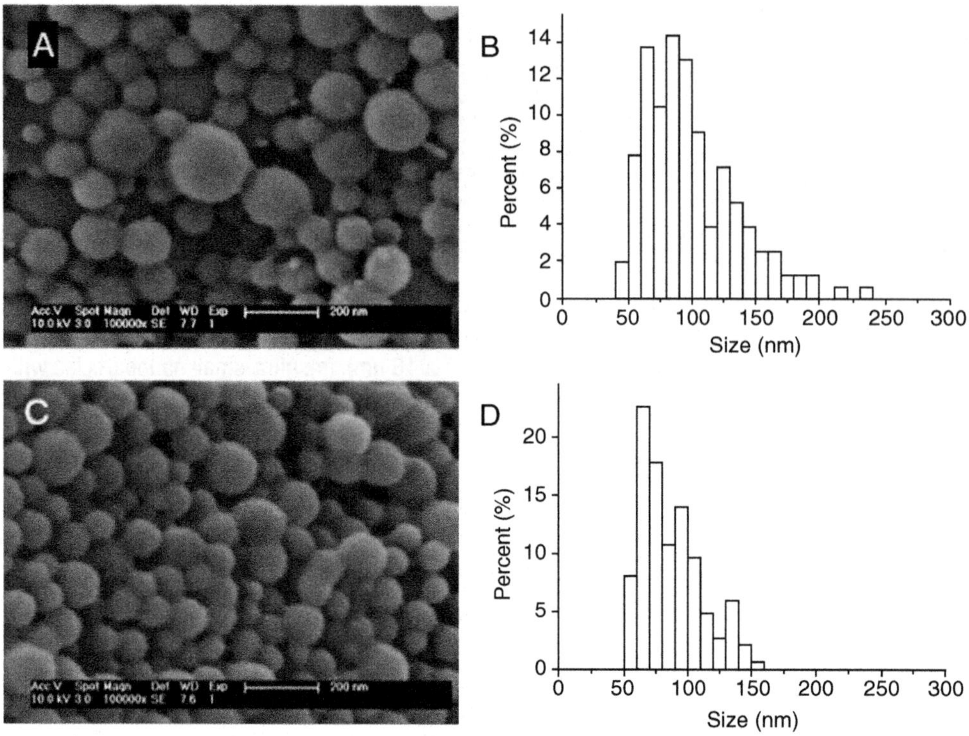

Fig. 3 Scanning electron microscopy images of PLGA nanoparticles demonstrating the impact of solvent choice on nanoparticle size. (**a**, **b**): PLGA nanoparticles fabricated using DCM as the solvent. (**c**, **d**): PLGA nanoparticles fabricated using EA as the solvent. Scale bars = 200 nm in panels **a** and **c**

A relatively higher initial centrifugation speed will pellet more large- and medium-sized nanoparticles, which will subsequently be discarded. This will result in a more homogenous population of ultra-small nanoparticles at the end of the fabrication process. However, a higher initial centrifugation speed will also result in a lower total batch yield, as more nanoparticles will be pelleted and removed during this step.

7. A high-speed ultracentrifuge is critical for collecting the ultra-small nanoparticles. We used the Sorvall Ultra Pro 80 centrifuge (at 24,000 rpm; 100,000 × *g*).
8. This step is to remove residual PVA from the surface of the nanoparticles.
9. Perform SEM on the reserved nanoparticle sample that does not contain trehalose. Once the trehalose is added, the nanoparticles become quite dispersed, making SEM more difficult. Samples were mounted on carbon tape and sputter-coated under vacuum with gold in an argon atmosphere using a Dynavac Mini Coater set at 40 mA current (Dynavac). SEM was carried out using a Philips XL30 SEM and a LaB electron gun with an accelerating voltage of 3 kV. Mean particle diameters and size distributions were determined by image

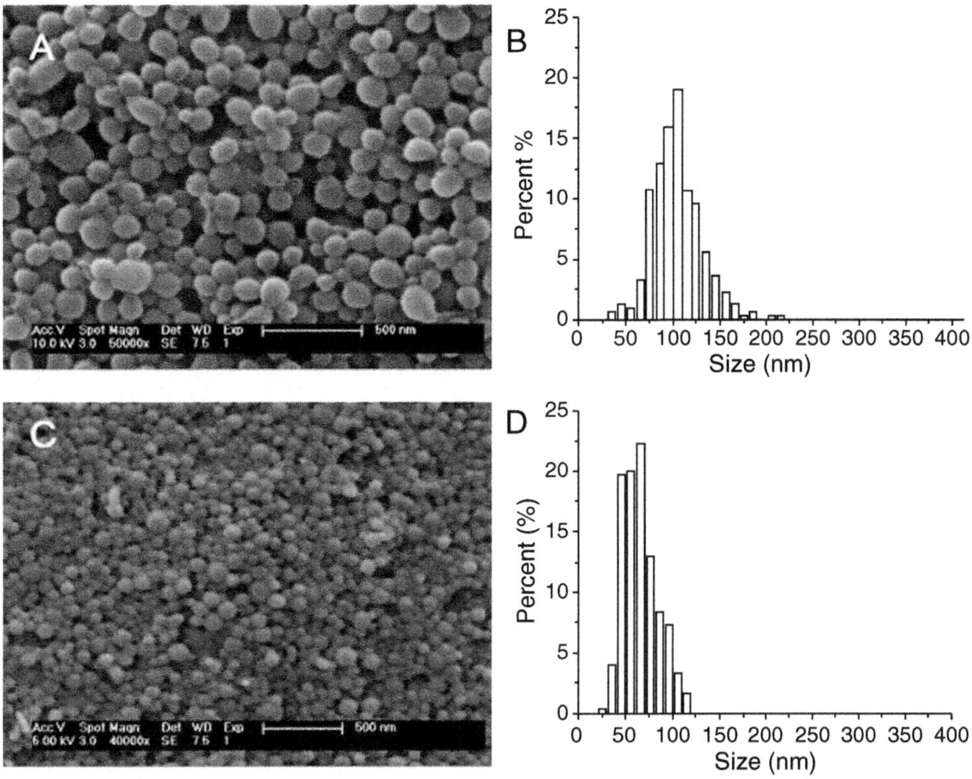

Fig. 4 Scanning electron microscopy images of PLGA nanoparticles synthesized using probe sonicators with different energy inputs and collected with different centrifuges. (**a**, **b**): PLGA nanoparticles synthesized using the Tekmar Ultrasonic Processor (400 W input) and collected with the Fisher Scientific Marathon 21000r centrifuge at 12,000 rpm (~15,000 × *g*). (**c**, **d**): PLGA nanoparticles synthesized using the Tekmar Ultrasonic Processor (600 W input) and collected with the Sorvall Ultra Pro 80 centrifuge at 24,000 rpm (100,000 × *g*). Scale bars = 500 nm in panels **a** and **c**

analysis of ~200 particles using ImageJ (National Institutes of Health). The same images were used to qualitatively assess particle morphology.

Acknowledgments

This work was supported by NIH Grants NS095817, NS095147, the State of Connecticut (J.Z.) and a discovery grant from the American Brain Tumor Association (J.Z.).

References

1. Patel T, Zhou J, Piepmeier JM, Saltzman WM (2012) Polymeric nanoparticles for drug delivery to the central nervous system. Adv Drug Deliv Rev 64:701–705
2. Zhou J, Atsina KB, Himes BT, Strohbehn GW, Saltzman WM (2012) Novel delivery strategies for glioblastoma. Cancer J 18:89–99

3. Zhou J, Patel TR, Fu M, Bertram JP, Saltzman WM (2012) Octa-functional PLGA nanoparticles for targeted and efficient siRNA delivery to tumors. Biomaterials 33:583–591
4. Thorne RG, Nicholson C (2006) In vivo diffusion analysis with quantum dots and dextrans predicts the width of brain extracellular space. Proc Natl Acad Sci U S A 103:5567–5572
5. Hobbs SK, Monsky WL, Yuan F, Roberts WG, Griffith L, Torchilin VP, Jain RK (1998) Regulation of transport pathways in tumor vessels: role of tumor type and microenvironment. Proc Natl Acad Sci U S A 95:4607–4612
6. Zhou J, Patel TR, Sirianni RW, Strohbehn G, Zheng M-Q, Duong N, Schafbauer T, Huttner AJ, Huang Y, Carson RE, Zhang Y, Sullivan DJ Jr, Piepmeier JM, Saltzman WM (2013) Highly penetrative, drug-loaded nanocarriers improve treatment of glioblastoma. Proc Natl Acad Sci U S A 110:11751–11756

Chapter 3

Construction of Bacteria-Based Cargo Carriers for Targeted Cancer Therapy

Mahama A. Traore, Ali Sahari, and Bahareh Behkam

Abstract

Despite significant recent progress in nanomedicine, drug delivery to solid tumors remains a formidable challenge often associated with low delivery efficiency and limited penetration of the drug in poorly vascularized regions of solid tumors. Attenuated strains of facultative anaerobes have been demonstrated to have exceptionally high selectivity to primary tumors and metastatic cancer, a good safety profile, and superior intratumoral penetration performance. However, bacteria have rarely been able to completely inhibit tumor growth in immunocompetent hosts solely by their presence in the tumor. We have developed a *Nano*scale *B*acteria-*E*nabled *A*utonomous Drug *D*elivery *S*ystem (NanoBEADS) in which the functional capabilities of tumor-targeting bacteria are interfaced with chemotherapeutic-loaded nanoparticles, an approach that would amplify the therapeutic potential of both modalities. Here, we describe two biomanufacturing techniques to construct NanoBEADS by linking different bacterial species with polymeric theranostic vehicles. NanoBEADS are envisioned to significantly impact current practices in cancer theranostics through improved targeting and intratumoral transport properties.

Key words Bacteria, Bacteria-based therapy, Self-assembly, Nanoparticle, Surface functionalization, Biomanufacturing, Intratumoral transport, Cancer

1 Introduction

Systemic chemotherapy is a major therapeutic approach for nearly all types and stages of cancer. Success of this treatment depends on the efficacy of therapeutics as well as the transport of drug to all tumor cells in sufficient concentrations. Despite significant recent progress in nanomedicine, treatment of solid tumors is thwarted by the low intravenous delivery efficiency and limited intratumoral transport [1, 2]. Only a minute fraction of intravenously delivered nanomedicine (typically less than 1%) is transported to the tumor site through extravasation from blood circulation [2–4]. The low delivery efficiency challenge is further exacerbated by the microenvironment-mediated drug resistance [1, 5]. Rapid growth of cancer cells combined with the unusually high fraction of

Rachael W. Sirianni and Bahareh Behkam (eds.), *Targeted Drug Delivery: Methods and Protocols*, Methods in Molecular Biology, vol. 1831, https://doi.org/10.1007/978-1-4939-8661-3_3,

stromal cells, dense extracellular matrix, and lack of lymphatic drainage lead to elevated interstitial fluid pressure and accumulated solid stress both of which significantly hinder the transport of nanomedicine in tumors, precluding deep penetration [5, 6]. New delivery strategies are presently needed in order to overcome the aforementioned challenges and improve the efficacy of drug delivery to solid tumors.

Bacteria are unicellular microorganisms with a characteristic size on the order of 1 μm and possess a host of attributes that make them uniquely advantageous as drug delivery vectors. Attenuated bacterial strains evade the immune responses while retaining high selectivity in targeting primary tumor and metastatic cancer, preferentially colonize tumors, effectively translocate in tumor interstitium, and treat cancers that are not responsive to conventional radio and chemotherapy [7]. Since the nineteenth century, bacteria and bacterial products have been shown to have therapeutic effects on cancer [8, 9]. Safety of attenuated bacteria has been extensively established in the recent decades [10–14]. Thus, bacterial vectors are emerging as a frontier of drug delivery [15]. It has been demonstrated that administration of both obligate [16–20] and facultative anaerobic bacteria [9, 21–27] treat transplanted tumors in immunocompromised mice; however, complete tumor eradication solely by the presence of bacteria in immunocompetent hosts has not been achieved [28]. These results suggest that there is a need for an improved system to achieve more efficacious bacteria-mediated cancer treatment.

We envision that a combinatorial therapy approach based on integrating tumor-targeting bacteria with chemotherapeutics-loaded nanoparticles will amplify the therapeutic potential of both modalities. Thus, we have developed a *Nano*scale *B*acteria-*E*nabled *A*utonomous Drug *D*elivery *S*ystem (NanoBEADS) in which the functional capabilities of tumor-targeting bacteria are interfaced with chemotherapeutic-loaded nanoparticles [29]. Each NanoBEADS agent is constructed by interfacing a bacterium with an ensemble of polymeric theranostics vehicles. Here, we describe two biomanufacturing techniques for controlled self-assembly of different bacterial species (e.g., *Salmonella* Typhimurium or *Escherichia coli*) with these nanoscale particles. The bacteria-particle assembly process relies on either specific (i.e., biotin-streptavidin) or nonspecific (i.e., electrostatic) interactions. NanoBEADS are envisioned to significantly impact current practices in theranostics through improved targeting and intratumoral transport properties.

2 Materials

All reagents and solutions should be prepared using autoclaved deionized (DI) water (R = 18 MΩ•cm at 25 °C) at room temperature. All media to be used in the experiment should be at neutral pH (pH = 7.0). All the labware used to culture bacteria and to prepare growth media should be sterile or should be autoclaved and kept sterile. All waste should be disposed of according to the institutional biosafety regulations.

2.1 Bacterial Culture

1. *Escherichia coli* MG1655 (ATCC 700926, American Type Culture Collection, Manassas, VA).
2. *Salmonella enterica* serovar Typhimurium VNP20009 (ATCC 202165, American Type Culture Collection, Manassas, VA).
3. Sterile inoculating loop.
4. 125 ml flask.
5. Sterile Petri dish, 100 mm diameter.
6. Orbital incubator shaker.
7. Microbiological incubator.
8. UV/Vis spectrophotometer.

2.2 Growth/ Motility Media

1. Lysogeny Broth (LB) growth medium: 1% (w/v) tryptone, 0.5% (w/v) yeast extract, 0.5% (w/v) NaCl in autoclaved DI water.
2. Motility buffer for *E. coli*: 0.01 M potassium phosphate, 0.067 M sodium chloride, 0.1 mM ethylenediaminetetraacetic acid (EDTA), 0.01 M glucose, and 0.002% (v/v) Tween-20, pH 7.0 [30] (*see* **Note 1**).
3. Motility buffer for *S.* Typhimurium: 6.4 mM K_2HPO_4, 3.5 mM KH_2PO_4, 0.1 mM EDTA, 1 μM L-methionine, 10 mM DL-lactate, 2 mM $MgSO_4$, 2 mM $CaCl_2$, pH 7.0 [31] (*see* **Note 1**).

2.3 Spherical and Non-spherical Particles

1. Carboxylate polystyrene (PS) particles (*see* **Note 2**).
2. Isopropyl alcohol (IPA).
3. Polyvinyl alcohol (PVA).
4. Mineral oil.
5. Toluene.
6. Glycerol.
7. Custom-made 2D mechanical stretcher [32, 33].

2.4 NanoBEADS Construction Using PLL

1. 0.005% (w/v) Poly-L-lysine (PLL) in DI water.
2. 1.5 ml centrifuge tube.
3. Microcentrifuge.
4. Vortex mixer.

2.5 NanoBEADS Construction Using Streptavidin-Biotin

1. Phosphate-buffered saline (PBS).
2. EZ-Link Sulfo-NHS-Biotinylation Kit (Thermo Fisher Scientific).
3. 1 mg/ml streptavidin-Cy3 buffered aqueous solution.
4. Biotin-conjugated goat polyclonal anti-lipid A LPS antibody.
5. PolyLink protein coupling kit (Polysciences, Warrington, PA, USA).
6. 1.5 ml centrifuge tube.
7. Microcentrifuge.
8. Vortex mixer.

3 Methods

3.1 NanoBEADS Construction Using PLL

Assembly of particles and bacteria through PLL relies on the non-specific (i.e., electrostatic) interactions between the positively charged PLL-coated particles and bacteria with negatively charged outer membranes [33].

1. Inoculate 10 ml of LB in a 125 ml flask with *E. coli* from a frozen stock and grow overnight (14–16 h) in an orbital shaker at 30 °C and 150 rpm (*see* **Note 3**).
2. Inoculate 5 ml of LB with 1% (v/v) of the overnight culture to make a fresh bacterial culture. Grow the bacteria at 30 °C and 150 rpm until the optical density (OD_{600}) reaches 0.5 (~2.5×10^8 CFU/ml).
3. Add 10 μl of 1% (w/v) PS micro/nano-particles to 1 ml 30% (v/v) IPA in DI water.
4. Centrifuge the particle suspension for 5 min at 3000 × *g* at room temperature (*see* **Note 4**).
5. Aspirate the supernatant gently to leave the particle pellet intact.
6. Resuspend the pellet in 30% (v/v) IPA in DI water.
7. Repeat the wash **steps 4–6** two more times to remove surfactants or other stabilizers from the surface of the particles (*see* **Note 5**).
8. After the final centrifugation, resuspend the particles in the PLL solution and gyrate on a vortex mixer for 1 h at 500 rpm

and room temperature to promote PLL adsorption to the particle surface.

9. Harvest 1 ml of the bacterial culture and centrifuge for 5 min at 1700 × *g* at room temperature in a 1.5 ml centrifuge vial.
10. Remove the supernatant and resuspend the bacteria in 1 ml of motility buffer. Briefly (~3–5 s) vortex mix the suspension a few times to ensure a homogenous distribution.
11. Centrifuge the PLL-coated particles from **step 10** for 5 min at 3000 × *g* at room temperature. Aspirate and discard the supernatant.
12. Transfer the bacterial suspension to the particle pellet. Mix by gentle repeated pipetting of the vial content.
13. Gyrate the bacteria/particles solution on a vortex mixer for 20 min at 500 rpm and room temperature to promote the assembly of the bacteria to the PLL-coated particles (*see* **Note 6**).
14. Prepare a 1:100 dilution of the NanoBEADS suspension in motility buffer for microscopy.

3.2 NanoBEADS Construction Using Biotin-Streptavidin Interaction

This method of NanoBEADS biomanufacturing takes advantage of the strong non-covalent interactions between biotin and streptavidin, which is essentially irreversible under physiologically relevant conditions (Fig. 1a). It relies on the specific interactions between bacteria decorated with a biotinylated cell membrane-specific antibody and streptavidin-coated particles [29, 34].

1. Inoculate 10 ml of LB in 125 ml flask with *E. coli* from a frozen stock and grow overnight (14–16 h) in an orbital shaker at 30 °C and 150 rpm (*see* **Note 3**).
2. Inoculate 5 ml of LB with 1% (v/v) of the overnight culture to make a fresh bacterial culture. Grow the bacteria at 30 °C and 150 rpm until the optical density (OD_{600}) reaches 0.5 (~2.5×10^8 CFU/ml).

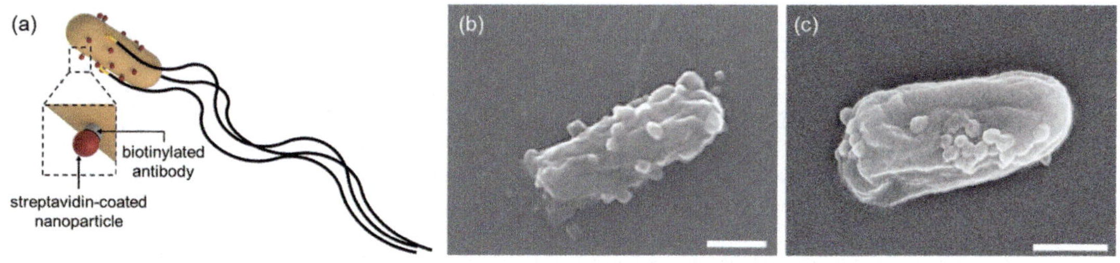

Fig. 1 Biomanufacturing of NanoBEADS using specific interactions. (**a**) NanoBEADS are constructed through high-affinity interactions between bacteria coated with biotinylated cell membrane-specific antibody and nanoparticles coated with streptavidin (**b**, **c**) Scanning electron microscopy (SEM) images of 110 nm particles attached to bacteria. All scale bars are 500 nm

3. Harvest 1 ml of the bacterial culture and centrifuge for 5 min at 1700 × *g* at room temperature in a 1.5 ml centrifuge vial.
4. Remove the supernatant and add 1 ml of motility buffer. Briefly (~3–5 s) vortex mix the suspension a few times to ensure that the bacteria are homogenously suspended.
5. Repeat the bacterial wash one more time and resuspend the final pellet in 1 ml of motility buffer.
6. Add 10 μg of goat polyclonal anti-LPS antibody to the bacterial suspension and gyrate on a vortex mixer at 500 rpm and room temperature for 1 h (*see* **Note 6**).
7. Centrifuge the bacterial solution for 5 min at 1700 × *g* at room temperature. Remove the free antibody by discarding the supernatant.
8. Resuspend the bacteria in 1 ml of motility buffer and mix gently to ensure that the bacteria are well distributed in the vial.
9. Add 2.5 × 10^{10} carboxylate polystyrene nanoparticles to 1 ml of 30% (v/v) IPA in DI water.
10. Centrifuge the suspension at 16,000 × *g* at room temperature for 10 min and remove the supernatant. A pellet of particles should be visible. If not, centrifugal acceleration and duration should be adjusted (*see* **Note 4**).
11. Aspirate the supernatant gently to leave the particle pellet intact.
12. Resuspend the pellet in 30% (v/v) IPA in DI water.
13. Repeat the **steps 10–12** two more times.
14. Suspend ~2.5 × 10^{10} nanoparticles in 200 μl PBS in a 1.5 ml centrifuge tube and centrifuge down to a pellet at 16,000 × *g* for 10 min.
15. Aspirate the supernatant and resuspend the particles in 200 μl of the coupling buffer. Ensure homogenous suspension by gently pipetting up and down followed by short vortex mixing.
16. Dilute the streptavidin-Cy3 stock solution to a final concentration of 100 μg/ml using the coupling buffer in the PolyLink protein coupling kit.
17. Separately dissolve 4 mg of 1-Ethyl-3-(3-dimethylaminopropyl) carbodiimide (EDAC) in the coupling buffer at 200 mg/ml (*see* **Note 7**).
18. Mix 10 μl of the diluted streptavidin-Cy3 solution and 20 μl of the EDAC solution with an additional 170 μl of the coupling buffer.
19. Combine the 200 μl solution prepared in **step 18** with the particle suspension prepared in **step 15** and gyrate on a vortex

mixer at 500 rpm and room temperature for 3 h to allow for sufficient coupling (*see* **Note 8**).

20. Centrifuge the particle solution for 10 min at 16,000 × *g*. Remove the free streptavidin by discarding the supernatant.
21. Resuspend the particles in 100 μl of motility buffer.
22. Add the bacteria solution to the pellet of streptavidin-coated particles at a bacteria-to-particle ratio of 1:100. Mix by gentle, repeated pipetting of the tube content.
23. Gyrate on a vortex mixer at 500 rpm and room temperature for 30 min (*see* **Note 6**).
24. Make a 1:100 dilution of the NanoBEADS solution in motility buffer for microscopy (Fig. 1b, c).

3.3 Non-spherical NanoBEADS Construction

Non-spherical polystyrene particles are fabricated using a high-throughput particle casting and mechanical stretching technique, as shown in Fig. 2a [32, 33].

1. Wash carboxylate polystyrene particles suspended in 30% (v/v) IPA in DI water by centrifugation at 3000 × *g* for 5 min at room temperature. A pellet of particles should be visible at the bottom of the vial (*see* **Note 4**).

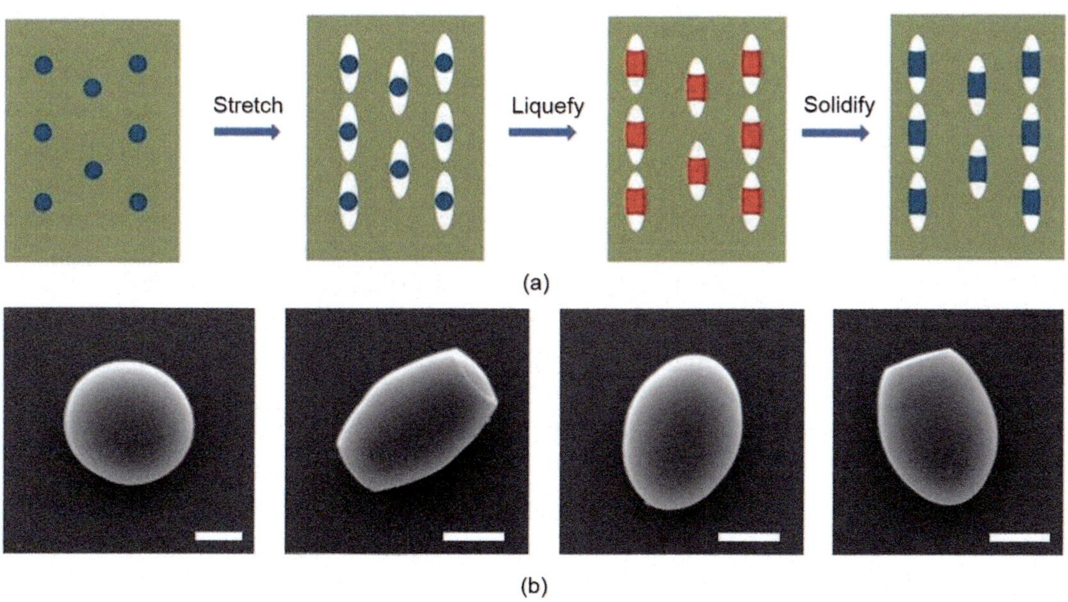

Fig. 2 Fabrication of non-spherical polystyrene (PS) particles. (**a**) Fabrication process flow for making non-spherical PS particles. Particles embedded in a PVA film are stretched in one dimension, liquefied in an oil bath, and then solidified at room temperature. (**b**) Scanning electron microscopy (SEM) images of spherical and non-spherical PS particles. All scale bars are 2 μm. Reproduced with permission from Springer [33]

Table 1
Experimental parameters for fabrication of non-spherical particles

Particle shape	Stretching aspect ratio	Liquefaction method	Plasticizer (Glycerol)
Prolate spheroid	1.2–1.3, 2.0	130 °C (Oil)	Yes
Barrel	1.1–1.3	130 °C (Oil)	No
Bullet	1.1–1.3	140 °C (Oil)	No
Elliptical disk	2.0	Toluene	Yes

2. Aspirate the supernatant gently to leave the particle pellet intact.
3. Resuspend the pellet in 30% (v/v) IPA in DI water.
4. Repeat **steps 1–3** two more times.
5. Resuspend the particle pellet in a 4 ml solution of 5% (w/v) PVA in DI water at 90 °C.
6. Add 2% (v/v) glycerol, as a plasticizer, to the PVA/particle solution.
7. After dissolving the PVA, pour the solution into a 100 mm Petri dish to let the film cast at room temperature overnight (~14 h). The result will be a 35 μm-thick film.
8. After the film sets, cut it into a square-shaped piece, mount it on an axial stretcher, and stretch it uniformly in one dimension to a desired aspect ratio.
9. Immerse the stretched film (while in the stretcher) in a bath of either toluene at room temperature for 3 h for making elliptical disks or hot mineral oil for making bullets, barrels, and prolate spheroids (*see* Table 1 for experimental parameters).
10. Let the film dry for 10 h if a bath of toluene was used. Let the film cool down for approximately 1 h if a bath of hot mineral oil was used.
11. Dissolve the PVA film in 30% (v/v) IPA:DI water overnight at 65 °C.
12. Wash the particles by centrifugation in 30% (v/v) IPA:DI water three times to extract the residual toluene/oil and purify the particle solution (Fig. 2b).
13. Follow the protocol described in Subheadings 3.1 or 3.2 to construct the NanoBEADS.

4 Notes

1. The motility buffer should be sterilized by filtration not autoclaving. Sterilize the motility buffer using a 0.25 μm or smaller pore size filter.
2. Negatively charged micro/nanoparticles made of other biocompatible materials (e.g., gold, PLGA, etc.) can also be used in this protocol. The protocols reported here were tested for 50 nm to 10 μm-diameter polystyrene particles, 100–200 nm PLGA particles, and 40 nm gold particles.
3. The prescribed bacterial growth temperature can be adjusted to match the needs of specific bacterial strains. Human pathogens such as *S*. Typhimurium are typically cultured at 37 °C [31].
4. The centrifugation acceleration and time needs to be adjusted based on the particle size and settling velocity [35]. Excess centrifugation may result in resuspension difficulties. To estimate the appropriate centrifugation duration, settling velocity of the particle is calculated using the Stokes' Law, $V = 2.\ G.\ r^2(\rho_p - \rho_m)/9\mu$, where V is the velocity (cm/s), G is the relative gravitational acceleration (cm/s^2), ρ_p and ρ_m are the density of the particle and suspending medium (g/cm^3), respectively, μ is the dynamic viscosity (gm/cm•s), and r is the particle radius (cm). The resultant velocity and the height of the centrifuge tube are then used to estimate the centrifugation time.
5. The purpose of this step is to remove the stabilizing surfactant from the particles and make the functional surface available for assembly. This step must be performed carefully as excess centrifugation leads to particle aggregation and resuspension difficulties. If the pellet cannot be resuspended, this step needs to be repeated with fewer rounds. Short and periodic water bath sonication pulses (for 15–20 s every 5 min) may also be attempted to break up the pellet and fully resuspend the particles.
6. Gyration on a vortex mixer may not produce an optimal shear rate for the assembly of 100 nm or smaller particles onto bacteria. In some strains of bacteria, the flagella may shear off if exposed to prolonged gyration at a high shear rate. The former can be assessed by SEM inspection of bacteria-particle complexes and the latter can be assessed by conducting a swimming motility assay after the completion of the assembly process. If either of the aforementioned problems arises, alternative mixing methods using an end-over-end mixer or a belly dancer shaker are recommended.
7. EDC is very labile in aqueous solutions especially in slightly acidic conditions such as the coupling buffer (pH 5.2). Thus,

the EDAC solution should be prepared as needed and not stored in solution.

8. For nanoparticles (particles less than 1 μm in diameter), aggregation may occur while using the coupling buffer. Avoid aggregation by adding 0.0005–0.005% Tween-20 or Triton X-100 to the coupling buffer. Furthermore, short and periodic sonication pulses (for 15–20 s every 20 min) can be used to break up the aggregates, if needed.

Acknowledgments

The authors would like to thank Samir Mitragotri Laboratory for invaluable discussions regarding the particle stretching technique and Eric Leaman for help with the CAD schematic. This work was supported by the National Science Foundation (IIS-117519 and CAREER award, CBET-1454226).

References

1. Minchinton AI, Tannock IF (2006) Drug penetration in solid tumours. Nat Rev Cancer 6:583–592
2. Wilhelm S, Tavares AJ, Dai Q, Ohta S, Audet J, Dvorak HF, Chan WCW (2016) Analysis of nanoparticle delivery to tumours. Nat Rev Mater 1:16014
3. Han Bae Y, Park K, Bae YH, Park K (2011) Targeted drug delivery to tumors: myths, reality and possibility. J Control Release 153:198–205
4. Dvorak HF, Nagy JA, Dvorak JT, Dvorak AM (1988) Identification and characterization of the blood vessels of solid tumors that are leaky to circulating macromolecules. Am J Pathol 133:95–109
5. Chauhan VP, Stylianopoulos T, Boucher Y, Jain RK (2011) Delivery of molecular and nanoscale medicine to tumors: transport barriers and strategies. Annu Rev Chem Biomol Eng 2:281–298
6. Nia HT, Liu H, Seano G et al (2016) Solid stress and elastic energy as measures of tumour mechanopathology. Nat Biomed Eng 1:4
7. Forbes NS (2006) Profile of a bacterial tumor killer. Nat Biotechnol 24:1484–1485
8. Coley WB (1991) The treatment of malignant tumors by repeated inoculations of erysipelas. With a report of ten original cases. 1893. Clin Orthop Relat Res 262:3–11
9. Pawelek JM, Low KB, Bermudes D (2003) Bacteria as tumour-targeting vectors. Lancet Oncol 4:548–556
10. Clairmont C, Lee KC, Pike J, Ittensohn M, Low KB, Pawelek J, Bermudes D, Brecher SM, Margitich D, Turnier J, Li Z, Luo X, King I, Zheng LM (2000) Biodistribution and genetic stability of the novel antitumor agent VNP20009, a genetically modified strain of *Salmonella typhimurium*. J Infect Dis 181:1996–2002
11. Thamm DH, Kurzman ID, King I, Li Z, Sznol M, Dubielzig RR, Vail DM, MacEwen EG (2005) Systemic administration of an attenuated, tumor-targeting *Salmonella typhimurium* to dogs with spontaneous neoplasia: phase I evaluation. Clin Cancer Res 11:4827–4834
12. Toso Gill V, Hwu P, Marincola F, Restifo N, Schwartzentruber D, Sherry R, Topalian S, Yang J, Stock F, Freezer L, Morton K, Seipp C, Haworth L, Mavroukakis S, White D, MacDonald S, Mao J, Sznol M, Rosenberg SJ (2002) Phase I study of the intravenous administration of attenuated *Salmonella typhimurium* to patients with metastatic melanoma. J Clin Oncol 20:142–152
13. Maciaga Radulovicb S, Rothmana JP (2009) The first clinical use of a live-attenuated *Listeria monocytogenes* vaccine: a phase I safety study of Lm-LLO-E7 in patients with advanced carcinoma of the cervix. Vaccine 27:3975–3983
14. Kramer MG, Masner M, Ferreira FA, Hoffman RM (2018) Bacterial therapy of cancer: promises, limitations, and insights for future directions. Front Microbiol 9:16

15. Curran CS, Rasooly A, He M, Prickril B, Thurin M, Sharon E (2018) Report on the NCI microbial-based cancer therapy conference. Cancer Immunol Res 6:122–126
16. Bettegowda C, Dang LH, Abrams R, Huso DL, Dillehay L, Cheong I, Agrawal N, Borzillary S, McCaffery JM, Watson EL, Lin K-S, Bunz F, Baidoo K, Pomper MG, Kinzler KW, Vogelstein B, Zhou S (2003) Overcoming the hypoxic barrier to radiation therapy with anaerobic bacteria. Proc Natl Acad Sci U S A 100:15083–15088
17. Yazawa Fujimori M, Amano J, Kano Y, Taniguchi SK (2000) *Bifidobacterium longum* as a delivery system for cancer gene therapy: selective localization and growth in hypoxic tumors. Cancer Gene Ther 7:269–274
18. Nuyts S, Van Mellaert L, Theys J, Landuyt W, Lambin P, Anné J (2002) *Clostridium* spores for tumor-specific drug delivery. Anti-Cancer Drugs 13:115–125
19. Borden JR, Papoutsakis ET (2007) Dynamics of genomic-library enrichment and identification of solvent tolerance genes for *Clostridium acetobutylicum*. Appl Env Microbiol 73:3061–3068
20. Minton NP (2003) Clostridia in cancer therapy. Nat Rev Microbiol 1:237–242
21. Zhao M, Yang M, Li X-M, Jiang P, Baranov E, Li S, Xu M, Penman S, Hoffman RM (2005) Tumor-targeting bacterial therapy with amino acid auxotrophs of GFP-expressing *Salmonella typhimurium*. Proc Natl Acad Sci U S A 102:755–760
22. Stritzker J, Weibel S, Seubert C, Götz A, Tresch A, van Rooijen N, Oelschlaeger TA, Hill PJ, Gentschev I, Szalay AA (2010) Enterobacterial tumor colonization in mice depends on bacterial metabolism and macrophages but is independent of chemotaxis and motility. Int J Med Microbiol 300:449–456
23. Zhao M, Yang M, Ma H, Li X, Tan X, Li S, Yang Z, Hoffman RM (2006) Targeted therapy with a *Salmonella typhimurium* leucine-arginine auxotroph cures orthotopic human breast tumors in nude mice. Cancer Res 66:7647–7652
24. Zhao M, Geller J, Ma H, Yang M, Penman S, Hoffman RM (2007) Monotherapy with a tumor-targeting mutant of *Salmonella typhimurium* cures orthotopic metastatic mouse models of human prostate cancer. Proc Natl Acad Sci U S A 104:10170–10174
25. Low KB, Ittensohn M, Le T, Platt J, Sodi S, Amoss M, Ash O, Carmichael E, Chakraborty A, Fischer J, Lin SL, Luo X, Miller SI, Zheng L, King I, Pawelek JM, Bermudes D (1999) Lipid A mutant *Salmonella* with suppressed virulence and TNFα induction retain tumor-targeting in vivo. Nat Biotechnol 17:37–41
26. Forbes NS, Munn LL, Fukumura D, Jain RK (2003) Sparse initial entrapment of systemically injected *Salmonella typhimurium* leads to heterogeneous accumulation within tumors. Cancer Res 63:5188–5193
27. Pawelek JM, Low KB, Bermudes D (1997) Tumor-targeted *Salmonella* as a novel anticancer vector. Cancer Res 57:4537–4544
28. Westphal K, Leschner S, Jablonska J, Loessner H, Weiss S (2008) Containment of tumor-colonizing bacteria by host neutrophils. Cancer Res 68:2952–2960
29. Traore MA, Damico CM, Behkam B (2014) Biomanufacturing and self-propulsion dynamics of nanoscale bacteria-enabled autonomous delivery systems. Appl Phys Lett 105:173702
30. Darnton N, Turner L, Breuer K, Berg H (2004) Moving fluid with bacterial carpets. Biophyiscal J 86:1863–1870
31. Broadway KM, Suh S, Behkam B, Scharf BE (2017) Optimizing the restored chemotactic behavior of anticancer agent *Salmonella enterica* serovar Typhimurium VNP20009. J Biotechnol 251:76–83
32. Champion JA, Katare YK, Mitragotri S (2007) Making polymeric micro- and nanoparticles of complex shapes. Proc Natl Acad Sci U S A 104:11901–11904
33. Sahari A, Headen D, Behkam B (2012) Effect of body shape on the motile behavior of bacteria-powered swimming microrobots (BacteriaBots). Biomed Microdevices 14:999–1007
34. Sahari A, Traore MA, Scharf BE, Behkam B (2014) Directed transport of bacteria-based drug delivery vehicles: bacterial chemotaxis dominates particle shape. Biomed Microdevices 16:717–725
35. Graham JM. (2001). Biological centrifugation. Bios Scientific Publishers Limited, Oxford, UK

Chapter 4

Production of Extracellular Vesicles Loaded with Therapeutic Cargo

Tek N. Lamichhane and Steven M. Jay

Abstract

Extracellular vesicles (EVs) are biological nanoparticles comprising exosomes, microvesicles, and other heterogeneous nanoscopic vesicle populations that are produced by most cell types. In addition to their putative roles as critical mediators of intercellular communication, EVs have begun to be harnessed as drug delivery vehicles, with early evidence indicating they may have significant advantages over synthetic nanoparticle delivery systems for particular applications. Targeted delivery of EV-encapsulated cargo has already been realized and may have broad applicability; however, methods for producing and purifying EVs and loading them with therapeutic molecules have yet to be standardized. In this chapter, we outline steps for EV isolation and characterization and compare current methods for active and passive loading of EVs with payloads of short interfering RNA (siRNA) or small molecules, with the results revealing that active loading via electroporation increases loading efficiency of siRNA but not of Rhodamine B, a model for a small molecule drug, in HEK293T-derived EVs. The methods described here may inform future design of targeted delivery of nucleic acids or small molecules via EVs.

Key words Extracellular vesicles (EVs), Exosomes, siRNA, Small molecules, Electroporation, Drug delivery, Cancer therapeutics

1 Introduction

Extracellular vesicles (EVs) are natural nanoscopic particles produced by most cells that hold immense promise for utilization as drug carriers. EVs include exosomes (30–120 nm), which are released to the extracellular environment upon fusion of multivesicular endosomes with the plasma membrane, as well as microvesicles (50–1000 nm), which are produced by the outward budding of membrane vesicles from the cell surface [1, 2]. Exosomes and microvesicles have similar properties and are difficult to completely separate with current isolation methods, thus we refer them here as EVs following the recommendations laid out by the International Society for Extracellular Vesicles [3].

Rachael W. Sirianni and Bahareh Behkam (eds.), *Targeted Drug Delivery: Methods and Protocols*, Methods in Molecular Biology, vol. 1831, https://doi.org/10.1007/978-1-4939-8661-3_4,

EVs play significant roles in intercellular communication via cell-cell transfer of proteins and especially nucleic acids such as microRNAs (miRNAs), long noncoding RNAs (lncRNAs), and mRNAs [4, 5]. The status of EVs as native nucleic acid carriers prompted investigation of their utility for short interfering RNA (siRNA) delivery, and a seminal study by Wood and colleagues demonstrated that exosomes could be targeted to the brain for delivery of therapeutic siRNA [6]. Additional work has shown that EVs can be utilized for targeted delivery of microRNA (miRNA) [7] and small molecule drugs [8] to combat cancer, opening a pathway for EVs to be applied as drug carriers for treatment of numerous diseases as well as in a variety of tissue repair and regeneration applications [9].

However, one limiting factor in further development of EV-based therapeutics is a lack of standardized methods for EV isolation and for loading EVs with therapeutic cargo. This chapter focuses on methods for loading of EVs with siRNA and small molecules; reviews of EV isolation methodologies are available elsewhere [10, 11]. In the study by Wood and colleagues, EVs were loaded with siRNA via electroporation [6, 12], a common molecular biology technique that has been used to deliver DNA, drugs or chemicals into prokaryotic or eukaryotic cells [13, 14]. However, other studies have reported an inability to efficiently load EVs with siRNA [15] or miRNA [7] using this approach, potentially due to electric field-induced aggregation of these short RNA molecules. Here, using HEK293T-derived EVs, we detail an approach for siRNA loading into EVs via electroporation that addresses siRNA aggregation and also define parameters for siRNA loading capacity in EVs.

In addition, we report on methods for loading EVs with small molecules. Small molecule drugs such as curcumin and doxorubicin have been successfully loaded into EVs by different methods [8, 16]. Passive loading, i.e., incubation of EVs with drug in solution with no additional stimulation, is sufficient for EVs to encapsulate curcumin [16]. Alternatively, electroporation has been employed to incorporate doxorubicin into EVs [8]. We have compared these passive and active loading methods using Rhodamine B as a model small molecule drug. Overall, this chapter provides an overview of various methods that could be used to incorporate therapeutic cargo into EVs for a wide variety of targeted delivery applications.

2 Materials

All aqueous solutions of reagents should be prepared using ultrapure water and filter-sterilized through a 0.22 μm filter into sterile container.

2.1 Cell Culture

1. EV producing cells: HEK293T cells (ThermoScientific HCL4517).

2. Cell culture media: DMEM high glucose with sodium pyruvate (110 mg/ml) + L-glutamine (6 mM) + penicillin (100 units/ml) + streptomycin (100 μg/ml) + 10% fetal bovine serum (FBS) as final concentrations.

2.2 EV Isolation and Characterization

1. Ultracentrifuge with rotor capable of 100,000 × *g* spins: Beckman Optima L-90K ultracentrifuge with T70i rotor.
2. Ultracentrifuge tubes: Optiseal tubes (Beckman 41121703).
3. Nanoparticle imaging apparatus with 50 nm sensitivity: Nanosight LM10 with Nanoparticle Tracking Analysis (NTA) software.

2.3 Cargo Preparation

1. siRNA.
   (a) Purified siRNA: sequence: GGUGCCAGUUC UCCAAGAUUdTdT (Dharmacon GE Life Sciences CTM-120916). Resuspend into ultrapure RNase-free water to make a final concentration of 200 pmol/μl (200 μM).
2. Small molecules.
   (a) Purified hydrophobic molecules less than 1000 Da: Rhodamine B (Sigma 83689-1G). Prepare 10 mM stock solution in DI H_2O and store at room temperature with protection from light.

2.4 Electroporation

1. Electroporation buffer: 1.15 mM potassium phosphate pH 7.2, 25 mM potassium chloride, 21% Optiprep, as described in Alvarez-Erviti et al. [6].
2. Electroporator and cuvettes: GenePulser Xcell electroporator (Biorad) with Gene Pulser/Micropulser Cuvettes (Biorad 165-2089).
3. 300 kDa MWCO filter: Pall Nanosep centrifugal device with Omega membrane, MWCO 300 kDa (OD300C33).

2.5 Loaded Cargo Detection

1. Kit that can detect nucleic acid concentration at picogram sensitivity: Quant-it PicoGreen Assay kit (Life Technologies P7589).
2. Labeling buffer: 0.5% DMSO in 1× TE (10 mM Tris, pH 7.5 and 1 mM EDTA, pH 8.0.
3. Black-walled clear bottom non-treated polystyrene 96-well plates.
4. 0.5 ml centrifuge tubes, 0.2 ml thin walled, nuclease-free PCR tubes.
5. Microplate reader with fluorescence capability (or any other modality needed for small molecule quantification): Molecular Devices SpectraMax M5.

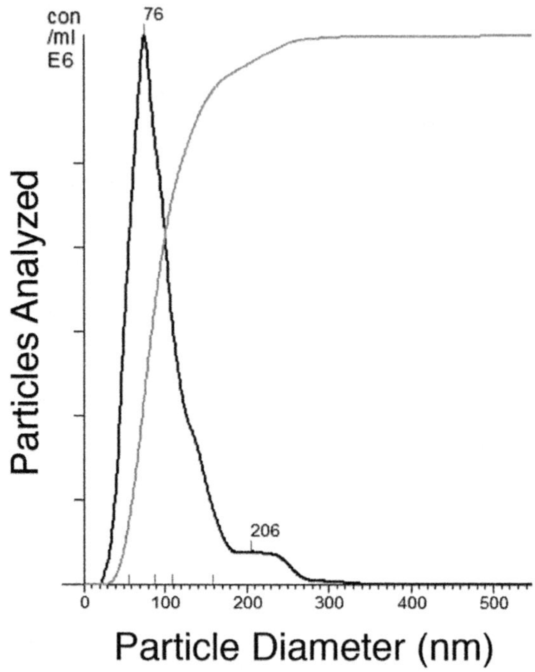

Fig. 1 EV size distribution. Size distribution of HEK293T-derived EVs as measured by NanoTracking Analysis reveals a peak at 76 nm in diameter, with the majority of isolated EVs being less than 200 nm in diameter

3 Methods

3.1 Measurement of EV Concentration and Size

1. Grow cells in EV-depleted media (*see* **Note 1**) in T150 flasks.
2. Isolate EVs using differential centrifugation method as described previously [17]. In brief, collect media from cultured cells and centrifuge at 300 × *g* for 10 min. Transfer supernatant into a new tube and centrifuge again at 2000 × *g* for 20 min and then 10,000 × *g* for 30 min to remove larger vesicles and debris. Finally, transfer the supernatant into ultracentrifuge tubes and centrifuge at 100,000 × *g* for 2 h to pellet EVs consisting primarily of exosome and microvesicle fractions.
3. Discard the supernatant and resuspend EVs into ice-cold 1× PBS (*see* **Note 2**).
4. Determine size and concentration of EVs (Fig. 1) (*see* **Note 3**).
5. For electroporation, resuspend EVs into electroporation buffer (EB) and, if not immediately used, store EVs either at −20 or −80 °C (*see* **Note 4**). For passive loading, resuspend EVs into 1× PBS and, if not immediately used, store EVs either at −20 or −80 °C.

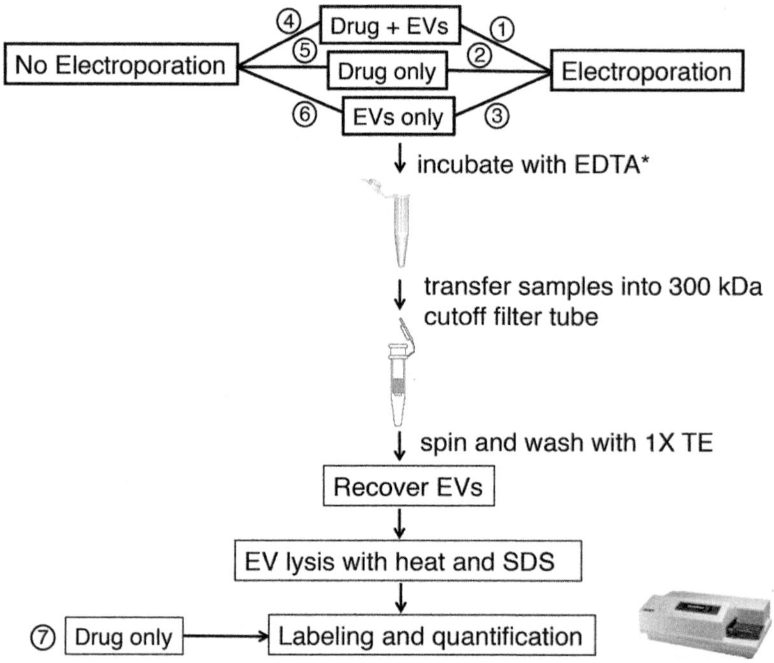

Fig. 2 Schematic for controlled experiments to assess active and/or passive loading of EVs. Sample preparation is described in **Notes 5** and **6**. Model drugs (drug) used included siRNA and Rhodamine B. Asterisk indicates this step is relevant for siRNA loading only

3.2 Passive and Active Loading

1. Prepare samples for loading using the appropriate proportions for each drug molecule type listed below. Examples of appropriate controls are indicated in Figs. 2 and 3 (*see* **Notes 5** and **6**).
   (a) siRNA: 10 μl of 1 μg/μl EVs (~3.2×10^8 vesicles for HEK293T) + 5 μl of 200 pmol/μl siRNA + 25 μl 2× electroporation buffer (or PBS for passive loading) + 10 μl DI H_2O (nuclease free).
   (b) Rhodamine B: 10 μl of 1 μg/μl EVs (~3.2×10^8 vesicles for HEK293T) + 10 μl of 10 mM Rhodamine B (*see* **Note 7**) + 25 μl 2× electroporation buffer (or PBS for passive loading) + 5 μl DI H_2O (nuclease free).
2. Perform loading step.
   (a) Active loading: Transfer samples (samples 1, 2, and 3 in Fig. 2) into ice chilled cuvettes and electroporate each sample at 400 V and 125 μF with two pulses.
   (b) Passive loading: Incubate samples at room temperature for 15 min (samples 4, 5, and 6 in Fig. 2).
3. Transfer each electroporated sample from its cuvette into a 0.5 ml tube.

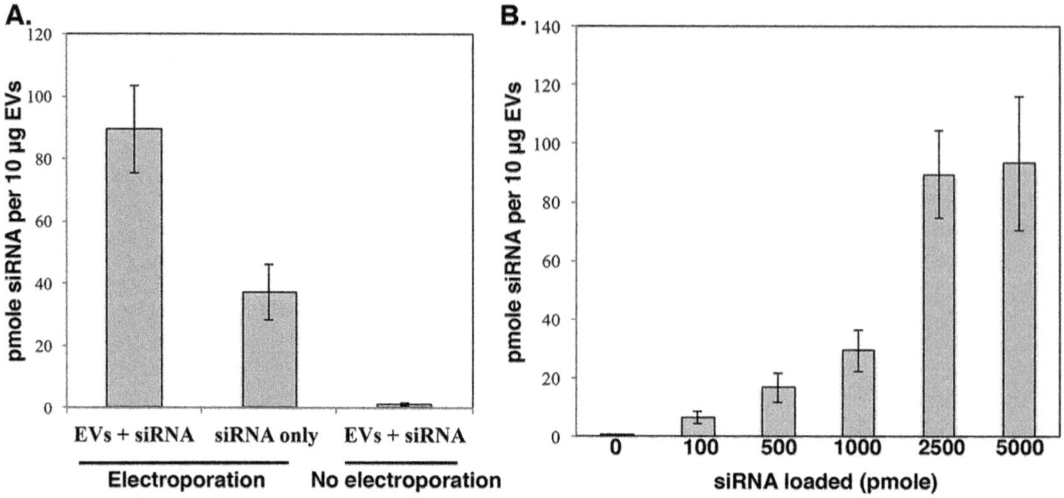

Fig. 3 siRNA incorporation into EVs. (**a**) siRNA is detectable from EVs that were electroporated in the presence of siRNA following extensive washing and filtration to remove unassociated molecules. Electroporation of siRNA alone does cause positive signal, potentially as the result of aggregation. EVs incubated passively with siRNA do not retain detectable amounts. (**b**) siRNA associated with EVs is influenced by the initial loading amount until saturation between 2500 and 5000 pmol loaded. These data were normalized to the background signal generated by electroporated siRNA at each loading amount. Note: 10 µg of EVs corresponds to ~3.2×10^8 vesicles

4. Recover the residual sample from each cuvette by adding 100 µl of 1× TE, pipetting up and down and transferring to the appropriate 0.5 ml tube.
5. For siRNA only, add EDTA to a final concentration of 1 mM to alleviate siRNA aggregation and incubate for 15 min at room temperature.
6. Transfer the sample to a 300 kDa MWCO filter tube. This filter retains EVs but small molecules and buffers that have not been incorporated into EVs will pass through the filter during washing steps.
7. Centrifuge samples at 5000 × *g* at 4 °C for 5 min to remove buffer and unincorporated cargo.
8. Discard flow through, add 500 µl of 1× TE into each tube, and centrifuge again at 5000 × *g* at 4 °C for 5 min.
9. Repeat **step 8** two times for a total of three washes.
10. Add 50 µl of 1× TE into the same filter tube, pipette up and down, and transfer the sample into a fresh 0.5 ml tube.
11. Add additional 45 µl of 1× TE to recover residual amount of sample from filter tube and transfer total volume of sample, i.e., 95 µl into a 0.2 ml thin walled PCR tube (*see* **Note 8**).

3.2.1 siRNA Quantification

1. To lyse EVs and release incorporated siRNA, add 5 μl of 0.4% SDS into 95 μl of EVs mixture, mix well, and incubate in a thermocycler for 15 min at 85 °C (*see* **Note 9**).
2. Prepare working solution (0.5% DMSO in 1× TE buffer). 10 μl of Quant-iT PicoGreen dye is added to 450 μl of working solution to make dye reagent (*see* **Note 10**). Protect dye from light by covering with foil or placing in the dark, as the dye is susceptible to photodegradation. Freshly prepare these solutions immediately prior to the labeling reaction.
3. Add equal volume of dye reagent to each sample prepared from **step 1** of this section. Dye reagent (100 μl) is added to 100 μl of each sample to make final volume of 200 μl.
4. Prepare a control that contains siRNA only (sample 7, Fig. 2). Mix 10 pmol of siRNA (10 μl, 1 pmol/μl) with 85 μl of 1× TE and 5 μl of 0.2% SDS. Finally, combine this solution with 100 μl of dye reagent to make final 200 μl final volume (*see* **Note 11**).
5. Transfer samples into 96-well plates (*see* **Note 12**) and incubate at room temperature for 10 min away from light (cover with aluminum foil). Measure the sample fluorescence using a fluorescence microplate reader (excitation ~480 nm, emission ~520 nm).
6. Measure the fluorescence value from 1× TE with 0.01% SDS as background and subtract this value from all samples (1–7).
7. After subtraction from background, almost no signal should be detected from samples 3, 5, and 6. No signal from sample 5 means that washing conditions are good enough to remove siRNA from the filter tube. Example data is shown in Fig. 3a (*see* **Note 13**).

3.2.2 Small Molecule Quantification

1. Lyse EVs by following **step 1** of Subheading 3.2.1 as described previously.
2. Prepare a control that contains Rhodamine B only (sample 7, Fig. 2). Mix 10 μl of Rhodamine B (1 nmol, 100 pmol/μl) with 85 μl of 1× TE and 5 μl of 0.2% SDS.
3. Transfer samples into 96-well plates and measure fluorescence using excitation and emission wavelengths of 540 and 625 nm respectively.
4. Measure the fluorescence value from 1× TE with 0.01% SDS at these wavelengths as background and subtract this value from all samples (1–7).
5. After subtraction from background, almost no signal should be detected from samples 3, 5, and 6. No signal from sample 5 means that washing conditions are good enough to remove Rhodamine B from the filter tube. Example data is shown in Fig. 4a (*see* **Note 14**).

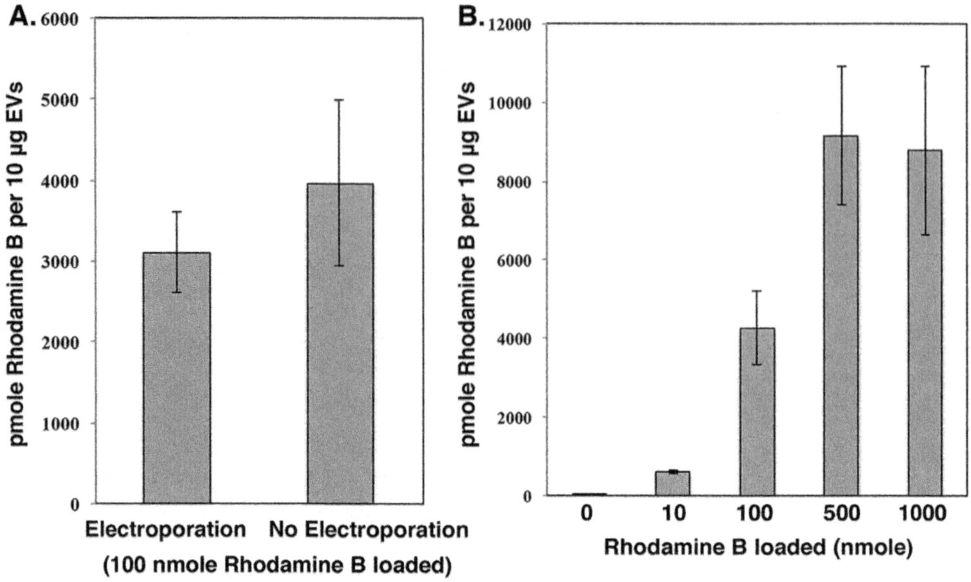

Fig. 4 Small molecule incorporation into EVs. (**a**) Rhodamine B is detectable from EVs that were electroporated or incubated in the presence of Rhodamine B after extensive washing and filtration to remove unassociated molecules. Unlike siRNA, there appears to be no increase in Rhodamine B incorporation into EVs associated with electroporation. (**b**) Rhodamine B associated with EVs is influenced by the initial loading amount until saturation between 500 and 1000 nmol loaded. These data were normalized to the background signal generated by non-electroporated Rhodamine B at each loading point. Note: 10 μg of EVs corresponds to ~3.2×10^8 vesicles

4 Notes

1. Prepare EV-depleted media by centrifuging complete media at 100,000 × *g* for 12 h. EVs included with serum are pelleted out and the supernatant (EV-depleted media) is transferred into a new container and filter sterilized before adding to cells.
2. EVs that are isolated from cells grown on T150 flasks (collected from 40 ml EV-depleted media) are resuspended into 1 ml of ice-cold, sterile 1× PBS. The concentration of EVs is also determined using the BCA assay.
3. Dilute EV samples at least 40-fold in 1× PBS to measure by Nanosight. 10 μl of sample is diluted with 390 μl of 1× PBS since approximate 400 μl sample volume is required for Nanosight measurement.
4. Aliquot EVs into 50 μl (final concentration is ~1 μg/μl) in 0.5 ml tubes to avoid multiple freezing and thawing. Store aliquoted tubes at −80 °C.

5. The composition of samples for siRNA loading, following the schematic described in Fig. 2, is:
   (a) Samples 1 and 4 contain 10 μl of EVs (10 μg, i.e., ~3.2×10^8 vesicles) + 5 μl of siRNA (200 pmol/μl) + 25 μl of 2× electroporation buffer + 10 μl of pure water.
   (b) Samples 2 and 5 are siRNA only, i.e., no EVs and the composition of mixture is 5 μl of siRNA (200 pmol/μl) + 25 μl of 2× electroporation buffer +20 μl of pure water.
   (c) Samples 3 and 6 are EVs only, i.e., without siRNA, the composition of mixture is 10 μl of EVs (10 μg, i.e., ~3.2×10^8 vesicles) + 25 μl of 2× electroporation buffer + 15 μl of pure water.

Sample 2 is used to determine if electroporation causes any siRNA aggregation and sample 5 is used to determine background siRNA levels after the filtration procedure.

6. The composition of samples for Rhodamine B loading, following the schematic described in Fig. 2, is:
   (a) Samples 1 and 4 contain 10 μl of EVs (10 μg, i.e., ~3.2×10^8 vesicles) + 10 μl of Rhodamine B + 25 μl of 2× electroporation buffer +5 μl of water.
   (b) Samples 2 and 5 do not contain EVs and the composition of the solutions is 10 μl of Rhodamine B + 25 μl of 2× electroporation buffer +15 μl of water.
   (c) Samples 3 and 6 do not contain Rhodamine B and the composition of the solutions is 10 μl of EVs (10 μg, i.e., ~3.2×10^8 vesicles) + 25 μl of 2× electroporation buffer +15 μl of water.

Sample 2 is used to determine if electroporation causes any Rhodamine B aggregation or other positive signal and sample 5 is used to determine background Rhodamine B levels after the filtration procedure.

7. Stock solution of Rhodamine B is 10 mM. Higher concentration of Rhodamine B may result in significant adhesion with filter tips and might result in inaccurate concentration measurement.
8. Sample is mixed by pipetting up and down multiple times with 1× TE to ensure that EVs are completely retrieved from the membrane of filter tube.
9. The concentration of SDS will be 0.02% during lysis, which is not inhibitory for the subsequent labeling reaction.
10. The ratio of dye to working solution is 1:50, modified from a suggested 1:200 ratio from the kit instructions.

11. SDS is also added to siRNA alone (sample 7, Fig. 2) to make the same final concentration of SDS as with other samples. The value obtained here is used in the determination of the amount of siRNA associated with EVs.
12. Transfer samples gently into 96-well plates because the presence of SDS can create bubbles easily that hinders fluorescence measurement.
13. The amount of siRNA loaded can be controlled up to a saturation point by varying the initial amount loaded, as indicated in Fig. 3b.
14. The amount of Rhodamine B loaded can be controlled up to a saturation point by varying the initial amount loaded, as indicated in Fig. 4b.

Acknowledgments

This work was supported by NIH R00 grant HL112905, by an ORAU Ralph E. Power Junior Faculty Enhancement Award, and by two University of Maryland Tier 1 seed grants (all to S.M.J.). The authors thank Rini Pek, Navein Arumugasaamy and Anjana Jeyaram for their helpful contributions.

References

1. Gyorgy B, Szabo TG, Pasztoi M, Pal Z, Misjak P, Aradi B, Laszlo V, Pallinger E, Pap E, Kittel A, Nagy G, Falus A, Buzas EI (2011) Membrane vesicles, current state-of-the-art: emerging role of extracellular vesicles. Cell Mol Life Sci 68:2667–2688
2. Colombo M, Raposo G, Thery C (2014) Biogenesis, secretion, and intercellular interactions of exosomes and other extracellular vesicles. Annu Rev Cell Dev Biol 30:255–289
3. Gould SJ, Raposo G (2013) As we wait: coping with an imperfect nomenclature for extracellular vesicles. J Extracell Vesicles 2:eCollection 2013
4. Valadi H, Ekstrom K, Bossios A, Sjostrand M, Lee JJ, Lotvall JO (2007) Exosome-mediated transfer of mRNAs and microRNAs is a novel mechanism of genetic exchange between cells. Nat Cell Biol 9:654–659
5. Ludwig AK, Giebel B (2012) Exosomes: small vesicles participating in intercellular communication. Int J Biochem Cell Biol 44:11–15
6. Alvarez-Erviti L, Seow Y, Yin H, Betts C, Lakhal S, Wood MJ (2011) Delivery of siRNA to the mouse brain by systemic injection of targeted exosomes. Nat Biotechnol 29:341–345
7. Ohno S, Takanashi M, Sudo K, Ueda S, Ishikawa A, Matsuyama N, Fujita K, Mizutani T, Ohgi T, Ochiya T, Gotoh N, Kuroda M (2013) Systemically injected exosomes targeted to EGFR deliver antitumor microRNA to breast cancer cells. Mol Ther 21:185–191
8. Tian Y, Li S, Song J, Ji T, Zhu M, Anderson GJ, Wei J, Nie G (2014) A doxorubicin delivery platform using engineered natural membrane vesicle exosomes for targeted tumor therapy. Biomaterials 35:2383–2390
9. Lamichhane TN, Sokic S, Schardt JS, Raiker RS, Lin JW, Jay SM (2015) Emerging roles for extracellular vesicles in tissue engineering and regenerative medicine. Tissue Eng Part B Rev 21:45–54
10. Taylor DD, Zacharias W, Gercel-Taylor C (2011) Exosome isolation for proteomic analyses and RNA profiling. Methods Mol Biol 728:235–246
11. Rani S, O'Brien K, Kelleher FC, Corcoran C, Germano S, Radomski MW, Crown J,

O'Driscoll L (2011) Isolation of exosomes for subsequent mRNA, MicroRNA, and protein profiling. Methods Mol Biol 784:181–195

12. El-Andaloussi S, Lee Y, Lakhal-Littleton S, Li J, Seow Y, Gardiner C, Alvarez-Erviti L, Sargent IL, Wood MJ (2012) Exosome-mediated delivery of siRNA in vitro and in vivo. Nat Protoc 7:2112–2126
13. Neumann E, Schaefer-Ridder M, Wang Y, Hofschneider PH (1982) Gene transfer into mouse lyoma cells by electroporation in high electric fields. EMBO J 1:841–845
14. Sugar IP, Neumann E (1984) Stochastic model for electric field-induced membrane pores electroporation. Biophys Chem 19:211–225
15. Kooijmans SA, Stremersch S, Braeckmans K, de Smedt SC, Hendrix A, Wood MJ, Schiffelers RM, Raemdonck K, Vader P (2013) Electroporation-induced siRNA precipitation obscures the efficiency of siRNA loading into extracellular vesicles. J Control Release 172:229–238
16. Sun D, Zhuang X, Xiang X, Liu Y, Zhang S, Liu C, Barnes S, Grizzle W, Miller D, Zhang HG (2010) A novel nanoparticle drug delivery system: the anti-inflammatory activity of curcumin is enhanced when encapsulated in exosomes. Mol Ther 18:1606–1614
17. Tauro BJ, Greening DW, Mathias RA, Ji H, Mathivanan S, Scott AM, Simpson RJ (2012) Comparison of ultracentrifugation, density gradient separation, and immunoaffinity capture methods for isolating human colon cancer cell line LIM1863-derived exosomes. Methods 56:293–304

Chapter 5

Delivery of Cytotoxic Mesenchymal Stem Cells with Biodegradable Scaffolds for Treatment of Postoperative Brain Cancer

Kevin T. Sheets, Juli R. Bagó, and Shawn D. Hingtgen

Abstract

Engineered stem cells have recently entered clinical trials as therapeutic agents for treating glioblastoma foci that remain after primary brain tumor resection. However, efficient delivery of anti-cancer mesenchymal stem cells (MSCs) into the resection cavity remains a potential obstacle to therapeutic efficacy in humans. Direct injection quickly leads to significant stem cell loss and poor tumor killing. Recent reports have shown that biodegradable scaffolds improve MSC persistence and restore therapeutic potential. Here, we describe a method for the delivery of therapeutic MSCs on biodegradable fibrin scaffolds into the resection cavity to treat postoperative brain cancer.

Key words Mesenchymal stem cell, Glioblastoma, Fibrin scaffold, Bioluminescence imaging, Cancer

1 Introduction

The stage IV brain cancer glioblastoma (GBM) remains incurable, with an average life expectancy of just over one year following diagnosis [1]. The current standard-of-care treatment regimen, consisting of surgical resection followed by adjuvant chemotherapy and radiation, inevitably results in tumor recurrence due to the highly aggressive and infiltrative phenotypes of the oncogenic astrocytes responsible for this disease [2–4]. Recently, a new therapeutic paradigm has emerged which uses engineered mesenchymal stem cells (MSCs) to chase down evasive tumor cells and deliver targeted payloads, such as the therapeutic agent TNF-α related apoptosis inducing ligand (TRAIL) [5–7]. However, delivery of these cells into the resection cavity has proven to be a difficult task because stem cells that are directly injected are lost within several days, preventing them from colocalizing with and secreting therapies into evasive tumor deposits [8]. To overcome this effect, cells can first be seeded onto a supportive scaffolding material prior to implantation in the

Rachael W. Sirianni and Bahareh Behkam (eds.), *Targeted Drug Delivery: Methods and Protocols*, Methods in Molecular Biology, vol. 1831, https://doi.org/10.1007/978-1-4939-8661-3_5,

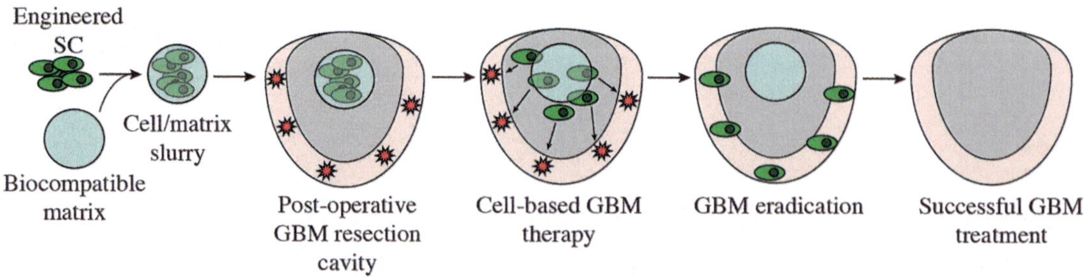

Fig. 1 Overall schematic of the use of a scaffolding material to improve retention, persistence, and therapeutic potential of stem cells (SCs) in the postoperative glioblastoma resection cavity. MSCs are loaded into the scaffold in vitro, which is then implanted in vivo. Over time, the MSCs emerge from the scaffold and migrate toward and colocalize with remnant tumor foci, where they continuously deliver cytotoxic payloads to reduce tumor burden

resection cavity (Fig. 1). The following protocol provides a method for the delivery of therapeutic MSCs on biodegradable polymeric fibrin scaffolds, which prevents early MSC loss, increases MSC persistence, and restores therapeutic efficacy [9].

2 Materials

2.1 Cell Lines and Culture Reagents

* It is beyond the scope of the current work to provide a detailed protocol for lentiviral engineering of diagnostic and therapeutic cell lines. Interested parties are directed to in-depth protocols by Salmon [10] as well as Segura et al. [11] for more information.

1. Engineered mesenchymal stem cells: Human mesenchymal stem cells stably expressing therapeutic protein (in this case secreted TRAIL) with GFP fluorescent marker and renilla luciferase bioluminescent marker (hMSC-sTR GFP-Rluc).
2. Cancer cells: U87 glioma cells stably expressing mCherry fluorescent marker and firefly luciferase bioluminescent marker (U87 mCherry-Fluc).
3. Cell culture media: DMEM supplemented with 10% heat-inactivated fetal bovine serum, 100 μg/ml penicillin, and 100 μg/ml streptomycin.

2.2 Synthetic ECM Polymer Scaffold

1. Fibrinogen (67–106 mg/ml) and thrombin (400–625 units/ml).

Note* One way to obtain these components is by extracting as-received TISSEEL (Baxter, Deerfield, IL), a clinically used biologic tissue sealant.

2.3 In Vivo Mouse Studies

1. Nude mice (6–8 weeks of age) (Jackson Labs, Bar Harbor, ME).
2. Stereotaxic injector (Stoelting Co., Wood Dale, IL).
3. Analgesic: 5 mg/kg carprofen.
4. Anesthetic: inhaled isoflurane.

5. Ophthalmic ointment.
6. Heating pad.
7. Webcol alcohol preps.
8. Betadine.
9. Gauze pads.
10. PBS (500 ml).
11. Syringe, 5 ml capacity.
12. Needles, 23 G and 18 G.
13. Forceps and surgical scissors.
14. Surgical drill.
15. Surgicel (Johnson and Johnson, New Brunswick, NJ).
16. Gastight syringe, 10 μl capacity (Hamilton Company, Reno, NV).
17. Vetbond tissue adhesive (3 M, St. Paul, MN).
18. D-Luciferin.
19. Insulin syringes, 28 G × ½ in.

3 Methods

3.1 Cranial Window

* Prior to initiating any animal studies, adapt an IACUC-approved protocol at your research institution and appropriately train animal handling personnel.

* The following volumes are provided on a per-mouse basis. Multiply as needed for additional mice.

* *See* **Note 1**

1. Administer 5 mg/kg carprofen approximately 30 min prior to the first incision.
2. Place the mouse in an induction chamber and expose the animal to 3–4% isoflurane, until consciousness is lost. Secure the mouse in the stereotaxic frame and reduce anesthesia to 2–3% isoflurane, adjusting as necessary to maintain proper depth of anesthesia.
3. Ensure proper anesthetization by performing a toe pinch on each limb and confirming negative reflex response.
4. Apply ophthalmic ointment to the eyes to protect the cornea from drying out.
5. Sterilize the incision site of the scalp by alternating alcohol and betadine wipes three times.
6. Pinch and lift the scalp with forceps and make a midline rostral-caudal incision spanning from the base of the eye to the top of the ear (no longer than 1 cm; *see* Fig. 4b) using surgical scissors. Irrigate the incision site with PBS. The subdermal fat layer can be cleaned from the surface of the skull by scraping with forceps or the flat edge of a scalpel blade if necessary.

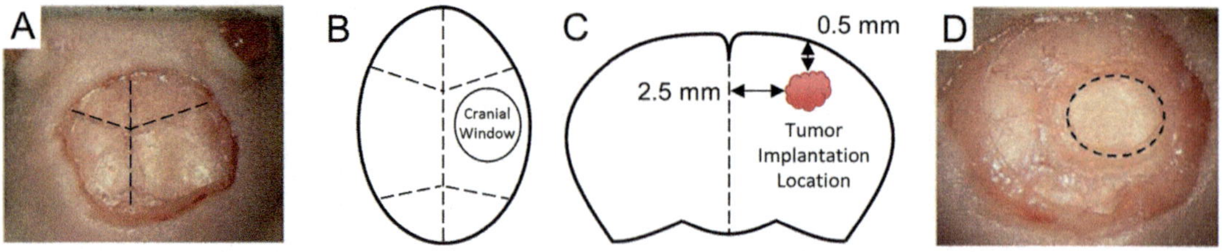

Fig. 2 (**a**) Light image of the mouse skull with skin removed. (**b**) Top-down and (**c**) coronal section views of tumor implantation coordinates. (**d**) Drilled rim around the cranial window. Dashed circle indicates the tumor growing area in the cranial window. Adapted with permission from Nature Publishing Group [8]

7. Scribe a cranial window in the skull using the micro drill. Use the drill to thin the bone on the edges of the window that covers a region large enough for tumor removal (Fig. 2a, b). Drill down through the entire skull thickness and stop just above the dura. When completely scribed, the window will detach and may be removed with forceps. Control bleeding with PBS irrigation and Surgicel as needed.
8. Close the skin and apply Vetbond to seal the wound. Remove the animal from inhaled anesthetic and transport to heated recovery. Return to cage once ambulatory. Continue to administer analgesic on IACUC-approved schedule.

3.2 Tumor Implantation

1. Allow at least 3 days following cranial window procedure prior to implanting tumors. This allows the animal to adequately recover from the previous surgery.
2. Trypsinize and pellet U87 mCherry-Fluc cells. Resuspend to a final concentration of 3.3×10^4 cells per μl media and pipette into a 2 ml vial. Keep the vial on ice until the cells can be injected.
3. Prepare the animal for tumor implantation surgery by following Subheading 3.1 **steps 1–6**. The skin incision should be made in the same location as the original wound. While leaving the dura intact, remove any subdermal fat, scar tissue, or remnant glue that may interfere with access to the implantation site.
4. Load a 10 μl Hamilton syringe with 5 μl U87 mCherry-Fluc cells into the stereotaxic injector (*see* **Note 2**).
5. Insert the syringe 2.5 mm lateral from the bregma and penetrate the dura and parenchyma to a 0.5 mm depth (Fig. 2c, d). Inject cells at a rate of 1 μl/min for 3 min. After injection, pause for 5 min to allow the cells to settle. Retract the syringe slowly.
6. Close the skin and apply Vetbond sealant to glue the wound back together. Remove the animal from inhaled anesthetic and transport to heated recovery. Return to cage once ambulatory. Continue to administer analgesic on IACUC-approved schedule.

3.3 Postoperative Tumor Growth Tracking

1. Using the 28 G insulin syringe, inject mice IP with 150 mg/kg luciferin. After injection, allow 10 min for the luciferin to circulate throughout the body and react with the engineered

cells in the brain prior to imaging. Place mice in a bioluminescent imaging system during this time.

2. Under anesthesia, image mice using sufficient exposure times to determine relative tumor size. A 5 min exposure time is typically used, however this may be adjusted (seconds to minutes) depending on tumor size. Using the manufacturer's software, draw a region of interest around the tumor signal and measure the flux (photons/s, *see* **Note 3**). Imaging every 2–4 days will enable accurate monitoring of the rate of tumor growth.
3. When tumor has reached appreciable size (*see* **Note 4**), schedule the mice for tumor resection and scaffold implantation surgery.

3.4 Seeding Fibrin Scaffolds

* The following volumes are provided on a per-scaffold basis. Multiply quantities as needed for additional scaffolds.

1. Trypsinize and pellet 1.0–5.0 × 10^5 MSCs for each scaffold.
2. Aspirate supernatant and resuspend MSCs in 8 μl fibrinogen component.
3. Cross-link by adding 8 μl thrombin and physically mix using a micropipette tip for 30 s to create "droplets".
4. If desired, scaffold droplets can be flattened into "surface patches" approximately 1 mm thick through application of physical pressure using a sterile conical tube. This altered scaffold morphology allows the cells to be delivered as a lining that leaves the interior of the surgical cavity empty to accommodate fluid accumulation or allow for delivery of additional scaffolds.
5. Cover the scaffolds in DMEM media and incubate for 24–48 h prior to implantation (Fig. 3).

3.5 Fluorescence-Guided Resection and Scaffold Implantation

1. Follow the procedure outlined in Subheading 3.1 **steps 1–6** to prepare mice for resection (Fig. 4).
2. With an 18 G needle, gently and slowly puncture the dura near the border of the cranial window. Repeat this motion such that a contiguous incision is made circumferentially around the window. Using forceps, peel and remove the dura, revealing the underlying tumor.
3. Using fluorescence guidance and a vacuum pump, aspirate the tumor. This can be accomplished using a normal stereotax setup that is placed under a stereomicroscope with fluorescent illumination. Control bleeding with copious PBS irrigation and surgicel if necessary (*see* **Note 5**).
4. Implant an MSC-loaded scaffold into the resection cavity. Add 1 μl fibrinogen followed by 1 μl thrombin to secure the scaffold in place (*see* **Note 6**).

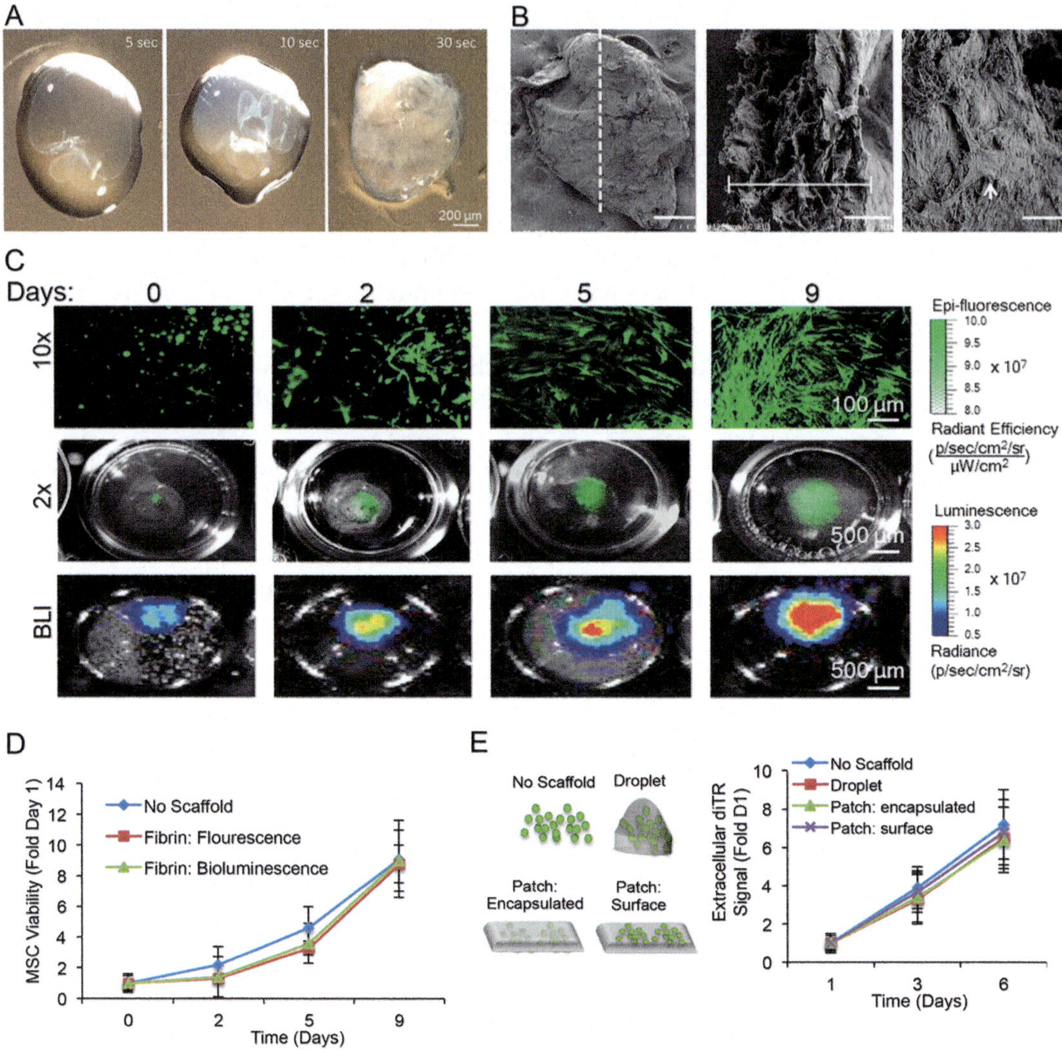

Fig. 3 Characterization of cytotoxic hMSCs within fibrin matrices. (**a**) Representative white-light images demonstrating the rapid gelation of fibrinogen 5, 10, and 30 s after the addition of thrombin to create encapsulated cytotoxic stem cells. (**b**) SEM images showing fibrin matrices encapsulating engineered hMSCs. Cross-sectional analysis revealed the presence of hMSCs within the fibrin matrix (indicated with arrowhead). Dotted line depicts site of cross section. (**c**) Representative fluorescent and bioluminescent imaging (BLI) data depicting the growth of hMSC in fibrin over time. Fluorescent images are captured at 10× to depict cellular morphology and 2× to demonstrate overall cell growth. Simultaneous BLI was performed to validate cell volumes. (**d**) Summary graph showing statistically similar growth of hMSC-sTR cultured with or without Fibrin ($P > 0.05$ value by Two-Way ANOVA). (**e**) Summary data showing the levels of cytotoxic protein secreted by hMSC-diTR grown in different fibrin matrices or without scaffolds. "Droplet" formation was created by suspending and polymerizing stem cells in a droplet of fibrin. The "encapsulated patch" was created by encapsulating stem cells in a fibrin droplet that was pressed into a flat sheet. The "surface patch" was created by seeding stem cells onto the surface of a fibrin scaffold that was polymerized and flattened. TRAIL secretion was determined by BLI on media samples collected 1, 3, and 6 days after seeding. Data in **d** and **e** are mean ± SEM and represent three different experiments performed in triplicate. Scale bar in **b** from left to right are 250 µm, 50 µm, and 10 µm. Adapted with permission from Elsevier [9]

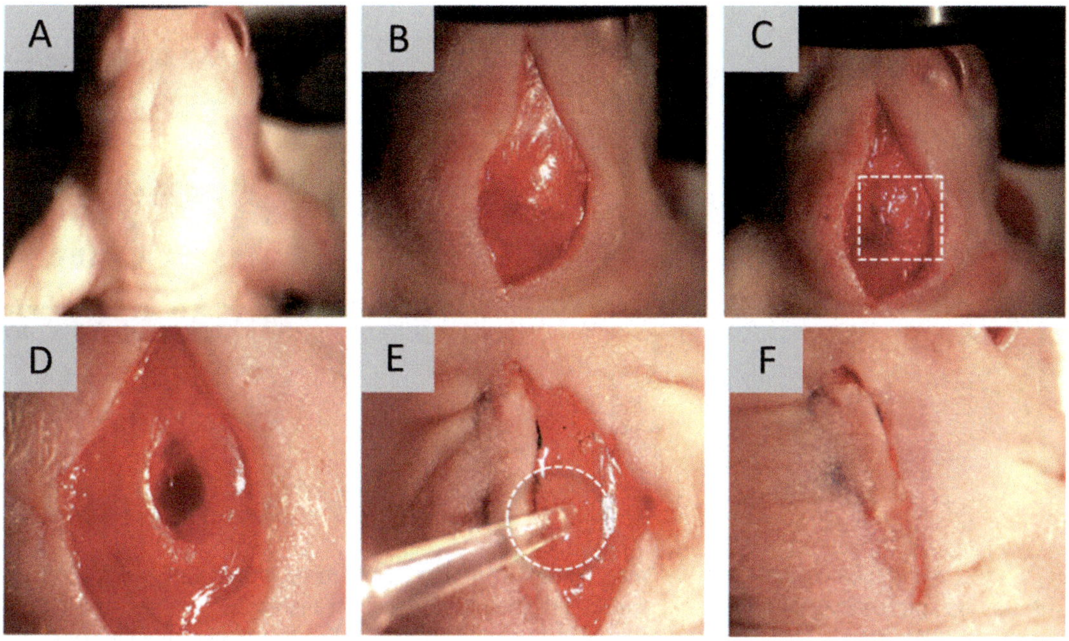

Fig. 4 Intra-operative images showing the seeding of engineered hMSCs encapsulated in fibrin matrices within the post-surgical cavity. Mice were immobilized on stereotactic devices (**a**) and an incision was made in the scalp (**b**). A craniotomy was performed to expose the underlying tumor (dashed square) (**c**) that was resected using image-guided microsurgery to create a resection cavity (**d**). Engineered hMSCs were seeded into the cavity in fibrin (dashed circle) (**e**). The skin was then closed over the resection cavity (**f**). Adapted with permission from Elsevier [9]

5. Close the skin and apply Vetbond tissue sealant to glue to wound back together. Remove the animal from inhaled anesthetic and transport to heated recovery. Return to cage once ambulatory. Continue to administer analgesic on IACUC-approved schedule.

3.6 Postoperative Imaging and Cytototxic Stem Cell Administration

1. Repeat imaging procedure outlined in Subheading 3.3 as needed to determine the growth of the primary tumor while continuing to monitor overall animal health. The MSCs will continuously secrete TRAIL, suppressing tumor growth. We find that imaging every 4–5 days provides sufficient temporal resolution for tumor growth when exposed to therapy.
2. Sacrifice mice and collect tissues for analysis when predetermined endp3oints outlined in IACUC protocol have been met (Fig. 5).

4 Notes

1. If desired, tumors may be implanted prior to establishing the cranial window. In this case, the tumor is established by passing the needle carrying tumor cells through a burr hole in the skull. Tumor growth is then tracked by bioluminescence. The full

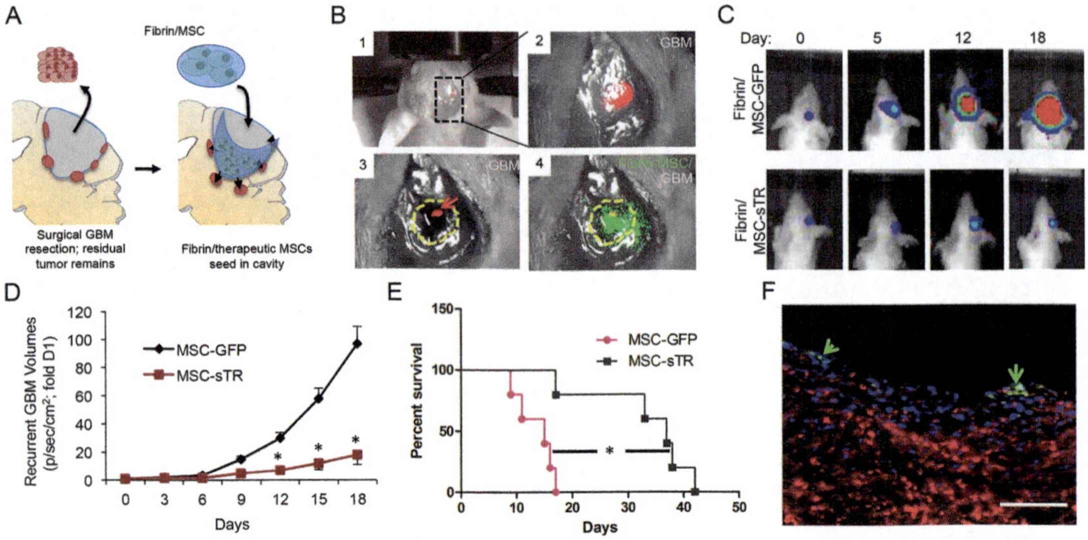

Fig. 5 Cytotoxic hMSCs delivered into the resection cavity in fibrin delay re-growth of post-surgical residual GBM. (**a**) To mimic clinical fibrin-delivered stem cell therapy for surgically resected GBM, established intracranial human GBMs were surgically debulked in mice. Therapeutic stem cells were transplanted into the post-operative cavity in fibrin patches. (**b**) Representative images showing pre-resection mCherry + GBMs, the post-surgical GBM cavity, and GFP + hMSC-sTR in fibrin seeded in the resection cavity. The dotted line indicates the resection cavity. The arrowhead indicates residual GBM foci. (**c**, **d**) Representative images (**c**) and summary graph (**d**) of serial BLI showing a significant reduction in GBM regrowth in hMSC-sTR-treated animals compared to control-treated animals. Significantly smaller tumor volumes were observed in hMSC-sTR-treated tumors across multiple time points. $^*P < 0.01$ by repeated measures ANOVA. (**e**) Kaplan-Meyer survival analysis showing the survival of animals with resected GBMs treated with hMSC-sTR therapy or control hMSC-GFPRLuc. Median survival was 36 days for hMSC-sTR treated animals vs. 15 days for control-treated mice. $^*P < 0.01$ by log-rank test. (**f**) Fluorescent images of post-mortem tissue sections showing the presence of GFP + hMSCs (green) along the border of the recurrent GBM (red). Nuclei were counterstained with Hoechst (blue). Data in **d** are mean ± SEM. Scale bar in **f** is 100 μm. Adapted with permission from Elsevier [9]

cranial window can then be created over the existing tumor prior to resection. We choose to create the window first so that the tumor's bioluminescent intensity is both brighter and more consistent among pre- and post-resection time points, but the impact of this decision is insignificant toward overall therapeutic efficacy and animal survival.

2. To maximize consistency of tumor volumes that are implanted, it is critical that the vial containing the U87s is well mixed prior to drawing cells into the Hamilton syringe. We find that using a pipette set to half of the overall cell mixture volume works well for this purpose. Since the cells should be placed on ice when not in use, they tend to quickly settle at the bottom of the vial. Therefore, it is important to triturate this vial prior to each loading of the syringe.
3. Bioluminescence imaging is used to track tumor growth (or MSC persistence) by counting the number of photons that are

emitted from luciferase+ cells during a given exposure time. As tumors grow, they become brighter and require shorter exposure times to gather the same number of photons and prevent signal saturation. For this reason, instead of photon (p) counts, the light emitted per second per area or "radiance" (p/s/cm^2) is used. Radiance allows for comparison of tumor signal across time points independent of exposure time.

4. Timing between tumor implantation and resection is critical for obtaining high-fidelity results when using mice to model dynamics of human tumors. Depending on tumor morphology and number of cells initially given, this gap is reported to vary from 1 to 4 weeks [12–14]. For example, U87s grow as a solid tumor mass and as such, timing between implantation and resection can be more forgiving. Other glioma lines, such as those obtained from patient-derived xenografts, grow in diffuse and highly infiltrative morphologies. If a diffuse tumor model is selected, a larger number of initial cells (5.0×10^5) can be used while simultaneously waiting a shorter period of time (3–4 days) prior to resection and scaffold implantation. This creates a scenario where the tumor is both large enough to visualize and condensed enough to mimic human tumor spreading. For the U87 model shown here, we typically resect 7–10 days after implantation of 1.0×10^5 cells, at which point the tumor's average radiance approaches 1×10^8 p/s/cm^2. Several days beyond this point, subjects will begin to become moribund. However, since radiance is affected by a number of factors, this benchmark should be confirmed when starting a new model and should not be relied upon as the sole deciding factor on when to initiate resection.
5. In our experience, the rate-limiting step of each surgery is controlling bleeding. Irrigation with room-temperature saline can partially slow bleeding, but it is important to use a hemostatic agent as well in situations where bleeding cannot be controlled within several minutes. We use Surgicel for this purpose. We cut a Surgicel sheet into resection cavity-sized snips and place in the cavity for 2–3 min. If after this time bleeding continues, we replace with a new snip of Surgicel. Once the bleeding has stopped, remove as much of the remnant Surgicel from the resection cavity as possible, and irrigate the cavity with PBS to restore physiological pH to the cavity tissue.
6. Use fibrinogen/thrombin to ensure that the scaffold remains in the resection cavity following surgery. Brain swelling following resection tends to push the scaffold outward, potentially removing it from the parenchyma if it is not temporarily held in place with a tissue sealant. Fibrin will stay intact long enough to hold the scaffold in place but will dissolve in time to permit MSC migration.

Acknowledgment

This work was supported by the UNC Lineberger Comprehensive Cancer Center's University Cancer Research Fund and the UNC Translational and Clinical Sciences Institute (KL2TR001109, UL1TR001111).

References

1. Dolecek T, Propp J, Stroup N, Kruchko C (2012) CBTRUS statistical report: primary brain and central nervous system tumors diagnosed in the United States in 2005–2009. Neuro-Oncology 14:v1–v49. https://doi.org/10.1093/neuonc/nos218
2. Agnihotri S, Burrell K, Wolf A et al (2012) Glioblastoma, a brief review of history, molecular genetics, animal models and novel therapeutic strategies. Arch Immunol Ther Exp 61:25–41. https://doi.org/10.1007/s00005-012-0203-0
3. Stupp R, Mason WP, van den Bent MJ et al (2005) Radiotherapy plus concomitant and adjuvant temozolomide for glioblastoma. N Engl J Med 352:987–996. https://doi.org/10.1056/NEJMoa043330
4. Omuro A, DeAngelis L (2013) Glioblastoma and other malignant gliomas: a clinical review. JAMA 310:1842–1850. https://doi.org/10.1001/jama.2013.280319
5. Aboody K, Najbauer J, Metz M et al (2013) Neural stem cell-mediated enzyme/prodrug therapy for glioma: preclinical studies. Sci Transl Med 5:184ra59. https://doi.org/10.1126/scitranslmed.3005365
6. Kim K, Kim P et al (2006) Human neural stem cells target experimental intracranial medulloblastoma and deliver a therapeutic gene leading to tumor regression. Clin Cancer Res 12:55505556. https://doi.org/10.1158/1078-0432.CCR-05-2508
7. Balyasnikova I, Ferguson S, Han Y et al (2011) Therapeutic effect of neural stem cells expressing TRAIL and bortezomib in mice with glioma xenografts. Cancer Lett 310:148–159. https://doi.org/10.1016/j.canlet.2011.06.029
8. Kauer T, Figueiredo J-L, Hingtgen S, Shah K (2011) Encapsulated therapeutic stem cells implanted in the tumor resection cavity induce cell death in gliomas. Nat Neurosci 15:197–204. https://doi.org/10.1038/nn.3019
9. Bagó J, Pegna G, Okolie O, Hingtgen S (2016) Fibrin matrices enhance the transplant and efficacy of cytotoxic stem cell therapy for post-surgical cancer. Biomaterials 84:42–53. https://doi.org/10.1016/j.biomaterials.2016.01.007
10. Salmon P (2013) Generation of human cell lines using lentiviral-mediated genetic engineering. Methods Mol Biol 945:417–448. https://doi.org/10.1007/978-1-62703-125-7_25
11. Segura MMM, Garnier A, Durocher Y et al (2010) New protocol for lentiviral vector mass production. Methods Mol Biol 614:39–52. https://doi.org/10.1007/978-1-60761-533-0_2
12. Martinez-Quintanilla J, He D, Wakimoto H et al (2015) Encapsulated stem cells loaded with hyaluronidase-expressing oncolytic virus for brain tumor therapy. Mol Ther 23:108–118. https://doi.org/10.1038/mt.2014.204
13. Redjal N, Zhu Y, Shah K (2015) Combination of systemic chemotherapy with local stem cell delivered S-TRAIL in resected brain tumors. Stem Cells 33:101–110. https://doi.org/10.1002/stem.1834
14. Hingtgen S, Figueiredo J-L, Farrar C et al (2012) Real-time multi-modality imaging of glioblastoma tumor resection and recurrence. J Neuro-Oncol 111:153–161. https://doi.org/10.1007/s11060-012-1008-z

Chapter 6

Nanoparticles for Targeted Drug Delivery to Cancer Stem Cells and Tumor

Hai Wang and Xiaoming He

Abstract

Due to the drug resistance of cancer stem cells (CSCs), CSC-targeted delivery of multiple drugs in nanoparticle-based drug delivery system holds great potential for the destruction of the CSCs and Tumor. In this chapter, we describe the preparation of multi-layered pH-responsive polymeric nanoparticles (NPs) by multiple emulsifications to encapsulate multiple hydrophilic and hydrophobic theranostic agents for controlled and sequenced release. Hyaluronic acid (HA) is used for not only actively targeting the CSCs to reduce their drug resistance due to dormancy (i.e., slow metabolism), but also replacing the commonly used poly (vinyl alcohol) (PVA) as a stabilizing agent to synthesize the nanoparticles.

Key words Nanoparticles, Cancer stem cells, Polymer, Controlled release, Combination therapy, Responsiveness, Active targeting

1 Introduction

Cancer stem cells (CSCs) are rare subpopulations of cancer cells that can initiate and/or reinitiate the formation of tumors including metastasis after the conventional radio and chemotherapy [1, 2]. Because of their resistance to chemotherapeutic drugs, the CSCs have attracted a great deal of attention in the field of oncology in the past ~10 years [3, 4]. One of the major strategies for overcoming drug resistance of CSCs is combination therapy, which is the combined use of two or more chemotherapeutic agents with different anticancer mechanisms or multiple treatment modalities [5–7]. However, due to the vast difference in physiochemical and pharmacokinetic properties of different chemotherapeutic drugs including solubility, biodistribution, circulation time in blood, and cell membrane transport properties, the current practice of simply using multiple free agents with no control of their delivery and release is far from being optimal in making use of the therapeutic capacity of the agents for cancer treatment. Therefore, it is

Rachael W. Sirianni and Bahareh Behkam (eds.), *Targeted Drug Delivery: Methods and Protocols*, Methods in Molecular Biology, vol. 1831, https://doi.org/10.1007/978-1-4939-8661-3_6,

important to develop a vehicle for delivering all the different chemotherapeutic drugs together in a controlled fashion [8, 9].

Amphiphilic block copolymer-based nanoparticles have attracted much attention for the delivery of chemotherapeutic drugs for several decades [10, 11]. The emulsion-solvent evaporation method is usually used for encapsulating hydrophobic drugs in the polymeric nanoparticles by fabricating an "oil-in-water" configuration [12]. The double emulsion method is the commonly used approach to form a "water-in-oil-in-water" configuration for encapsulating hydrophilic drugs [13, 14]. Both methods have been extensively utilized to encapsulate chemotherapeutic drugs for cancer treatment. However, for most studies using the two methods, either hydrophobic or hydrophilic agent (but not both) has been encapsulated in the nanoparticles for delivery. In this chapter, we report a series of emulsion-based methods for assembling multi-layered core-shell polymeric nanoparticles to encapsulate one or more hydrophilic and hydrophobic agents for co-delivery.

Furthermore, in order to actively target the CSCs, we have developed the method by using hyaluronic acid (HA) instead of poly (vinyl alcohol) (PVA) during the preparation of the multi-layered core–shell polymeric nanoparticles. Since HA can bind to the variant CD44 antigen commonly overexpressed on the surface of many types of CSCs [15, 16], the resultant nanoparticles can be used to specifically co-deliver multiple drugs into the CSCs. In this protocol, curcumin (CUR, hydrophobic), doxorubicin hydrochloride (DOX, hydrophilic), irinotecan or camptothecin (CPT, hydrophobic), and indocyanine green (ICG, hydrophilic) were used as the model agents. The nanoparticles are prepared with four polymers that are approved by the US Food and Drug Administration (FDA) for medical use: Poly(d,l-lactide-co-glycolide) (PLGA), Pluronic F127 (PF127 with and without chitosan modification), chitosan, and HA. By combining PLGA and PF127 together, more stable and uniform-sized nanoparticles can be obtained than using PLGA or PF127 alone. Chitosan has also been shown to specifically bind to the variant CD44 overexpressed on the CSCs [17].

2 Materials

2.1 Nanoparticle Synthesis

1. PLGA (lactide:glycolide: 75:25, Mw: 4000–15,000).
2. Pluronic F127 (PF127).
3. Hyaluronic acid (HA, Mw: 66–90 kDa).
4. Polyvinyl alcohol (PVA, Mw: 100 kDa).
5. Chitosan oligosaccharide of pharmaceutical grade (Mw: 1.2 kDa, 95% deacetylation).
6. Irinotecan/camptothecin.

2.2 Preparation of Drug Solutions

1. For DOX, weigh the desired amount of DOX (1–10 mg/ml) and mix it with 5 ml of deionized water for 1 h. Store the solution at 4 °C for no more than 1 month before use and keep it away from light.
2. For ICG, mix it with deionized water for 0.5 h before use.
3. For hydrophobic drugs, dissolve in dichloromethane (DCM, 1–30 mg/ml) before use.

2.3 In Vitro Drug Release Study

1. Phosphate-buffered saline (PBS) buffer of pH 7.4 or 5.0.
2. Dialysis bags (MWCO: 20 kDa).

3 Methods

3.1 Preparation of Chitosan-Modified PF127 (Chitosan-PF127)

1. Add a total of 30 ml of PF127 solution (26 mM in benzene) dropwise into 30 ml of 4-nitrophenyl chloroformate (4-NPC) (160 mM in benzene) solution.
2. Stir the mixture for 3 h in N_2 atmosphere at room temperature to activate PF127.
3. Precipitate and filter the activated polymer in excess (ice-cold) diethyl ether for three times and dried under vacuum overnight.
4. Add a total of 10 ml of chitosan solution (200 mg/ml, in DI water) dropwise into 10 ml of the activated PF127 solution (400 mg/ml, in deionized water).
5. After stirring for 12 h, dialyze (MWCO: 7 kDa) the mixture against DI water for 24 h.
6. Freeze-dry the sample for 48 h to remove water to obtain dry chitosan-modified PF127 (chitosan-PF127).

3.2 Preparation of HA Solution

0.125% HA solution: Weigh 125 mg of HA and mix with 100 ml of deionized (DI) water (Resistivity >10 Ω.m) for 24 h. Store at 4 °C.

3.3 Preparation of PVA Solution

1. Slowly add PVA powder into DI water to fully disperse it in water.
2. Once the powder is fully dispersed (~2 h), heat the suspension to the temperature at which the polymer is soluble (temperature from 90 °C to 95 °C is suitable).
3. Stir the sample at this temperature until fully solubilizing the PVA (~5 h). Store the solution at room temperature for no more than 1 month before use.

3.4 Particle Fabrication Using the Single-Emulsion Method

1. Dissolve 10 mg of PLGA, 10 mg of PF127, and the desired amount of CUR (starting from 1 mg, and the amount can be adjusted according to the drug encapsulation efficiency and the desired amount of drug in the nanoparticles) in 1 ml of DCM. Transfer this solution together with 10 ml of the aqueous

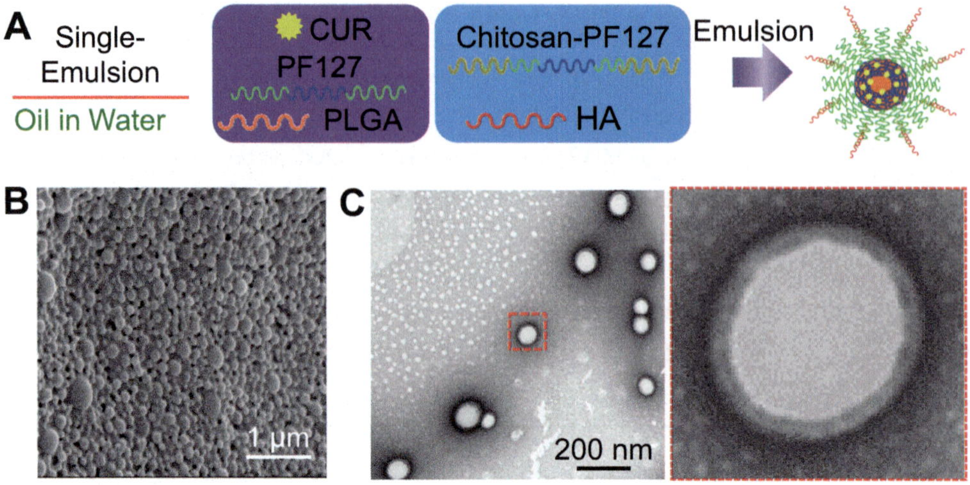

Fig. 1 (**A**) A schematic illustration of the single-emulsion method. (**B**) Scanning electron microscopy (SEM) and (**C**) transmission electron microscopy (TEM) images of the resultant nanoparticles. The inset in (**C**) is a zoom-in view of the nanoparticle showing its core-shell morphology (reproduced from [9] with permission from Royal Society of Chemistry)

solution of chitosan-PF127 (10 mg) and HA into a centrifuge tube and emulsify the two immiscible solutions by sonication for 2 min using Ultrasonic Liquid Sonicators (*see* **Note 1**).

2. Remove the DCM by rotary evaporation of the resultant emulsion for 15 min (*see* **Note 2**).
3. Collect the nanoparticles by centrifugation at 13,800 × *g* for 10 min at room temperature and washing twice with deionized water.
4. Suspend the nanoparticles at the desired concentration for further use.

In summary, the single-emulsion method can be used for encapsulating one or more hydrophobic agents. A schematic illustration of the procedure of single-emulsion method and the characterization of the resultant nanoparticles are summarized in Fig. 1 (*see* **Note 3**). The nanoparticles can be used immediately or store at −20 °C for ~1 month.

3.5 Particle Fabrication Using the Double-Emulsion Method

1. Transfer a total of 0.4 ml of DOX solution (in deionized water) at the desired concentration, together with 2 ml of DCM containing 10 mg of PLGA, 10 mg of PF127, and the desired amount of CUR (same as that in Subheading 3.4) into a centrifuge tube and emulsify the two immiscible solutions by sonication for 2 min using Ultrasonic Liquid Sonicators (*see* **Note 1**).
2. Mix the first emulsion with 10 ml of aqueous solution of chitosan-PF127 and HA.
3. Emulsify the mixture by sonication for 2 min (*see* **Note 4**).

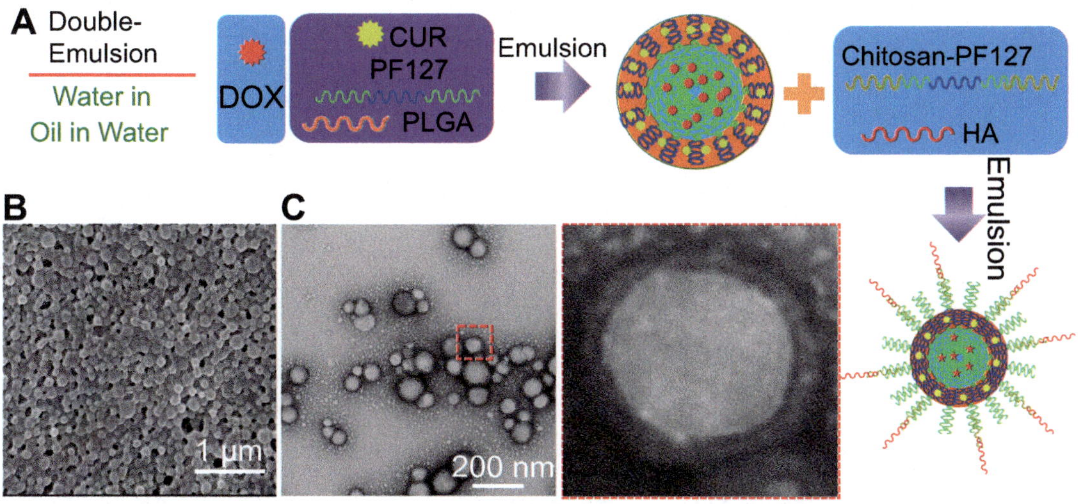

Fig. 2 (**A**) A schematic illustration of the double-emulsion method. (**B**) SEM and (**C**) TEM images of the resultant nanoparticles. The inset in (**C**) is a zoom-in view of the resultant nanoparticle showing its core-shell morphology (reproduced from [9] with permission from Royal Society of Chemistry)

4. Remove DCM by rotary evaporation of the resultant emulsion for 15 min (*see* **Note 2**).
5. Collect nanoparticles by centrifugation at 13,800 × *g* for 10 min at room temperature and wash twice with deionized water.
6. Suspend the nanoparticles in a desired solution (e.g., culture medium) for further use.

In summary, the double-emulsion method can be used for encapsulating both hydrophobic and hydrophilic agents. A schematic illustration of the procedure of the double-emulsion method and the characterization of the resultant nanoparticles are given in Fig. 2 (*see* **Note 3**). The nanoparticles can be used immediately or store at −20 °C for ~1 month.

3.6 Particle Fabrication Using the Triple-Emulsion Method

1. Dissolve a total of 10 mg of PLGA, 10 mg of PF127, and the desired amount of CUR (same as that in Subheading 3.4) in 0.5 ml of DCM. Then, transfer this solution together with 2 ml of 2% PVA solution (in deionized water) into a centrifuge tube, and emulsify the two immiscible solutions by sonication for 1 min (*see* **Note 1**).
2. Mix the first emulsion with 100 μl of DOX solution (in deionized water).
3. Add a total of 4 ml of DCM with PLGA and PF127 (10 mg for both PLGA and PF127) and emulsified by sonication for 2 min.
4. Mix the second emulsion with 100 μl of CPT solution (in DCM).
5. Add a total of 10 ml of aqueous solution of chitosan-PF127 and HA and emulsify the mixture by sonication for 2 min (*see* **Note 5**).

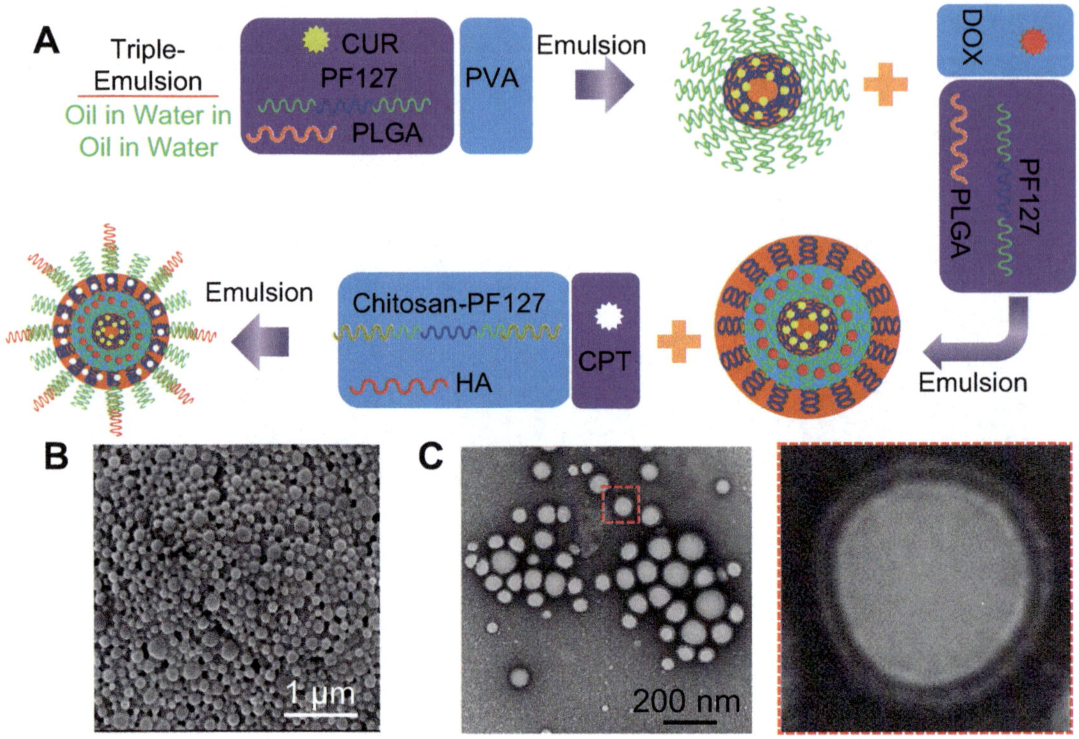

Fig. 3 (**A**) A schematic illustration of the triple-emulsion method. (**B**) SEM and (**C**) TEM images of the resultant nanoparticles. The inset in (**C**) is a zoom-in view of the resultant nanoparticle showing its core and two-layered morphology (reproduced from [9] with permission from Royal Society of Chemistry)

6. Remove DCM by rotary evaporation of the resultant emulsion for 15 min (*see* **Note 2**).
7. Collect nanoparticles by centrifugation at 13,800 × *g* for 10 min at room temperature and wash twice with deionized water.
8. Suspend the nanoparticles in a desired solution (e.g., culture medium) for further use.

In summary, both hydrophobic and hydrophilic agents can be encapsulated into the multi-layered nanoparticles produced by the triple-emulsion method. The hydrophobic agents can be encapsulated in the core or the outer hydrophobic layer. The hydrophilic agents can be encapsulated in the middle hydrophilic layer. A schematic illustration of the procedure of the triple-emulsion method and the characterization of the resultant nanoparticles are given in Fig. 3 (*see* **Note 3**). The nanoparticles can be used immediately or store at −20 °C for ~1 month.

3.7 Particle Fabrication Using the Quadruple-Emulsion Method

1. Dissolve 10 mg of PLGA and 10 mg of PF127 in 1 ml of DCM (*see* **Note 1**).
2. After adding 0.2 ml of DOX solution (in deionized water), emulsify the immiscible solutions by sonication for 1 min.

3. Mix this first emulsion with 100 μl of CUR solution (in DCM).
4. Add a total of 2 ml of 2% PVA solution (in deionized water) and the mixture emulsified by sonication for 2 min.
5. Mix the second emulsion with 100 μl of ICG solution (in deionized water).
6. Add a total of 4 ml of DCM with PLGA and PF127 and emulsify the mixture by sonication for 2 min.
7. Mix the third emulsion with 100 μl of CPT solution (in DCM).
8. Add a total of 15 ml of chitosan-PF127 and HA solution (in deionized water) and emulsify the mixture by sonication for 2 min.
9. Remove DCM by rotary evaporation of the resultant emulsion for 15 min (*see* **Note 2**).
10. Collect the nanoparticles by centrifugation at 13,800 × *g* for 10 min at room temperature and wash twice with deionized water.
11. Suspend the nanoparticles in a desired solution (e.g., culture medium) for further use.

In summary, both hydrophilic and hydrophobic agents can be encapsulated into the multi-layered nanoparticles produced by the quadruple-emulsion method. The hydrophilic agents can be encapsulated in the core or the middle hydrophilic layer, while hydrophobic agents can be encapsulated in the middle or outer hydrophobic layer. A schematic illustration of the procedure of the quadruple-emulsion method and the characterization of the resultant nanoparticles are given in Fig. 4 (*see* **Note 3**). The nanoparticles can be used immediately or store at −20 °C for ~1 month.

3.8 In Vitro Drug Release Study

1. Drug-laden nanoparticles (20–30 mg) are dissolved in PBS (5 ml, pH 5 or 7.4).
2. Transfer the nanoparticles solution into dialysis bags (MWCO: 20 kDa).
3. Put the dialysis bags in 30 ml of the same PBS at 37 °C and stir at 110 rpm using a mini-stir bar.
4. At appropriate time points, 100 μl of the dialysate is collected, and the sample is replenished with the same amount of fresh PBS.
5. The concentration of the released agents/drugs in the removed dialysate is determined using UV-Vis spectrophotometry based on the absorbance of drug (*see* **Note 6**).

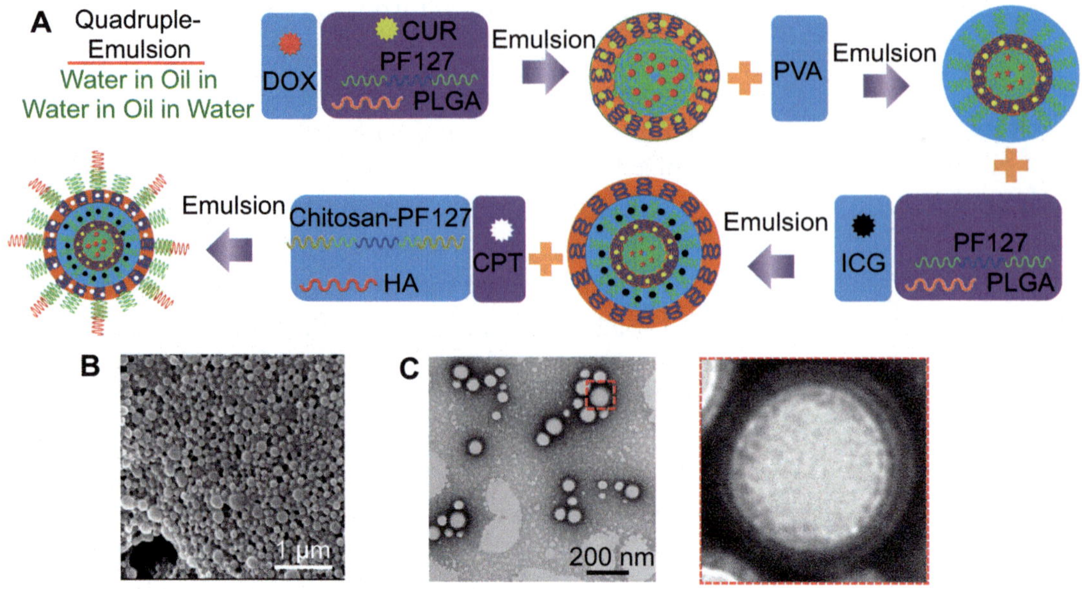

Fig. 4 (**A**) A schematic illustration of the quadruple-emulsion method. (**B**) SEM and (**C**) TEM images of the nanoparticles. The inset in (**C**) is a zoom-in view of the nanoparticle showing its core and three-layered morphology (reproduced from [9] with permission from Royal Society of Chemistry)

4 Notes

1. The amount of polymers and drugs can be adjusted. The volume of oil (i.e., organic solvent) and aqueous solution can be adjusted to make nanoparticles of different sizes in the core and shell(s). The power and time of the ultrasound for emulsification can be changed also to make nanoparticles of different sizes.
2. Complete removal of organic solvent is crucial to obtain small-sized nanoparticles and minimize the potential toxicity of the resultant nanoparticles. Usually, no bubble formation in the mixture indicates complete removal of organic solvent.
3. The polydispersity of the resulting particles is mainly dependent on the sonication process. A better polydispersity can be achieved if the emulsion is more homogeneous during sonication. The size of the nanoparticles is also associated with the sonication process. Under higher power, the size of the nanoparticles is smaller compared with the ones made with lower power.
4. To minimize overheating during the emulsification, the tube with the mixture can be placed in the ice or water bath to control the temperature.
5. At the last emulsion, the total volume of the sample is large compared with previous emulsions. Therefore, in order to

achieve homogenous emulsion, the solution can be divided and emulsified at a higher power.

6. High-performance liquid chromatography (HLPC) can also be used to determine the amount of the agents/drugs, which is not affected by the polymers in the nanoparticles.

Acknowledgment

This work was supported by an American Cancer Society (ACS) Research Scholar Grant (No. 120936-RSG-11-109-01-CDD) and an NIH grant (R01CA206366) to X.H., and a Pelotonia Postdoctoral Fellowship to H.W.

Reference

1. Clevers H (2011) The cancer stem cell: premises, promises and challenges. Nat Med 17:313–319
2. Rosen JM, Jordan CT (2009) The increasing complexity of the cancer stem cell paradigm. Science 324:1670–1673
3. Dean M, Fojo T, Bates S (2005) Tumour stem cells and drug resistance. Nat Rev Cancer 5:275–284
4. Donnenberg VS, Donnenberg AD (2005) Multiple drug resistance in cancer revisited: the cancer stem cell hypothesis. J Clin Pharmacol 45:872–877
5. Wang H, Agarwal P, Zhao S, Xu RX, Yu J, Lu X, He X (2015) Hyaluronic acid-decorated dual responsive nanoparticles of Pluronic F127, PLGA, and chitosan for targeted co-delivery of doxorubicin and irinotecan to eliminate cancer stem-like cells. Biomaterials 72:74–89
6. Reya T, Morrison SJ, Clarke MF, Weissman IL (2001) Stem cells, cancer, and cancer stem cells. Nature 414:105–111
7. Lonardo E, Hermann PC, Mueller M-T, Huber S, Balic A, Miranda-Lorenzo I, Zagorac S, Alcala S, Rodriguez-Arabaolaza I, Ramirez JC (2011) Nodal/Activin signaling drives self-renewal and tumorigenicity of pancreatic cancer stem cells and provides a target for combined drug therapy. Cell Stem Cell 9:433–446
8. Wang H, Yu J, Lu X, He X (2016) Nanoparticle systems reduce systemic toxicity in cancer treatment. Nanomedicine 11:103–106
9. Wang H, Zhao S, Agarwal P, Dumbleton J, Yu J, Lu X, He X (2015) Multi-layered polymeric nanoparticles for pH-responsive and sequenced release of theranostic agents. Chem Commun 51:7733–7736
10. Kataoka K, Harada A, Nagasaki Y (2001) Block copolymer micelles for drug delivery: design, characterization and biological significance. Adv Drug Deliv Rev 47:113–131
11. Rösler A, Vandermeulen GW, Klok H-A (2012) Advanced drug delivery devices via self-assembly of amphiphilic block copolymers. Adv Drug Deliv Rev 64:270–279
12. Kim B, Hwang S, Park J, Park HJ (2002) Preparation and characterization of drug-loaded polymethacrylate microspheres by an emulsion solvent evaporation method. J Microencapsul 19:811–822
13. Zambaux M, Bonneaux F, Gref R, Maincent P, Dellacherie E, Alonso M, Labrude P, Vigneron C (1998) Influence of experimental parameters on the characteristics of poly (lactic acid) nanoparticles prepared by a double emulsion method. J Control Release 50:31–40
14. Wang H, Zhao Y, Wu Y, Hu Y-l, Nan K, Nie G, Chen H (2011) Enhanced anti-tumor efficacy by co-delivery of doxorubicin and paclitaxel with amphiphilic methoxy PEG-PLGA copolymer nanoparticles. Biomaterials 32:8281–8290
15. Avigdor A, Goichberg P, Shivtiel S, Dar A, Peled A, Samira S, Kollet O, Hershkoviz R, Alon R, Hardan I (2004) CD44 and hyaluronic acid cooperate with SDF-1 in the trafficking of human CD34+ stem/progenitor cells to bone marrow. Blood 103:2981–2989
16. Jin L, Hope KJ, Zhai Q, Smadja-Joffe F, Dick JE (2006) Targeting of CD44 eradicates human acute myeloid leukemic stem cells. Nat Med 12:1167–1174
17. Rao W, Wang H, Han J, Zhao S, Dumbleton J, Agarwal P, Zhang W, Zhao G, Yu J, Zynger DL, Lu X, He X (2015) Chitosan-decorated doxorubicin-encapsulated nanoparticle targets and eliminates tumor reinitiating cancer stem-like cells. ACS Nano 9:5725–5740

Part II

Passive and Active Targeting Methods

Chapter 7

Exploiting Phage Display for Development of Novel Cellular Targeting Strategies

William Marsh, Amanda Witten, and Sarah E. Stabenfeldt

Abstract

Targeting strategies for drug delivery applications rely on targeting moieties (i.e., peptide, antibody) specific to the desired cell surface receptor or protein of interest. However, current targeting strategies are limited to previously identified epitopes/ligand pairs. The field of phage display opens up the targeting moiety options whereby new epitope/ligand pairs may be discovered through well-designed biopanning assays for the target cell population of interest. Here, we provide a detailed protocol to perform phage biopanning assays on adherent cell cultures. The methods described here may be modified to user-specific targeting interests.

Key words Phage display, Single chain antibody fragment (scFv), Domain antibody (dAb), Astrocytes

1 Introduction

A critical component of an active targeted drug delivery system is the actual targeting motif, typically selected based on unique characteristics of the target cell/tissue system. For example, tumor angiogenesis is commonly marked by high levels of vascular endothelial cell growth factor receptor (VEGFR) motivating the development of VEGFR-based targeting strategies (*see* review [1]). However, many disease pathologies are more complex than the upregulation of a single receptor or cell surface protein. Therefore, epitope/ligand discovery tools such as phage display are essential for identifying new targeting motifs with high specificity to complex pathologies. Phage display is a molecular biology technique that exploits the ease of genetic manipulation of bacteriophage (phage) to generate large combinatorial phage libraries that present motifs on the outer coat proteins (i.e., short peptide sequences, single-domain antibody (sdAb), fragment antigen-binding region of monoclonal antibody (Fab), single chain antibody fragments (scFvs), and nucleic acid sequences) [2, 3].

Rachael W. Sirianni and Bahareh Behkam (eds.), *Targeted Drug Delivery: Methods and Protocols*, Methods in Molecular Biology, vol. 1831, https://doi.org/10.1007/978-1-4939-8661-3_7, © Springer Science+Business Media, LLC, part of Springer Nature 2018

Subsequent biopanning screens with phage libraries against a target of interest (e.g., tumor biopsy) facilitate discovery of a unique motif with high affinity and specificity.

Particular consideration should be given when selecting the type of targeting motif as a variety of options are available including monoclonal antibodies (full length), Fab, sdAb, scFv, nucleic acids, aptamers, short peptide sequences, and small molecules (*see* review [4]. Peptide and small molecules afford small size; however, these systems typically have an order of magnitude higher equilibrium binding dissociation constants (K_D) compared to antibody-based systems [5, 6]. Whereas approaches that employ full length antibody and even Fab systems trade affinity for larger size. ScFv and sdAb systems are unique as they are truncated antibodies composed of the variable heavy (VH) and/or variable light (VL) chains containing the critical epitope recognition regions (complementary determining regions; CDRs) thus maintaining high affinity without the size tradeoff [3].

Here, in this chapter, we outline in vitro biopanning phage display against viable, adherent cell cultures. We specifically describe methods with commercially available Domain antibody library and the Tomlinson I + J. Phage production, purification, biopanning, and scFv/sdAb production and purification outlined in this chapter are based on a compilation of previous publications and accompanying product documentation [3, 7, 8]. However, to our knowledge, we have uniquely modified the protocol to perform biopanning on viable, adherent cell cultures to identify subtle alterations between quiescent and activated cellular phenotypes. We use primary astrocyte cultures as our model system and developed scFv/sdAbs with high specificity and affinity to reactive astrocytes. This protocol may be modified to suit each user's experimental goals.

2 Materials

2.1 Bacteriophage Production and Purification (See Note 1)

1. Phage library (*see* **Note 2**).
2. 100 mm × 15 mm petri dishes.
3. 245 mm square bioassay dishes (Alternatively, four 100 mm × 15 mm petri dishes can be used as a substitute).
4. Bacterial cell spreader.
5. 2xTY medium: For 1 L stock, dissolve 16 g of bacto-tryptone, 10 g of yeast extract, and 5 g of NaCl 500 mL deionized water, bring final volume up to 1 L with deionized water, autoclave, let it cool to room temperature (RT; 25 °C), store at RT or 4 °C (*see* **Note 3**).

6. 20% Glucose solution: 200 g of glucose per 1 L of deionized water, sterile filter (0.2 μm filter), store at 4 °C.
7. Ampicillin stock (1000×): 100 mg/mL ampicillin in deionized water, sterile filter, and store in 1 mL aliquots at −20 °C. Recommend preparing 50–100 mL at a time. Ampicillin is light sensitive and should be stored in a dark container to avoid degradation.
8. Tryptone Yeast Extract (TYE) agar plates: For 1 L stock, dissolve 8 g of NaCl, 10 g of bacto-tryptone, and 5 g of yeast extract in 800 mL of deionized water, add 15 g of agar and bring final volume up to 1 L with deionized water. Autoclave and then cool down to 50 °C (*see* **Note 4**). Pour 20 mL of solution into 100 mm × 15 mm petri dishes. Place lid on dishes, cool for 1 h, store at 4 °C for up to 4 weeks.
9. TYE ampicillin glucose agar (TAG) plates: For 1 L stock, dissolve 8 g of NaCl, 10 g of bacto-tryptone and 5 g of yeast extract in 600 mL of deionized water, add 15 g of agar and bring final volume up to 800 mL with deionized water. Autoclave and then cool down to 50 °C (*see* **Note 4**), add 1 mL of ampicillin solution (light sensitive) and 200 mL of 20% glucose solution. Pour 20 mL of solution into 100 mm × 15 mm petri dishes. Place lid on dishes, cool for 1 h, store at 4 °C for up to 4 weeks. A separate batch of TAG should be made to prepare larger TAG plates (245 mm square bioassay dishes) for use in the screening process (Subheading 3.2).
10. Kanamycin stock (1000×): 50 mg/mL kanamycin dissolved in deionized water, sterile filter, and store in 1 mL aliquots at −20 °C. Recommend preparing 50–100 mL at a time. Kanamycin is light sensitive and should be stored in a dark container to avoid degradation.
11. 1× Phosphate buffer (PBS; pH 7.4): For 1 L stock, dissolve 8 g of NaCl (137 mM), 1.44 g of Na_2HPO_4 (10 mM), 0.2 g of KCl (1.8 mM), and 0.24 g of KH_2PO_4 (10 mM) in 900 mL of deionized water, adjust pH to 7.4, bring final volume to 1 L and autoclave. Store at RT.
12. 1× Tris Buffer (TBS; pH 7.4): For 1 L stock, dissolve 1.5 g of Trizma base (10 mM), 8 g of NaCl (137 mM) and 0.15 g CaCl2 (1 mM) in 900 mL of liter of deionized water, adjust pH to 7.4, bring final volume to 1 L and autoclave. Store at RT.
13. 25% PEG 6000, 2.5 M NaCl solution: For 500 mL stock, dissolve 125 g of PEG-6000 and 73 g of NaCl in 500 mL of deionized water (final volume). Autoclave, then stir continuously while cooling to RT. Store at RT.

14. Trypsin stock (100×): 10 mg/mL trypsin at 10 mg/mL in TBS, sterile filter, store in 100 μL aliquots at −20 °C. Recommend preparing 10 mL at a time (100× stock concentration).
15. 0.005 M EDTA, 0.1 mg/mL BSA in PBS (PBS/EDTA/BSA): Dissolve 4 mg of bovine serum albumin in 40 mL of 1× PBS supplemented with 5 mM EDTA, sterile filter and store at 4 °C.
16. 50% Glycerol: Dilute equal parts 100% glycerol with deionized water to obtain an end concentration of 50% glycerol solution.
17. Centrifuge that can house 250 mL centrifuge bottles and reach speeds up to 12,000 × *g*.
    (a) Example: Beckman Coulter Allegra 25R.
18. Bacterial shaker incubator.
19. 250 mL polypropylene centrifuge bottles.

2.1.1 Biopanning

1. 96-well polystyrene, flat, sterile tissue culture plates.
2. 96-well polystyrene, round bottom, untreated sterile plates.
3. Anti-M13 Antibody Biotinylated.
4. Streptavidin with HRP conjugate.
5. 1-Step Ultra-TMB-ELISA.

2.1.2 Cell Specific

1. Adherent cell line of interest.
2. Cell culture media.

2.1.3 Genetic Analysis

PCRss

1. GelRed™ Nucleic Acid Gel Stain.
2. 100 bp PCR molecular ladder.
3. GoTaq® PCR Core System I.
4. TAE Buffer: Prepare a 10× stock buffer by dissolving 48.4 g of Tris-base, 11.4 mL of glacial acetic acid (17.4 M) and 3.7 g of EDTA disodium salt in 900 mL of deionized water. Bring final volume to 1 L with deionized water; store at RT. When needed, dilute 100 mL of 10× TAE stock with 900 mL of deionized water to achieve a final working solution of 40 mM Tris, 20 mM acetic acid and 1 mM EDTA.
5. Primers (Custom order *see* Table 1).

2.1.4 DNA Sequencing

1. QIAprep Miniprep Kit.
2. Primers (Life Technologies, Custom order *see* Table 1).

2.1.5 scFv/dAb Production and Purification

1. 1 M Isopropyl-β-D-thiogalactopyranoside (IPTG): Dissolve 2.38 g of IPTG in 8.5 mL of deionized water. Bring final volume up to 10 mL, sterile filter, and store in 1 mL aliquots at −20 °C.

Table 1
Recommended primers for analyzing ScFv/dAb insert length (PCR + Electrophoresis) and sequence

Primer	Sequence	Use	References
LMB3	5′-CAGGAAACAGCTATG AC-3′	Forward primer for Tomlinson I + J and dAb libraries	
pHEN	5′-CTATGCGGCCCCATTCA-3′	Reverse primer for Tomlinson I + J libraries	
dAb Reverse	5′-GTTTTGTCGTCTTTCCAGACG-3′	Reverse primer for dAb library	Dudgeon et al. [7]

2. Pierce Protease Inhibitor Mini Tablets, EDTA-free.
3. Lysozyme.
4. Triton X-100.
5. 100 U/mL DNAse I stock: Dissolve DNase I in the appropriate volume of 10 mM Tris–HCl + 2 mM $CaCl_2$. Aliquot into 5 mL portions in 15 mL polypropylene centrifuge tubes and store at −20 °C.
6. Probe-based sonicator (for lysing cells).
7. FPLC or alternative protein purification method.
8. Protein-A or AG affinity FPLC column.
9. 0.2% NaN_3 stock solution: Dissolve 200 mg of NaN_3 in 100 mL of 1× PBS. Caution NaN_3 is *very toxic* and possesses explosive properties when exposed to metals. Use extreme caution when handling this product (even when dissolved at 0.2%). Collect all waste and dispose of via a proper chemical waste mechanism.

3 Methods

3.1 Bacteriophage Production and Purification (Modified from [3])

3.1.1 Production and Purification

1. Thaw an aliquot of frozen antibody stock library (dAb or scFv library) on ice.
2. Add phage library 1 mL aliquot to a sterile 2 L Erlenmeyer flask containing 500 mL 2xTY medium supplemented with 4% (wt/vol) glucose and 100 μg/mL of ampicillin (Use appropriate glucose and ampicillin stock solutions; *see* **Notes 5** and **6**).
3. Place the bacteria in a bacterial shaker incubator and culture at 37 °C and 250 rpm until reaching an optical density reading at 600 nm of 0.1 (OD600; *see* **Note 7**).
4. Transfer 250 mL of the bacterial culture to a new sterile 1 L Erlenmeyer flask (*see* **Note 8**).

5. Add 1×10^{12} KM13 helper phage to the 250 mL culture and incubate in a water bath at 37 °C for 30–45 min (*see* **Note 8**).
6. After incubation, spin cultures down at 3200 × *g* for 10 min at 4 °C in 250 mL autoclaved centrifuge bottles. Load a maximum of 200 mL per bottle.
7. Discard the supernatant.
8. Resuspend bacterial pellets in 500 mL of 2xTY medium supplemented with 0.1% (wt/vol) glucose, 100 μg/mL of ampicillin, and 50 μg/mL of kanamycin in a 2 L Erlenmeyer flask (Use appropriate prepared stock solutions; *see* **Notes 9** and **10**).
9. Grow culture overnight for 16–20 h at 25 °C and 250 rpm.

3.1.2 Phage PEG Purification

1. Spin down overnight cultures for 15 min at 10,800 × *g* at 4 °C in sterile 250 mL polypropylene centrifuge bottles.
2. Collect the supernatant and add 15% by volume of the 25% PEG 6000, 2.5 M NaCl solution.
3. Divide the supernatant/PEG solution equally between two to three autoclaved 250 mL polypropylene centrifuge bottles. Mix well by inverting bottles 50 times. Incubate for 2 h at 4 °C.
4. Spin down precipitated phage at 6000 × *g* for 45 min.
5. Discard the supernatant.
6. Resuspend the phage pellet in 15 mL of PBS (*see* **Note 11**). To aid resuspension, place the phage solution on a rocker at 4 °C for 30 min to 1 h at 50 rpm. If a rocker is unavailable, incubate the phage pellet at 4 °C for 1 h and then manually swirl the solution to resuspend the pellet. Do not vortex nor aspirate.
7. Combine phage solutions into a single 250 mL centrifuge bottle or 50 mL polypropylene centrifuge tube.
8. Add 15% by volume of the 25% PEG 6000, 2.5 M NaCl solution. Invert 50 times. Incubate at 4 °C overnight.
9. Spin down overnight incubation for 45 min at 6000 × *g* and 4 °C.
10. Discard the supernatant and resuspend phage pellet in 5 mL of PBS/EDTA/BSA solution (*see* **Note 12**).
11. Transfer suspension to a new 15 mL polypropylene centrifuge tube. Spin at 10,800 × *g* for 10 min to remove any remaining biological debris.
12. Transfer to a new 15 mL polypropylene centrifuge tube and store the supernatant at 4 °C. Use phage within 7 days.

3.1.3 Quantification of Phage Concentration (Colony Forming Units; CFU)

1. Streak out stock TG1 bacteria on TYE plates and culture at 37 °C overnight (*see* **Note 1**).
2. Transfer TG1 plates to 4 °C for storage. Use within 1 month. Prepare new plates as needed for experimental preparation.
3. Prepare an overnight, starved TG1 culture by inoculating 5 mL of 2xTY medium with a single TG1 colony pulled from the TG1 plate. Use vented capped tubes or loosely tape the cap onto a standard 50 mL centrifuge tube. Incubate in bacterial shaker overnight at 250 rpm and 37 °C.
4. The next day, prepare 100-fold dilution of overnight-starved bacteria with 10 mL of fresh 2xTY media. Incubate at 250 rpm and 37 °C until OD600 of 0.5 has reached (~1.5–2.5 h). Culture may be stored at 4 °C for up to 8 h until ready to complete the assay.
5. Prepare serial dilutions from purified phage sample to achieve the following dilutions: 10^{-5}, 10^{-7}, 10^{-9}, 10^{-11} in PBS. The most effective means of performing this series is to generate 10 mL of a 10^{-3} dilution (10 μL of phage stock + 10 mL of PBS) followed by 100-fold dilutions in PBS (10 μL + 990 μL of PBS) (*see* **Note 13**).
6. Using the appropriate number of 0.5 mL microcentrifuge tubes, transfer 90 μL of the starved TG1 culture each tube. Transfer 10 μL of the phage serial dilutions to each tube to achieve an end dilution set of 10^{-4}, 10^{-6}, 10^{-8}, 10^{-10}, 10^{-12}. Include a PBS only +TG1 cells control.
7. Incubate the inoculated phage+TG1 solution in a water bath set at 37 °C for 30–45 min.
8. During this incubation, place two to three TAG plates in the bacterial incubator for 15–30 min (37 °C). This step serves to dry any condensation that may have formed on the TAG plate. If numerous bubbles are observed in the agar after warming in an incubator, allow plates to slowly warm to RT before placing in an incubator.
9. On the back of the TAG plate, draw two lines to divide the plate into quarters with three small circles in each lane (*see* Fig. 1). It is recommended that each dilution is spotted in triplicates, but the pattern drawn on the plates can be modified to suit each individual's needs.
10. Pipette 10 μL of each dilution onto the TAG plate in triplicate (Fig. 1). Use the pre-drawn lanes and circles as guides. Place the lid on the plate once the plate is full.
11. Once the solution has absorbed into the TAG plates, seal the plate with a thin layer of Parafilm.

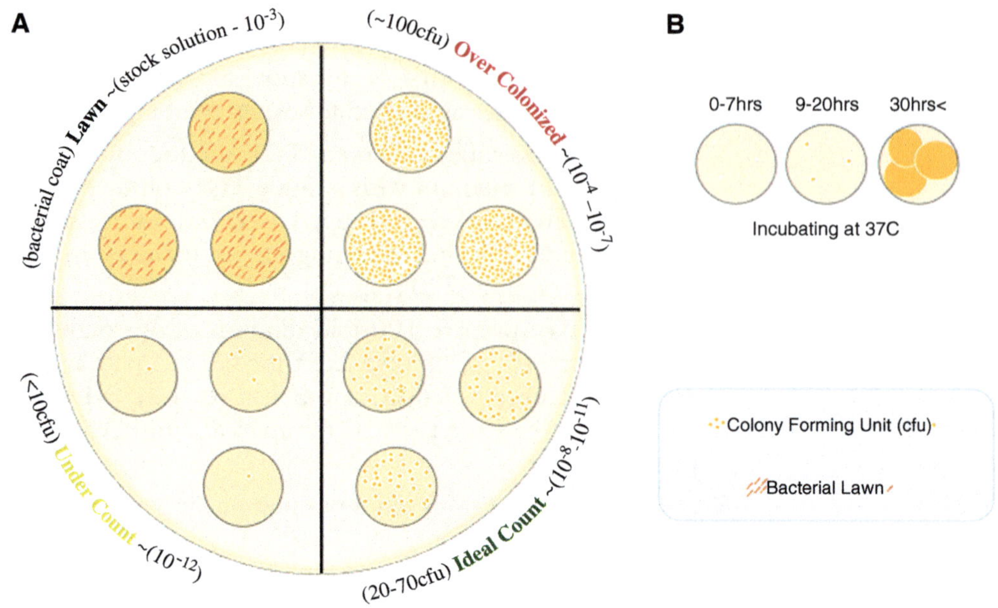

Fig. 1 Bacterial colony forming unit assay. (**a**) Schematic of TAG plate to determine the number of functional phage as measured by bacterial colony forming unit (CFU) assay. Each quadrant of the TAG plate represents various potential outcomes for this assay, lawn formation, colony overpopulation, ideal colony count, and low colony population. (**b**) Schematic of colony progression over time. If the incubation runs over the recommended 12–16 h time, distinct individual colonies will be difficult to identify

12. Place the plate on a stationary shelf upside down in a bacterial incubator or oven set to 37 °C for 9–16 h. Alternatively, incubate at 30 °C for 16–24 h.
13. After an appropriate incubation time frame, remove the plates, count and record the total number of colonies for each dilution (*see* Fig. 1 and **Note 14**).
14. Determine colony forming unit (CFU) concentration for phage sample with the following equation:

$$\text{CFU} / \text{mL} = (\text{Average colony count}) / (\text{Dilution} \times 0.01\,\text{mL}).$$

3.2 Biopanning on Adherent Cell Cultures

All cell culture steps prior to biopanning steps listed below should be performed using the standard tissue culture sterile technique. Once the biopanning steps begin and the phage particles are introduced to the cell cultures, do not return the cell cultures to the standard tissue culture working areas. Perform the remainder of the screen steps using aseptic techniques standard for bacterial work.

3.2.1 Basal Cell Culture

1. Culture cell line of interest according to the specified standard culture protocol in a T25 tissue culture flask. Prepare at least

three flasks for the negative screen and one flask for the positive screens.

   (a) Example: Primary astrocytes cultured in 10% FBS by volume of DMEM plated at 4 × 10^5 cells/cm^2 density and allowed to adhere and proliferate for 24–48 h.

2. If needed, apply appropriate signaling agents to induce targeted cell behavior for positive screens.

   (a) Example: Use TGF-β to induce phenotypic switch from quiescent to reactive astrocyte phenotype. Astrocytes are subjected to serum starvation for 12 h (DMEM without FBS). After 12 h of starvation, astrocytes are treated with standard medium supplemented with 10 ng/mL of TGF-β for 48 h. After 48 h of TGF-β supplementation, remove TGF-β supplemented media and return to basal media.

3. Perform the biopanning screen immediately after cells are ready.

3.2.2 Negative Screens

A negative screen against potential basal adherent cells or background factors (i.e., tissue culture polystyrene, adsorbed FBS, etc.) reduces the phage population with high affinity and specificity to such substrates. This step aids in eliminating phage clones with overlapping recognition to the cell type and/or phenotype of interests.

1. The evening prior to performing negative screen, prepare an overnight, starved TG1 culture by inoculating 5 mL of 2xTY medium with a single TG1 colony pulled from the stock TG1 plate. Use vented capped tubes or loosely tape the cap onto a standard 50 mL centrifuge tube. Incubate in bacterial shaker overnight at 250 rpm and 37 °C.
2. The following day (day of negative screen), prepare 100-fold dilution of overnight-starved bacteria and by transferring 1 mL into 99 mL of fresh 2xTY media. Incubate at 250 rpm and 37 °C until OD600 of 0.5 is reached (~1.5–2.5 h). Culture may be stored at 4 °C for up to 8 h until completion of the negative screen.
3. Prepare a 5 × 10^{12} phage particle solution by diluting stock phage (prepared in Subheading 3.1) in 5 mL of standard culture medium.
4. Take one T25 flask containing basal cells and aspirate the medium.
5. Place the phage solution (5 × 10^{12} phage 5 mL of culture medium) in the flask and incubate for 1 h at 50 rpm and 30 °C (use bacterial incubator).

6. After 1 h, remove the supernatant and transfer into a second flask of basal cells. Incubate for 1 h at 50 rpm and 30 °C (use a bacterial incubator).
7. Repeat **step 4** for a third basal culture.
8. At the end of the third and final negative screen, mix the final supernatant with 30 mL of starved TG1 bacterial cells prepared in **steps 1** and **2**. Recommend using a 50 mL polypropylene centrifuge tube.
9. Incubate for 30 min at 50 rpm at 37 °C (bacterial incubator).
10. During the same incubation, set one large TAG 245 mm square bioassay dish (or 4 × TAG petri dishes) in bacterial incubator stationary rack or oven set at 37 °C to dry the plate.
11. Spin down incubation at 3400 × *g* for 15 min.
12. Remove the supernatant and discard.
13. Resuspend pellet in 1 mL of 2xTY media.
14. Use a 1 mL pipette to evenly distribute the 1 mL cell suspension over the dried TAG 245 mm square bioassay dish (or 4 × TAG petri dishes). Spread the cell suspension gently across the entire surface of the dish with a sterile bacterial cell spreader. Place the lid on the dish.
15. Wait approximately 30 min for the cell solution to absorb into the TAG plate. Wrap dish in parafilm.
16. Incubate TAG dish at 37 °C overnight (16–24 h; bacterial incubator shelf or oven).
17. The following day, remove TAG dish/plates from the incubator. A lawn of bacteria should be observed.
18. Transfer 20 mL of fresh 2xTY media to the TAG dish and quickly use a sterile bacterial cell scraper to gently dislodge the bacteria. Collect the bacteria dense media and transfer into a 50 mL polypropylene centrifuge tube. Final volume will be ~10–13 mL as some of the media will adsorb into the TAG gel.
19. Add 15% by volume glycerol to bacteria dense media and store in 1 mL aliquots at −80 °C. These aliquots represent the negative screen stock and are used in the subsequent biopanning round instead of the stock library. Keep aliquots from each stage of the screen in case a screen needs to be repeated or modified.

3.2.3 Checking for dAb/scFv Inserts

A critical check point after each screen stage of phage biopanning is to randomly check for the over growth of wild type phage or mutations of the genetic coding for scFv/dAb inserts (e.g., frame shifts) (*see* **Note 15**). Two methods are recommended to monitor the stability of the scFv/dAb inserts, (1) Evaluate insert length (PCR and electrophoresis), and (2) DNA sequencing. Each of these methods is briefly outlined below and relies on a prior knowledge of PCR, electrophoresis, and DNA purification. Table 1 lists the recommended primers for each technique.

1. Dry four TAG plates in a bacterial incubator (37 °C) for 30 min.
2. Use a cotton swab or inoculation loop to obtain a small sample of frozen TG1 cells from the screen of interest. For example, if probing for alterations after the negative screen, one would streak out TG1 cells from the frozen aliquots obtained at the end of the negative screen.
3. Immediately streak out TG1 sample onto the four TAG plates.
4. Incubate TAG plates overnight upside down at 37 °C (~16 h).
5. Remove plates from the incubator and use immediately or place in 4 °C for storage up to 1 month.

Evaluate Insert Length (PCR and Electrophoresis)

1. Prepare enough working PCR solution for five 15 μL PCR reactions according to PCR Core and recommended forward and reverse primers (Table 1).
   (a) Recommended pairing for Tomlinson I + J library: LMB3 and pHEN. If scFv inserts are present, bands will appear around 900–950 bp. If no scFv inserts are present, bands will appear around 300–350 bp.
   (b) Recommended pairing for domain antibody library: LMB3 and dAb reverse. If dAb inserts are present, bands will appear around 600–700 bp. If no dAb inserts are present, bands will appear around 200–300 bp.
2. Aliquot 10 μL of working PCR solution into five PCR tubes.
3. Using a 10 μL pipettor with matching pipette tip, select one unique clone from the streaked plate and transfer to one PCR tube via titration.
4. Repeat **step 3** for the four remaining PCR samples.
5. Spin samples for ~10 s on a small pulse benchtop centrifuge.
6. Load samples into a thermocycler and run with the following PCR amplification settings:
   (a) Pre-denaturation: 9 min at 94 °C.
   (b) Denaturation, Annealing, and Extension: 30 cycles of 45 s at 95 °C, 45 s at 55 °C, 1 min at 72 °C; then 5 min at 72 °C. For Tomlinson I + J, set annealing for 1 min and extension for 2 min.
   (c) Hold at 4 °C (will maintain sample integrity until removed from the thermocycler).
7. During amplification, prepare a 3% agarose gel in 1× TAE buffer supplemented with Gel Red Nucleic Acid Stain.

8. After PCR amplification, load 10 μL of PCR samples in 3% agarose gel across five different lanes. Include an appropriate base-pair ladder for size reference. Run gel according to the manufacturer's directions.
9. Use a UV box or imager to evaluate the length of the inserts. If the scFv/dAb insert is lost in more than 60% of the samples (i.e., three out of five), then the previous screen step may need to be repeated.

Plasmid Purification and Sequencing

1. Prepare five bacterial culture tubes with 5 mL of 2xTY media.
2. Inoculate each tube with a single TG1 colony pulled from the previously streaked out plate from the screen of interest.
3. Incubate cultures in a bacterial shaker overnight at 250 rpm and 37 °C overnight (~16 h). Use vented capped tubes or loosely tape the cap onto a standard 50 mL centrifuge tube.
4. The following morning, use a Qiagen Miniprep Kit to purify plasmids from the overnight cultures according to the manufacturer's protocol.
5. Submit purified plasmid DNA to a DNA sequencing center for the analysis of the specific clones (*see* Table 1 for suggested primers).
6. Multiple software programs may be used to analyze the sequencing results. The freeware A plasmid Editor (ApE; University of Utah—M. Wayne Davis) is a useful program to quickly analyze results and determine presence or absence of inserts and mutations.

   (a) Tomlinson I + J libraries:
   - Open. seq file in ApE program.
   - Under "Enzyme" tab, use "Enzyme Selector" tool to highlight SfiI, SmlI, and NotI sites.
   - If SfiI is not present, this may indicate that you do not have an insert present. Sometimes, the NotI is not present due to a short or poor read.
   - Usually need to perform forward (LMB3 primer) and reverse (pHEN primer) reading to sequence whole insert.
   - Highlight sequence beginning right after the SfiI site (ATGG...) and ending about 120 nucleotides after NotI site.
   - Translate—Under "ORFs" tab, use "Translate" tool. Specify 10 AA per line and translate selection only.
   - Log sequence into Excel spreadsheet.

(b) Domain antibody library:
- Open. seq file in ApE program.
- Under "Enzyme" tab, use "Enzyme Selector" tool to highlight SfiI and NotI sites.
- If SfiI is not present, this may indicate that you do not have an insert present. Sometimes, the NotI is not present due to a short or poor read.
- Highlight sequence beginning right after the SfiI site (ATGG...) and ending about 120 nucleotides after NotI site.
- Translate—Under "ORFs" tab, use "Translate" tool. Specify 10 AA per line and translate selection only.
- Log sequence into Excel spreadsheet.

3.2.4 Positive Screens

Positive screens encompass successive biopanning rounds to generate an enriched phage population of high affinity to the target of interest. Here, an example of a reactive astrocyte phenotype is used as the target adherent cell type. It is recommended that at least three rounds of positive screens are performed. Additional rounds may be required if specificity and high affinity to the target of interest is not achieved.

1. The critical first step of a positive screen is coordination of the phage particle and target sample preparation. Samples and phage need to be prepared in parallel.
   (a) Phage particles obtained from the infected TG1 cells from the previous round need to be produced, purified, and quantified according to the steps outlined in Subheading 3.1. For instance, the first positive screen will use phage particles produced from a TG1 aliquot from the negative screen. Note that this process will take a minimum of 3 days; account for this time in experimental planning and preparation.
   (b) Prepare one adherent cell target of interest in a T25 flask. Be sure to account for sample maturation/treatment timelines in experimental planning and preparation. For example, a minimum of four days is required to generate a reactive astrocyte culture.
2. The evening prior to performing positive screen, prepare an overnight, starved TG1 culture by inoculating 5 mL of 2xTY medium with a single TG1 colony pulled from the stock TG1 plate. Incubate in a bacterial shaker overnight at 250 rpm and 37 °C.
3. The following day (day of screen), prepare 100-fold dilution of overnight-starved bacteria by transferring 1 mL into 99 mL of

fresh 2xTY media. Incubate at 250 rpm and 37 °C until OD600 of 0.5 is reached (about 1.5–2.5 h). Culture may be stored at 4 °C for up to 8 h until completion of the screen.

4. After preparing phage particles and adherent cell target of interest, prepare a 5×10^{12} phage particle solution by diluting concentrated phage in 5 mL of standard culture medium.
5. Aspirate culture media from T25 flask containing target cells of interest and place the 5 mL of phage/culture media solution onto the cells. Keep 200 μL of media/phage solution in a 1.5 mL microcentrifuge tube to verify total number of phage at the start of the screen.
6. Incubate the phage with the positive screen adherent cells for 1 h at 30 °C with agitation (~50 rpm) in a bacterial incubator.
7. Remove media and keep media to assess the number of unbound phage particles.
8. Rinse with 5 mL of PBS for 5 min with agitation (~50 rpm) three times. Each time collect the rinse to assess the number of phage particles removed during the rinse process.
9. After the three rinses, elute the phage by applying 2 mL of trypsin solution. Incubate at 30 °C for 15 min at 50 rpm (*see* **Note 16**).
10. Transfer 2 mL trypsin phage elution to a clean 15 mL centrifuge tube and spin down at 1120 × *g* for 5 min.
11. Transfer the supernatant (discard pellet) to 30 mL culture of overnight-starved TG1 cells (use 50 mL centrifuge tube) and incubate for 30 min at 37 °C and 50 rpm.
    (a) Dry out one large TAG bioassay dish (or 4 × TAG petri dishes) in the bacterial incubator or oven during this incubation.
12. Spin down the bacterial culture at 3400 × *g* for 15 min.
13. Discard the supernatant and resuspend the TG1 pellet in 1 mL of 2xTY media.
14. Use a 1 mL pipette to evenly distribute the 1 mL cell suspension over the dried TAG 245 mm square bioassay dish. Spread the cell suspension gently across the entire surface of the dish with a sterile bacterial cell spreader. Place the lid on the dish.
15. Wait approximately 30 min for the cell solution to absorb into the TAG gel. Wrap dish in parafilm.
16. Incubate TAG dish at 37 °C overnight upside down (16–24 h; bacterial incubator shelf or oven).
17. The following day, remove dish from the incubator. A lawn of bacteria should be observed.

18. Transfer 20 mL of fresh 2xTY media to the TAG dish and quickly use a sterile bacterial cell scraper to gently dislodge the bacteria. Collect the bacteria dense media (10–13 mL as some of the media will adsorb into the TAG gel) and transfer to a 50 mL polypropylene centrifuge tube.
19. Add 15% by volume glycerol to bacteria dense media and store in 1 mL aliquots at −80 °C. These aliquots now represent a positive screen stock for your screen. Keep aliquots from each stage of the screen in case a screen needs to be repeated or modified.
20. It is recommended to check for presence of scFv/dAb inserts after each round. Follow the steps outlined in Subheading 3.2.3. If inserts are still present, continue with next screen (i.e., repeat steps outline in this section with TG1 cells from the round that was just completed). After completing three rounds of positive screens, continue onto Subheading 3.3.

3.3 Identification of Potential High Affinity scFv/dAb via ELISA

The next phase entails identifying specific phage clones with high affinity and specificity to target of interest. To accomplish this goal, single clones will be produced in a high-throughput 96-well plate manner to evaluate single clone affinity via a modified enzyme-linked immunosorbant assay (ELISA).

3.3.1 Phage Clone Preparation (96-well plate format)

1. Dry eight TAG plates in a bacterial incubator (37 °C) for 30 min.
2. Use a cotton swab or inoculation loop to obtain a small sample of frozen TG1 cells from the third positive screen.
3. Immediately streak out TG1 sample onto four TAG plates.
4. Using a fresh cotton swab or inoculation loop, repeat **steps 2** and **3** on two TAG plates for the initial scFv/dAb stock library (required for negative control clones).
5. Using a fresh cotton swab or inoculation loop, repeat **steps 2** and **3** on the remaining two TAG plates for the anti-ubiquitin vial supplied by the phage library kit (required for positive control clones).
6. After parafilming, incubate TAG plates overnight upside down at 37 °C (~16 h).
7. Remove plates from the incubator and use immediately or place in 4 °C for storage up to 1 month.
8. Prep a 96-well round bottom plate with 200 μL of 2xTY supplemented with 4% glucose + 100 μg/mL ampicillin in each well (recommend preparing master solution of supplemented media and then dispensing 200 μL into each well).
9. Using the streaked out plates from the third positive screen, inoculate each well of the 96-well plate with a single colony

picked with a 10 μL pipette tip (supplemented with the media). It is recommended to pick at least 88 clones (11 columns). The remaining column (eight wells) should be inoculated with colonies from the original scFv/dAb library stock to serve as random controls and anti-ubiquitin stock to provide a positive control (four wells per). Place the lid on the plate when complete and parafilm the lid to the base plate.

10. Place the 96-well plate into 96-well plate racks in bacterial incubator. Grow overnight at 37 °C and 250 rpm.
11. After the overnight growth, prepare a fresh 96-well round bottom plate containing 200 μL of 2xTY + 4% glucose + 100 μg/mL ampicillin.
12. Transfer 5 μL of the overnight culture from each well to the matching corresponding well in the fresh 96-well plate; it is helpful to use a multi-channel pipettor for this process but be sure to use a clean pipette tip for each well.
    (a) Do not discard remainder of overnight 96-well plate. Add 55 μL of a 50% glycerol (100% glycerol diluted with 2xTY) to each well.
    (b) Place the lid on the plate and secure with Parafilm. Store at −80 °C. This plate serves as the single clone stock for the phage biopanning (*see* Subheading 3.4.3).
13. Secure the freshly inoculated plates in the bacterial incubator and incubate at 37 °C and 250 rpm for 4 h.
14. Add 50 μL of 2xTY containing 4×10^8 KM13 helper phage (8×10^9 phage/mL) to each well.
15. Secure the plate in a bacterial incubator and incubate at 37 °C and 50 rpm for 45 min.
16. Spin plate down at 3200 × *g* for 10 min.
17. Discard the supernatant by quickly inverting the plate over a wide-mouth collection bin.
18. Resuspend cell pellets in the bottom of each well in 2xTY + 0.1% glucose + 100 μg/mL ampicillin + 50 μg/mL kanamycin.
19. Secure the plate in a bacterial incubator and incubate overnight at 25 °C and 250 rpm for 16–24 h.
20. Spin down the plate at 3200 × *g* for 10 min.
21. Carefully transfer the supernatant to a new 96-well round bottom plate and store at 4 °C for use within 1 week. This supernatant contains the phage particles for the modified ELISA.

3.4 Modified ELISA Protocol

3.4.1 Adherent Cell Plate Prep

Prepare two 96-well plates for the modified ELISA. One plate consists of the basal non-targeted cell population prepared for the negative screen. The other plate will be prepared according to the target cell plating protocol used during the phage biopanning screens. The example outlined here details specifics for generating basal and reactive astrocytes.

1. Seed two 96-well cell culture plates with 40,000 cells/cm^2 and allow to grow for a minimum of 48 h in 10% FBS DMEM media.
2. After 48 h, serum-starve one plate (DMEM without FBS) for 12 h in preparation for treating the astrocytes with 10 ng/mL of TGF-β. The second plate will remain in DMEM +10% FBS.
3. After the 12 h starvation period, aspirate the starvation media and treat the cells with 10 ng/mL of TGF-β for a minimum of 48 h

3.4.2 Modified ELISA

1. Prepare diluted phage clone solutions in a new 96-well round bottom plate.
   (a) Dispense 185.5 μL of working astrocyte media (DMEM + 10% FBS) into each well.
   (b) Transfer 62.5 μL of phage supernatant acquired in Subheading 3.3.1 to each corresponding/matching well.
2. Remove media from the two 96-well adherent cultures (one basal and one reactive plate) by gently inverting the plate over a wide-mouth collection container.
3. Transfer 100 μL of diluted phage into each corresponding well of the adherent cell plates (one basal and one reactive plate).
4. Secure plates in bacterial incubator and incubate at 30 °C for 1 h at ~50 rpm.
5. Discard the supernatant by gently inverting plate over a wide-mouth collection container.
6. Wash the wells three times with PBS.
7. Add 100 μL of 1:2000 HRP-anti-M13 conjugate (diluted in working adherent culture media) to each well of both ELISA plates.
8. Secure plates in bacterial incubator and incubate at 30 °C and ~50 rpm.
9. Discard the supernatant by gently inverting the plate over a wide-mouth collection container.
10. Wash the wells three times again with PBS.
11. Add 65 μL of 1-Step Ultra-TMB-ELISA to each well.
12. Allow the solution to develop for approximately 30 min with gentle agitation on an orbital shaker at room temperature. A deep blue color should develop in the positive wells.
13. Stop the TMB-HRP reaction with 40 μL of 2 N sulfuric acid. The solution should turn yellow and enzymatic breakdown of TMB should cease.

14. Read the absorbance at 450 nm in the plate reader with reference wavelength of 560 nm.
15. Analyze the absorbance readings.
    (a) Subtract average blank absorbance readings (i.e., cell + no antibody phage + HRP-anti-M13 conjugate) from all wells on each plate.
    (b) Take note of the baseline response for each control random clone for each plate. This cell-based ELISA may generate very noisy results. Absorbance readings above the random clone baseline indicate preferential binding to the specific cell population.
    (c) Generate a ratio of active/basal absorbance for each phage clone.
    (d) Use bar graph to visually compare absorbance ratios.
    (e) Identify top ten clones with highest ratio of active/basal response.
16. Sequence the top ten clones using the methods outlined in Subheading "Plasmid Purification and Sequencing".

3.4.3 Concentration-Dependent Modified ELISA

The initial modified ELISA provides a high-throughput method for identifying clones of interest to characterize further. Here, the modified ELISA will be performed with a controlled concentration of phage particles for the top four to five clones identified in Subheading 3.4. In addition to four to five clones, it is recommended to also test one random initial stock control clone as a negative control and anti-ubiquitin clone as a positive control.

1. Generate stock aliquots of phage clones of interest by using frozen infected TG1 cells from the 96-well plate prepared in Subheading 3.3.1 **step 12**.
2. Inoculate 20 mL of 2xTY + 4% glucose +100 μg/mL of ampicillin with phage clone of interest pulled from stock 96-well plate (50 mL tube; loosely tape lid). Grow culture at 37 °C and 250 rpm for 3–4 h.
3. Add 2×10^{11} helper phage to 20 mL culture. Incubate in 37 °C water bath for 60 min.
4. Spin culture at 3200 × *g* for 10 min.
5. Discard the supernatant and resuspend pellet in 50 mL of 2xTY + 0.1% glucose + 100 μg/mL of ampicillin + 50 μg/mL kanamycin (250 mL Erlenmeyer flask).
6. Grow culture at 250 rpm and 30 °C for ~20 h.
7. Follow the standard PEG purification protocol as outlined in Subheading 3.1.2 and determine total phage CFU (Subheading 3.1.3).

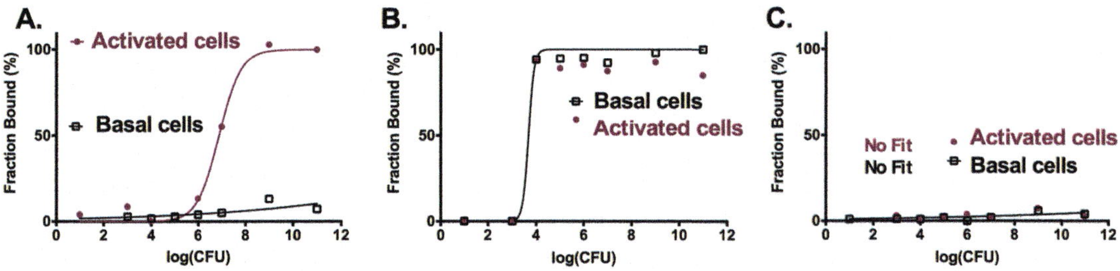

Fig. 2 Modified Klotz plot sample results. Concentration-dependent binding curves for three scFv clones to basal or activated cell targets. (**a**) scFv/dAb clone with affinity to activated cells. (**b**) scFv/dAb clone with comparable high affinity to both basal and activated cell targets. (**c**) Negative control scFv/dAb clone with no discernable affinity to either basal or activated cell targets

8. **Steps 1–7** may be performed in parallel for each clone of interest.
9. Prepare 96-well plates with basal and target cells as outlined in Subheading 3.3 (Plan according to prepare prior to running ELISA).
10. On the day of the ELISA, prepare diluted stock phage solutions for each clone in the appropriate cell culture medium to achieve a concentration of 1×10^{11} CFU/mL (5 mL).
11. Prepare serial dilutions with concentrations of 10^{11}, 10^{9}, 10^{7}, 10^{6}, 10^{5}, 10^{4}, 10^{3}, 10^{1} in the cell culture medium (1.5 mL each).
12. Obtain the prepared 96-well cell cultures. Aspirate medium out of wells.
13. Transfer 200 μL of phage dilution solution to three wells in the basal and targeted cell plates. Continue until all dilutions (including a non-phage control sample well) are dispensed on the plates.
14. Follow **steps 4–14** in Subheading 3.4 to complete the ELISA.
15. Analysis for the concentration-dependent ELISA entails generating a modified Klotz plot whereby the absorbance is plotted versus the phage CFU for each individual clone (*see* Fig. 2 for representative plot). This analysis enables relative comparisons of affinity characteristics across different clones.

4 Production of scFv/dAb

4.1 Generating HB2151 Stocks

The TG1 strain is a suppressor strain of bacteria that recognizes an amber stop codon as a glutamine residue, thus facilitating phage endowing an scFv/dAb fusion protein on the outer coat protein. However, non-suppressor strains such as HB2151 recognize the amber stop codon and enable the production of the scFv/dAb portion alone. Here, the basic outline for generating HB2151 stocks and basic production and purification of the scFv/dAb are provided (*see* **Note 17**).

1. Streak out HB2151 bacteria on TYE plates and culture at 37 °C overnight (*see* **Note 1**).
2. Transfer HB2151 plates to 4 °C for storage. Use within 1 month. Prepare new plates as needed for experimental preparation.
3. Generate phage for clones of interest by using frozen infected TGl cells from the 96-well plate prepared in Subheading 3.3.1 **step 12**.
4. Inoculate 20 mL of 2xTY + 4% glucose + 100 μg/mL of ampicillin with phage clone of interest pulled from stock 96-well plate (50 mL tube; loosely tape lid). Grow culture at 37 °C and 250 rpm for 3–4 h.
5. Add 2 × 10^{11} helper phage to 20 mL culture. Incubate in 37 °C water bath for 60 min.
6. Spin culture at 3200 × *g* for 10 min.
7. Discard the supernatant and resuspend the pellet in 50 mL of 2xTY + 0.1% glucose + 100 μg/mL of ampicillin + 50 μg/mL kanamycin (250 mL Erlenmeyer flask).
8. Grow culture at 250 rpm and 30 °C for ~20 h.
9. Follow the standard PEG purification protocol as outlined in Subheading 3.1.2 and determine total phage CFU (Subheading 3.1.3).
10. **Steps 1–9** may be performed in parallel for each clone of interest.
11. Prepare an overnight, starved HB2151 culture by inoculating 5 mL of 2xTY medium with a single HB2151 colony pulled from the stock HB2151 plate. Incubate in a bacterial shaker overnight at 250 rpm and 37 °C.
12. The following day, prepare 100-fold dilution of overnight-starved bacteria and by transferring 100 μL of starved culture in 10 mL of 2xTY (use 50 mL tube loosely tape lid to prevent it from unscrewing in the incubator). Incubate at 250 rpm and 37 °C until OD600 of 0.5 is reached (about 1.5–2.5 h). Prepare one 10 mL culture per clone.
13. At the same time, set one large bioassay TAG plate and one TAG petri dish in a bacterial incubator or oven to dry (one plate and dish per clone).
14. Add 100 μL of one phage clone to each 10 mL HB2151 culture and incubate in a water bath at 37 °C for 30 min.

15. Spin culture at 3200 × *g* for 5 min.
16. Discard the supernatant and resuspend the pellet in 0.5 mL of 2xTY.
17. Plate 450 μL of the concentrated cell solution one TAG bioassay dish. Spread evenly across plate surface with bacterial cell spreader. Grow overnight at 30–37 °C. Titer remaining cells at 10^2, 10^3, 10^4, 10^5 dilutions on the TAG petri dish.
18. Repeat **step 17** for all clones.
19. After overnight growth, add 10 mL of 2xTY medium per large biodish and gently dislodge cells with bacterial cell scraper/spreader. Use serological pipette to transfer cell suspension to a 50 mL centrifuge tube.
20. Add 100% glycerol to generated 15% glycerol final volume and aliquot into 1 mL aliquots. Freeze and store at −80 °C. Store the titer plate at 4 °C.
21. It is recommended to use four to six colonies from the titer plate to generate cultures for plasmid DNA extraction to send out for sequencing in order to verify clone homogeneity (*See* Subheading "Plasmid Purification and Sequencing").

4.2 Production of scFv/dAb

The final step in this process is to produce and purify the scFv/dAb for further characterization and eventual use for the desired application. Below are basic outlines for protein purification from the cell lysates and cell media, however, it is noted that as with any recombinant proteins, production rates and amounts vary from clone to clone. Optimal methods for purification may need to be performed for each clone.

1. Add 1 mL of HB2151 infected stock to 500 mL of 2xTY + 0.1% glucose + 100 μg/mL ampicillin (use 2 L Erlenmeyer flask). Grow at 37 °C and 250 rpm ~4 h.
2. Add 0.5 mL of 1 M IPTG to culture (induce scFv/dAb production) and grow overnight at 30 °C and 250 rpm.
3. Spin overnight culture at 8000 × *g* for 10 min. Recommend using a single 250 mL centrifuge bottle to collect the entire cell pellet. This may require multiple rounds of centrifugation using the same collection bottle.
4. Aspirate the supernatant and store in 500 mL bottle and keep cell pellet.

4.3 Purification of scFv/dAb: Cell Lysate

1. Prepare 45 mL of 1xPBS + one tablet of Protease Inhibitor Mini Tablet.
2. Use the 45 mL of PBS + Protease inhibitor to resuspend cell pellet.

3. Prepare 5–10 mL of 10 mg/mL lysozyme in 25 mM Tris–HCl, pH 8.0.
4. Add 5 mL of lysozyme solution to cell solution.
5. Use a probe sonicator to further lyse the cells (on ice). Suggested sonication sequence is 3–4 cycles of 20 s sonication at 40–50% maximum power and then off for 30 s. No foam should appear. Do not over sonicate.
6. Immediately add Triton X-100 and 100 U/mL of DNAse I to the cell lysate and bring the final concentration to 1% Triton X-100 and 10 U/mL of DNAse I.
7. Place on an orbital shaker to gently mix for 30 min.
8. Freeze lysate −20 °C for minimum of 6 h. The lysate may be stored at −20 °C for longer if lysate will not be purified immediately.
9. The day of purification, thaw lysate out at RT.
10. Spin the sample down for 15 min at 12,000 × *g*.
11. Filter the supernatant through a 0.22 μm pore filter and add 0.1% NaN_3 to generate a final concentration of 0.02% NaN_3.
12. Use preferred method of protein purification to extract scFv/dAb. The recommend method is Fast-Performance Liquid Chromotography (FPLC) with a Protein-A affinity column. In order to achieve optimal protein purification, it may be necessary to use alternative resin designed to capture specific types of antibody fragments.

4.4 Purification of scFv/dAb: Culture Supernatant

Some clones will readily produce the scFv/dAb as soluble proteins in the bacterial culture medium. The culture medium may be desalted and concentrated using a tangential flow filtration system. The resulting concentrated solution may then be purified using the same FPLC with a Protein-A affinity column recommended above in Subheading 4.3.

4.5 Further Characterization

After production and purification of scFv/dAb for clones of interest, perform concentration-dependent ELISAs to validate results obtained from the phage-based assays. Further characterization assays to include surface Plasmon resonance (SPR) and immunocytochemistry to determine dynamic binding constants and spatial location of epitopes.

5 Notes

1. Bacterial work (reagent preparation and subsequent phage biopanning steps) is best performed using aseptic techniques within 6–10 in. of a burning alcohol lamp. *See* reference for a

more thorough description of standard bacterial and aseptic techniques [9, 10].

2. Domain antibody library (dAb) or Tomlinson I + J single-chain variable fragment (scFv) antibody libraries, *Escherichia coli* TG1 TR strain, *E. coli* HB2151 strain, positive control clone (β-galactosidase-specific), negative control clone (phagemid) and KM13 helper phage (Source Bioscience, Nottingham, UK).
3. 2xTY medium is prone to contamination. Inspect medium visually before each use to verify the medium is clear and free of contamination.
4. Place the autoclaved agar solution in a water bath to 50 °C. Allow solution to equilibrate to 50 °C prior to pouring into petri dishes. However, if the temperature drops below 50 °C then agar will begin to gel prior to pouring into the petri dishes.
5. The optimal media volume for the Domain antibody library is 500 mL while Tomilinson I + J requires only 200 mL. Adjust the volume depending on which library is being used.
6. The presence of 4% glucose allowed the effective suppression of antibody expression during bacterial growth by preventing lactose permease production, thereby inhibiting the uptake of the disaccharide lactose by the host *E. coli* from the yeast extract present in TYE. Remaining intracellular lactose would be digested by the production of β-galactosidase produced by the LacZ gene. Without the presence of lactose, the Lac repressor successfully inhibits the LacO operon, thus suppressing expression of our scFv/dAb insert. Ampicillin kills off any bacterium which did not contain the synthetic library vector. *See* Genetic Analysis for insert detection and efficacy testing.
7. Growth of the culture to reach an OD600 of 0.1 typically takes about 1.5–2 h at 37 °C and 250 rpm.
8. The suggested volume and helper phage concentration is suggested for Domain Antibody Library. For the Tomlinson I + J, incubate 50 mL of the bacterial culture with 2×10^{11} KM13 helper phage in a water bath at 37 °C for 30–45 min.
9. For Tomlinson I + J, resuspend cell pellet in 100 mL of 2xTY supplemented with 0.1% glucose 100 μg/mL of ampicillin and 50 μg/mL of kanamycin.
10. The 0.1% glucose provides a food source for the overnight growth of bacteria without arresting phage expansion.
11. Carefully examine the bottle after centrifugation. The phage pellet will appear as a small white thin layer.

12. The EDTA acts as a chelating agent, most likely toward the remaining PEG. The BSA also acts as a protein preservative/protectant.
13. Recommend using 2 mL round bottom centrifuge tubes for the phage dilutions. After diluting each sample, close the cap and invert 3–5× to ensure complete mixing of each dilution.
14. Depending on the number of active phage, each dilution will give a range of CFUs (1–2 colonies to an uncountable lawn of bacteria). Use the intermediary dilutions with distinct colonies to calculate CFUs (i.e., ~20–80 colonies).
15. The stock library may have a high percentage of wild type phage that do not display an scFv/dAb fragment. Negative screens do not remove the wild type phage as efficiently as positive screens. After several rounds of positive screens, the prevalence of inserts should greatly increase.
16. Bound phage are eluted from the target cell cells via trypsin cleavage site between the phage body and scFv/dAb fragment.
17. HB2151 cells are not an optimal production line and therefore alternative expression/production lines will be required for large scale protein production.

References

1. Byrne JD, Betancourt T, Brannon-Peppas L (2008) Active targeting schemes for nanoparticle systems in cancer therapeutics. Adv Drug Deliv Rev 60:1615–1626. https://doi.org/10.1016/j.addr.2008.08.005
2. Paschke M (2005) Phage display systems and their applications. Appl Microbiol Biotechnol 70:2–11. https://doi.org/10.1007/s00253-005-0270-9
3. Lee CMY, Iorno N, Sierro F, Christ D (2007) Selection of human antibody fragments by phage display. Nat Protoc 2:3001–3008. https://doi.org/10.1038/nprot.2007.448
4. Bertrand N, Wu J, Xu X et al (2014) Cancer nanotechnology: the impact of passive and active targeting in the era of modern cancer biology. Adv Drug Deliv Rev 66:2–25. https://doi.org/10.1016/j.addr.2013.11.009
5. Stabenfeldt SE, Gossett JJ, Barker TH (2010) Building better fibrin knob mimics: an investigation of synthetic fibrin knob peptide structures in solution and their dynamic binding with fibrinogen/fibrin holes. Blood 116:1352–1359. https://doi.org/10.1182/blood-2009-11-251801
6. Brown AC, Stabenfeldt SE, Ahn B et al (2014) Ultrasoft microgels displaying emergent platelet-like behaviours. Nat Mater 13:1108–1114. https://doi.org/10.1038/nmat4066
7. Dudgeon K, Famm K, Christ D (2008) Sequence determinants of protein aggregation in human VH domains. Protein Eng Des Sel 22:217–220. https://doi.org/10.1093/protein/gzn059
8. Kvam E, Sierks MR, Shoemaker CB, Messer A (2010) Physico-chemical determinants of soluble intrabody expression in mammalian cell cytoplasm. Protein Eng Des Sel 23:489–498. https://doi.org/10.1093/protein/gzq022
9. Sanders ER (2012) Aseptic laboratory techniques: plating methods. JoVE. https://doi.org/10.3791/3064
10. Cote RJ (1998) Aseptic technique for cell culture. Curr Protoc Cell Biol:1–10

Chapter 8

CD44 Targeted Lipid Nanoparticles for MicroRNA Therapy

Stephen L. Hayward and Srivatsan Kidambi

Abstract

MicroRNAs are small noncoding RNAs that function as powerful endogenous regulators of gene expression. Dysregulation of MicroRNA biogenesis has been correlated with the onset and progression of many human diseases. MicroRNA therapy involves the re-equilibration of aberrant intracellular MicroRNA expression profiles for long-term disease management. Despite the significant potential of MicroRNA therapy, the utilization of MicroRNA-based therapeutics has been drastically hindered in practice by the lack of a targeted and translatable delivery vehicle. CD44 is a cell surface glycoprotein that facilitates cellular communication and motility through cell-cell and cell-extracellular matrix interactions. CD44 has been shown to be elevated in multiple disease states including cancer making it a potential diagnostic biomarker and an ideal receptor for targeted drug delivery systems. We describe a method for targeting CD44 using a lipid nanocarrier for the cytoplasmic delivery of active MicroRNA.

Key words Liposomes, MicroRNA, Hyaluronic acid, CD44, Gene therapy, Lipid nanoparticles, Active targeting

1 Introduction

MicroRNAs (miRs) are small ~22 nucleotide long noncoding RNAs of endogenous origin that perform post transcriptional gene regulation [1]. These highly conserved RNA molecules integrate and subsequently navigate the active protein-miR RNA induced silencing complex (RISC) to directly repress or degrade messenger RNAs as a function of base pair complementarity [2]. Current studies estimate that there are a total of 1500 different miRs in humans that cumulatively regulate more than half of all protein-coding genes [3, 4]. Consequently, it is logical that aberrant intracellular miR expression profiles have been found to promote abnormal cellular behavior and the onset and progression of disease states including cancer [5, 6] cardiovascular [7, 8], and liver disease [9]. Recently, the notion of re-equilibrating intracellular miR levels has led to the idea of miR-replacement or miR-quenching therapy as a promising therapeutic tool [10, 11]. However, the lack in the development of a translatable nanocarrier

Rachael W. Sirianni and Bahareh Behkam (eds.), *Targeted Drug Delivery: Methods and Protocols*, Methods in Molecular Biology, vol. 1831, https://doi.org/10.1007/978-1-4939-8661-3_8, © Springer Science+Business Media, LLC, part of Springer Nature 2018

that can mediate targeted delivery in a safe and reliable manner has greatly hindered miR-based therapeutics [12, 13].

In order to simultaneously reduce offsite toxicity and mitigate the dose required for an effective therapy, nanoscale drug and gene delivery platforms commonly employ active targeting mechanisms to achieve per-cell preferential uptake. Active targeting ligands range from antibodies and aptamers to peptides and polysaccharides, all of which are used to surface decorate nanocarriers to facilitate a specific interaction with an over-expressed cell surface receptor [14]. A promising ligand-receptor pair for targeted therapy is hyaluronic acid (HA)–CD44. CD44 is a cell surface receptor exploited for its significant up regulation in various cancer types such as breast, colorectal, and lung as opposed to basal expression in corresponding healthy tissue [15]. While HA coated nanocarriers have achieved success in the delivery of a range of cargo types including chemotherapeutic drugs [16, 17] and siRNA [18], minimal HA decorated nanocarriers have been developed for the targeted delivery of miR.

To harness the vast potential of CD44 driven targeting for nanoscale miR therapy, our lab has developed a highly effective delivery platform consisting of a biocompatible liposome core (LNP) followed by surface functionalization with high molecular weight HA (HALNP) [19–21]. Herein, we describe the synthesis process for the LNPs, surface decoration with HA, and purification steps necessary prior to application. We then use breast cancer as a model system to demonstrate the HALNP's targeting potential, ability to promote intracellular miR delivery, and robust potency in target mRNA silencing.

2 Materials

2.1 Lipid Nanoparticle (LNP) Synthesis

1. L α-Phosphatidylcholine (PC).
2. 1, 2-Dipalmitoyl-sn-Glycero-3-Phopshoethanolamine (DPPE).
3. Cholesterol (CHOL).
4. Boric Acid (H_3BO_3).
5. Glacial Acetic Acid (CH_3COOH).
6. HEPES Free Acid ($C_8H_{18}N_2O_4S$).
7. Sodium Acetate (CH_3COONa).
8. Sodium Chloride (NaCl).
9. Potassium Chloride (KCl).
10. Sodium Phosphate Dibasic (Na_2HPO_4).
11. Potassium Phosphate Monobasic (KH_2PO_4).
12. Rotary Evaporator.
13. Mini extruder apparatus (1 mL version) with 0.8, 0.4, 0.2, and 0.08 μm polycarbonate membranes and filter supports.

14. 20 mM HEPES Buffer pH 7.4: 4.77 g HEPES free acid, 800 mL ddH_2O, pH adjust with NaOH, Bring volume to 1 L with ddH_2O.
15. 100 mM Borate Buffer pH 8.6: 6.18 g Boric Acid, 800 mL ddH_2O, pH adjust with NaOH, Bring volume to 1 L with ddH_2O.
16. 1 M Acetic Acid: 5.75 mL Glacial Acetic Acid, 94.25 ddH_2O.
17. 100 mM Sodium Acetate Buffer pH 5: 8.2 g Sodium Acetate, 800 mL ddH_2O, pH adjust with 1 M Acetic Acid, Bring to 1 L with ddH_2O.
18. 1× PBS pH 7.4: 800 mL ddH_2O, 8 g NaCl, 0.2 g KCl, 1.44 g Na_2HPO_4, 0.24 g KH_2PO_4, adjust pH with HCl, Bring to 1 L with ddH_2O.
19. 1.65 MDa Hyaluronic Acid (HA).
20. 1-ethyl-3-(3-dimethylaminopropyl) carbomiide (EDC).
21. Ultracentrifuge.
22. Chamber Freeze Dry System Lyophilizer.
23. Shaker Table.

2.2 Lipid Nanoparticle (LNP) Characterization

1. Zeta potential and Dynamic Light Scattering Instrument.
2. 0.05× PBS pH 7.4: 950 mL ddH_2O, 50 mL 1× PBS (recipe shown above).
3. Transmission Electron Microscope.
4. Carbon Film on a Mesh Copper Grid.
5. Phosphotungstic Acid 2% Solution.

2.3 Cell Culture, Western Blot, and HALNP Uptake Analysis

1. MCF10A Cells (ATCC CRL-10317) human normal breast tissue cell line.
2. MCF10A Media: DMEM/F12 50/50 mix from Mediatech (Manassas, VA, USA) supplemented with 1% L-glutamine, 1% penicillin-streptomycin (PS), 5% Horse Serum, 0.1 ng/mL cholera toxin, 0.5 μg/mL hydrocortisone, 10 μg/mL insulin, and 0.02 ng/μL rhEGF.
3. 21MT-1 cells were a kind gift from Dr. Band at the University of Nebraska Medical Center. This human HER2 positive metastatic breast cancer cell line was derived from mammary tumor specimens isolated from the metastatic pleural effusion [22].
4. 21MT-1 Media: α-MEM supplemented with 5% fetal bovine serum (FBS), 1% PS, 1% L-glutamine, 20 mM HEPES, 1% non-essential amino acids, 1% sodium pyruvate, 12.5 ng/mL epidermal growth factor, and 1 μg/mL hydrocortisone.
5. Western Blot: Anti-CD44, and Anti-Tubulin antibodies.
6. 20 kDa FITC-tagged Dextran.

7. Fluorescent Plate Reader.
8. Inverted Microscope with Progress C3 camera.

2.4 MiR Entrapment Efficiency, Intracellular Delivery, and Potency Analysis

1. Human miRIDIAN miR125a-5p mature sequence: UCCCU GAGACCCUUUAACCUGUGA.
2. Quant-iT Ribogreen Nucleic Acid Binding Dye.
3. Lipofectamine 2000.
4. Human GAPDH Primer: (R: 5′-AGG-GGC-CAT-CCA-CAG-TCT-TC-3′), (F: 5′-AGA-AGG-CTG-GGG-CTC-ATT-TG-3′).
5. Human HER2 Primer: (R: 5′-TGA-TGA-GGA-TCC-CAA-AGA-CC-3′), (F: 5′-AAC-TGC-ACC-CAC-TCC-TGT-GT-3′).
6. FV500 Inverted Confocal Microscope.
7. Hoescht Nuclear Stain.
8. Confocal dishes (35 mm glass bottom).

3 Methods

3.1 LNP Fabrication, Surface Functionalization with HA (HALNP), and Purification Steps

Hyaluronic Acid coated Lipid Nanoparticles (HALNPs) are surface decorated nanoscale vesicles that can deliver both hydrophilic and hydrophobic cargo in a targeted manner with a high level of spatiotemporal control [19–21]. The synthesis of the HALNPs involves creating micron size multilamellar vesicles (MLVs) made from biocompatible lipid components, mechanical extrusion down to the nanoscale to form lipid nanoparticles (LNPs), and surface functionalization with high molecular weight HA via EDC-mediated amide bond formations to generate HALNPs (Fig. 1a).

1. Create MLVs comprising of PC: DPPE: CHOL in a 3:1:1 molar ratio respectively via the dry lipid film technique [23–26]. Briefly, combine 37 mg of total lipid mass in pure ethanol and mix in a rotating round bottom flask at 65 °C for 30 min until complete dissolution (*see* **Notes 1** and **2**). Rotary evaporate for 2 h at 65 °C (~350 mBar) followed by 30 min under complete vacuum (<100 mBar) to remove ethanol and create a dry lipid film. Run the dry lipid film under an indirect stream of nitrogen from a nitrogen gun for at least 10 min to remove trace ethanol prior to rehydration.
2. Hydrate the dry lipid film immediately following complete ethanol removal with any physiological buffer that can be used downstream with cell culture experiments such as 20 mM HEPES or 1× PBS to a final lipid concentration of 10 mg/mL (approximately 3.7 mL total volume).

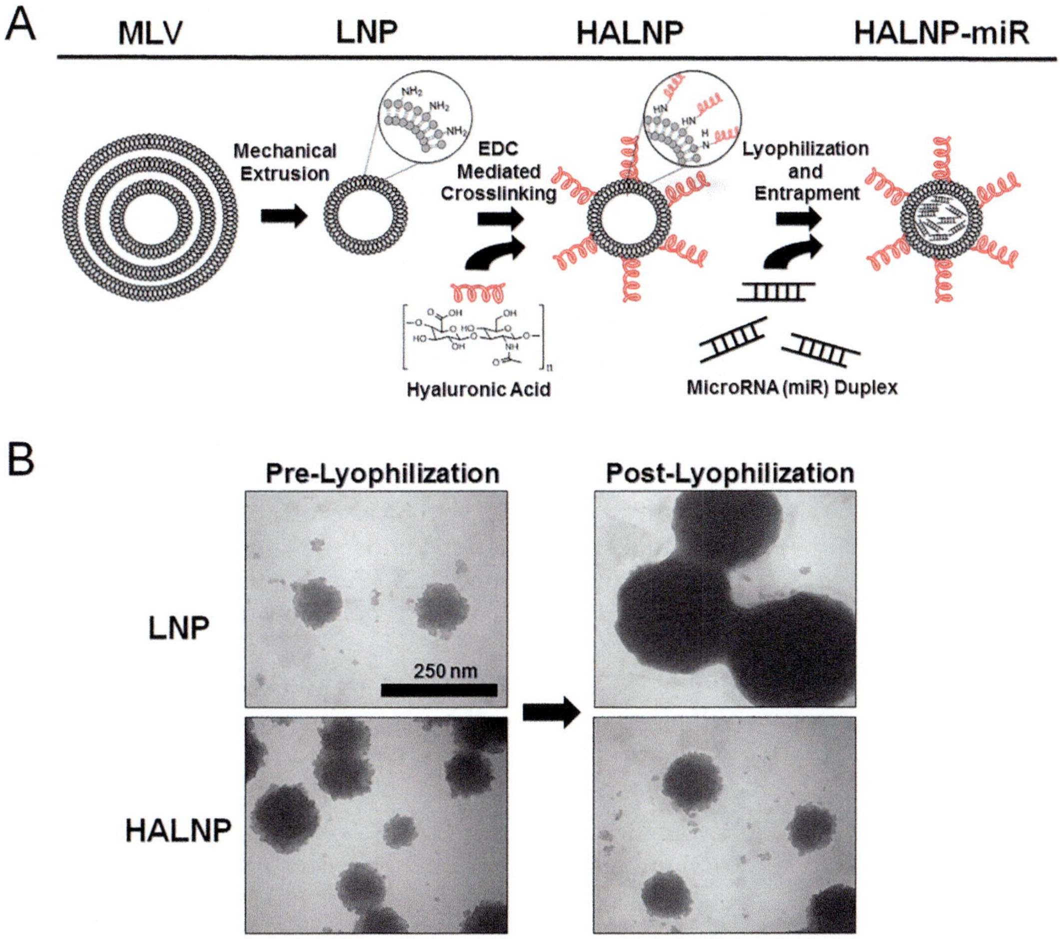

Fig. 1 Lipid Nanoparticle fabrication scheme and characterization. (**a**) Lipid Nanoparticle (LNP) synthesis, surface functionalization with hyaluronic acid (HALNP), and microRNA cargo entrapment (HALNP-miR). (**b**) Characterization of both LNPs and HALNPs pre and post the lyophilization and rehydration procedure by Transmission Electron Microscopy (TEM) using the negative stain method. The HA coating is a crucial aspect of the delivery scheme because it acts as a lyoprotectant by reducing rehydration fusion events and thereby simultaneously retaining the nanoscale dimensions of the particles while promoting high entrapment efficiency. Scale bar is 250 nm

3. Vortex the solution for 15 min at maximum intensity, and then store overnight at 4 °C (*see* **Note 3**).
4. Preheat the mini extruder apparatus to 65 °C. Pass 1 mL at a time of MLV volume through polycarbonate membranes to systematically reduce the number of lipid bilayers and overall nanoparticle size (in a decreasing stepwise fashion from 800 nm → 400 nm → 200 nm → 80 nm) to form the LNPs.
5. Pass the solution through each membrane 21 times, always ending on the opposite side as the initial MLV solution to achieve a homogeneous single particle distribution (*see* **Note 4**). Continue

to process in 1 mL increments with the rest of the MLV solution to achieve the LNP solution.

6. Store LNP solution at 4 °C for not more than 2 days before HA surface functionalization (*see* **Note 5**).
7. HA surface functionalization: Dissolve 40 mg of 1.65 MDa HA in sodium acetate buffer at a concentration of 2 mg/mL overnight on a low-speed shaker table at room temperature. Activate the HA by combining 4 mg HA (2 mL of HA solution) with 120 mg EDC (1–30 mass ratio of HA to EDC), bringing the solution to a pH of 4, and incubating for 2 h at 37 °C on a stir plate with low stir speed.
8. Purify the extruded 3.7 mL LNPs solution to remove lipid debris via ultracentrifugation (135,000 × *g*, 1.5 h, 4 °C) and resuspend in 3.7 mL borate buffer (pH 8.6).
9. Add the purified LNPs dropwise with a 200 μL pipette into the activated HA solution still under slow stir, bring the mixture to pH 7.4, and incubate for 2–3 h at 37 °C with slow stir speed. Adjust the pH to 8.4–8.8 and incubate overnight at 37 °C with slow stir speed.
10. Purify the HALNPs by three to four wash steps via ultracentrifugation (135,000 × *g*, 1.5 h, 4 °C) using 1× PBS as the washing buffer (*see* **Note 6**). Store the HALNP solution at 4 °C (*see* **Note 7**).
11. Lyophilization of the HALNPs: Aliquot the HALNPs solution into glass flat bottom lyophilizer vials (300 μL/tube) and snap freeze in a mixture of dry ice and ethanol for 30 min (*see* **Note 8**).
12. Transfer the tubes to a lyophilizer, and lyophilize for 48–60 h at −30 °C (primary drying), 0.5–1 h transition time to ramp up the temperature to 25 °C, and 4 h at 25 °C (secondary drying) followed by machine-assisted vial capping. Store the lyophilized aliquots at −80 °C until use.

3.2 Rehydration and Cargo Entrapment Procedure

1. Remove the vial from the −80 °C freezer and allow equilibration to room temperature before rehydration and cargo entrapment (*see* **Note 9**).
2. Add 30 μL (1/10th the original volume per vial) of the drug or gene cargo of choice to the vial (*see* **Note 10**).
3. Ensure the complete lipid film is hydrated by the solution, and then incubate for 30 min at room temperature to facilitate liposome re-assembly and cargo entrapment. Vortexing can be used to aid in rehydration of the lyophilized film; however, this should be very brief and at a very low intensity (750 rpm for less than 5 s).

4. Bring the vial to its original volume by adding (270 μL) sterile nuclease-free 1× PBS, and vortex very briefly (if needed; 750 rpm for less than 5 s) to disrupt any HALNP aggregation.
5. Determine encapsulation efficiency by one of two ways depending on the cargo type:
6. *Method 1.* For fluorescent non-nucleic acid-based cargoes such as FITC tagged Dextran (FD) and Doxorubicin (DOX), ultracentrifuge the rehydrated HALNPs to remove un-encapsulated drug in the supernatant (140,000 × *g*, 1.25 h, 4 °C), permeabilize the purified HALNPs with 0.1% triton by incubation at room temperature for 5 min followed by 2 min of maximum intensity vortexing, and utilize a known standard curve to determine total internal payload. Also quantify the fluorescent signal in the supernatant to validate conservation of mass.
7. *Method 2.* For nucleic acid cargoes such as miR, siRNA, shRNA, or DNA, use the Quant-iT Ribogreen Nucleic Acid Binding Dye to determine the ratio of encapsulated and non-encapsulated cargo. The binding dye is unable to penetrate intact lipid membranes, and therefore in the absence of triton detergent only the fluorescence of the un-entrapped nucleic acid cargo can be measured. But, in the presence of detergent, the total fluorescence can be measured to determine the percent encapsulation (*see* **Note 11**).

3.3 Nanocarrier Characterization

1. Dynamic Light Scattering and Zeta Potential Analysis (Table 1): Dilute a sample of LNP or HALNP solution 10–20× in 0.05× PBS (pH 7.4). Measure nanoparticle size at an angle of 90° with intensity distribution, and nanoparticle charge using the Smoluchowki model. Take all measurements at 25 °C.
2. Transmission Electron Microscopy and the Negative Stain Method: Add a drop of around 5–10 μL of the different nanoparticle solutions (at the same lipid concentrations) to a carbon copper grid, cover with 2% phosphotungstic acid solution, and allow it to air dry before visualization (Fig. 1b).

Table 1
Lipid nanoparticle size and charge analysis pre and post surface functionalization with high molecular weight hyaluronic acid

	Hydrodynamic diameter (nm)	Polydispersity index (PI)	Zeta potential (mV)
LNP	102.5 ± 0.1	0.116	−4.63 ± 0.59
HALNP	169.7 ± 2.1	0.190	−38.03 ± 2.33

3.4 Quantification of CD44 Targeting Potential of HALNPs

Fluorescent microscopy and plate reader quantification is used to confirm the preferential targeting of HALNPs to CD44 positive cells. Normal (MCF10A) and cancerous (21MT-1) breast cells are used as a model system [20]. This experiment is run in three sections: (1) probe the CD44 expression in each cell type, (2) encapsulate the model fluorescent therapeutic cargo, FITC-tagged dextran (FD), into HALNPs (HALNP-FD), and (3) incubate the HALNP-FDs with the cells and compare uptake.

1. Culture both MCF10A cells and 21MT-1 cells in their respective complete media, isolate protein following standard protocol, load 10 μg total protein per lane, and run western blot to probe for CD44 expression (Fig. 2a). It is beyond the scope of the current work to provide a detailed protocol for protein isolation and western blot assay. Interested parties are directed to in-depth protocols [27, 28].
2. Dissolve 20 mg of 20 kDa FD in 2 mL of 0.05× PBS, rehydrate a lyophilized vial of HALNP with 30 μL of the FD solution (total of 300 μg FD) and bring to 300 μL with 1× PBS, quantify total entrapped FD payload using Method 1 in Subheading 3.2, and filter sterilize through a 0.45 μm filter (*see* **Note 12**).
3. Seed MCF10A and 21MT-1 cells as monocultures in 12-well plates with a seeding density of 100,000 cells/well (1 mL media per well). Culture cells in complete media overnight at 37 °C, 5% CO_2.
4. Switch the complete media to analogous media without serum and PS, and add 70 pmol of FD per well in two different forms: (a) naked FD as an uptake control, and (b) FD encapsulated into HALNPs (HALNP-FD).
5. Incubate for 5 h, wash cells three times with 1× PBS, and then measure fluorescence qualitatively by fluorescent microscopy (Fig. 2b) and quantitatively with a plate reader (Fig. 2c) for both cell types (490 ex., 520 em).

3.5 Validation of Intracellular miR Delivered by HALNPs

MiR must be cytosolic to incorporate into the RNA-induced silencing (RISC) complex and reduce target mRNA levels. Confirmation of intracellular miR delivery is performed by tagging the miR cargo, encapsulating the tagged miR inside the HALNPs, incubating with cells, and then performing confocal microscopy.

1. Seed 21MT-1 cells at a density of 200,000 cells per 35 mm glass bottom confocal plate overnight to promote cell attachment (2 mL media per plate).
2. Mix 400 pmol miR125a-5p with 4 μL Quant-iT Ribogreen Nucleic Acid Binding Dye and incubate the solution for 10 min at room temperature to create miR-dye complexes (*see* **Note 13**).

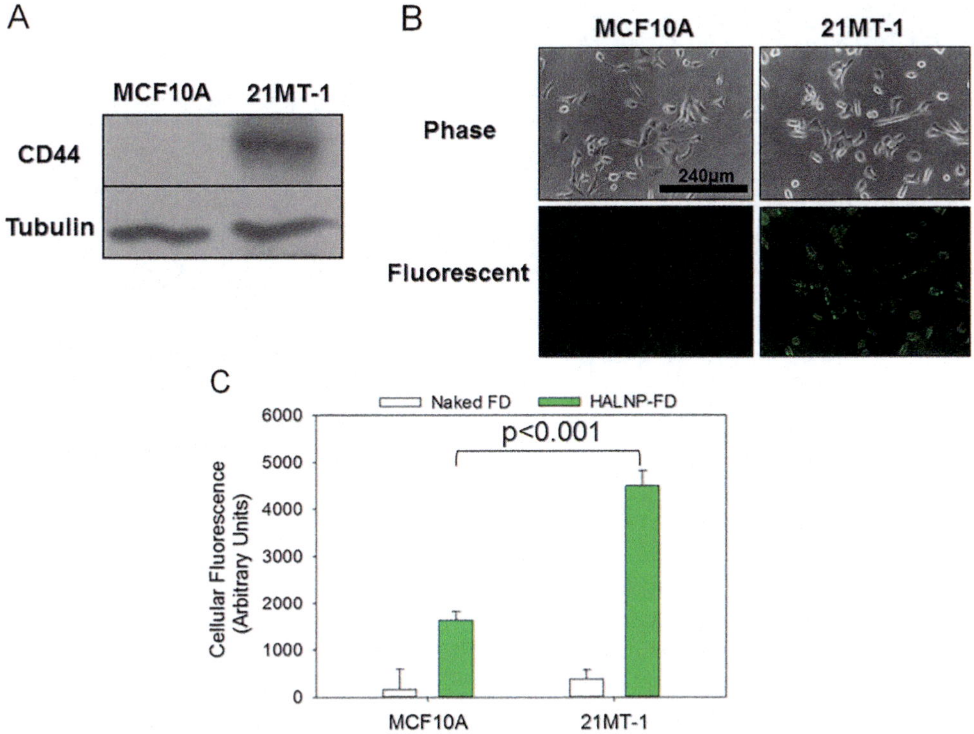

Fig. 2 Investigation of the targeting potential of HALNPs for CD44 overexpressing cells. Normal (MCF10A) and cancerous (21MT-1) human breast cells were chosen as a test system. (**a**) Western blot was used to measure the cell-specific CD44 protein levels. Following validation of differential CD44 expression, 20 kDa FITC-tagged dextran (FD) model drug was employed: (1) naked as an uptake control because FD is resistant to traversing cell membranes and (2) encapsulated inside HALNPs (HALNP-FD). (**b**) Fluorescent and phase contrast microscopy images of MCF10A cells and 21MT-1 cells after a 5 h incubation with HALNP-FDs. (**c**) Plate reader quantification of cellular fluorescence comparing naked FD and HALNP-FD following a 5 h incubation ($n = 3$). The significant difference in HALNP mediated per cell fluorescence between the 21MT-1 cells and MCF10A cells confirms the preferential targeting of HALNPs to CD44 positive cells. Scale bar for the fluorescent microscopy is 240 μm

3. Use this solution to rehydrate a vial of lyophilized HALNPs, remove un-encapsulated complexes via ultracentrifugation, filter sterilize through a 0.45 μm filter, and incubate the purified HALNPs with encapsulated miR-dye complexes with the 21MT-1 cells for 1 h (use media without serum and PS for this step) (*see* **Note 14**).
4. Wash the plate three times with 1× PBS, stain the cellular nucleus with Hoescht, and visualize the sample using live cell confocal microscopy (RNA Dye: 490 ex., 520 em; Hoerscht: 346 ex., 497 em). Figure 3 is an example with HALNP delivered miR125a-5p-dye complexes.

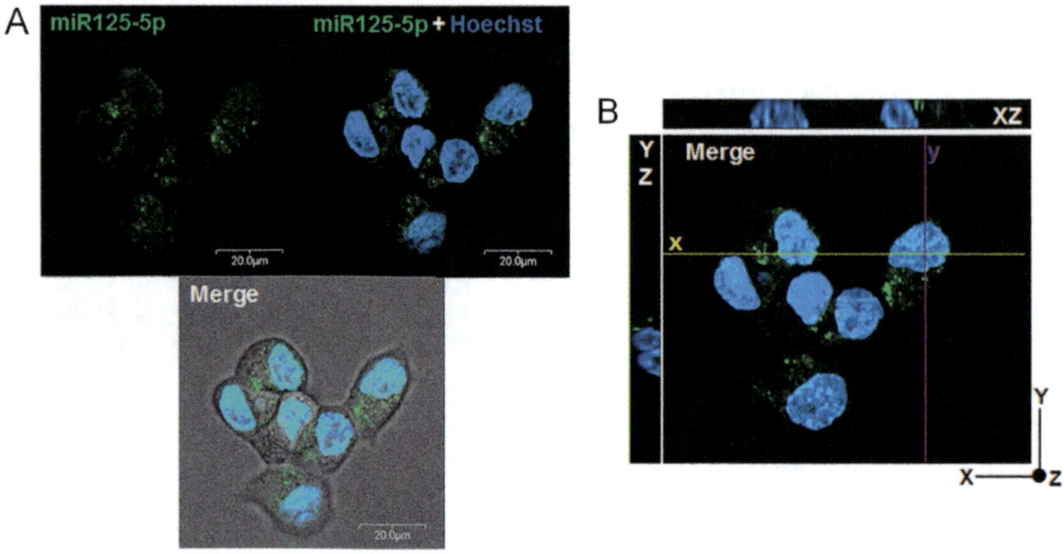

Fig. 3 Validation of intracellular miR delivery via HALNPs. MiR125a-5p was complexed with RNA binding dye, encapsulated inside HALNPs, and incubated with 21MT-1 cells for 1 h. (**a**) Live cell confocal microscopy demonstrated the intracellular delivery of HALNP-miR125a-5p which was confirmed by (**b**) a *z*-axis transformation utilizing the nucleus as an inter-cellular reference point (RNA Dye + miR complex: 490 ex. 520 em. Hoerscht: 346 ex., 497 em). The *XZ* and *YX* planes show the height and respective widths of the cell

3.6 Potent HER2 mRNA Knockdown with Active miR125a-5p Delivered via HALNPs

Human Epidermal Growth Factor Receptor 2 (HER2) is an oncogene commonly amplified in breast cancer [29]. HER2 was chosen as a model mRNA target to demonstrate the efficacy of the HALNP system to deliver active miR. MiR125a-5p, a tumor suppressor of HER2 [20, 30], was encapsulated into HALNPs, delivered into 21MT-1 cells, and HER2 mRNA expression was quantified by qRT-PCR (Fig. 4).

1. Seed 21MT-1 cells at 60,000 cells per well in a 12-well format in complete media (1 mL media per well). Culture overnight at 37 °C, 5% CO_2.
2. Rehydrate a vial of lyophilized HALNPs with 1500 pmol miR125a-5p and quantify entrapment with Method 2 in Subheading 3.2.
3. Remove un-encapsulated miR via ultracentrifugation and filter sterilize through a 0.45 μm filter (HALNP-miR125a-5p).
4. Employ a commercial transfection reagent such as Lipofectamine 2000 (LF2K) as a positive control for miR silencing of HER2. For 50 pmol miR transfection, dilute 50 pmol miR125a-5p in 100 μL media with no PS or serum (Solution A). Additionally, dilute 3 μL of LF2K reagent in 100 μL media with no PS or serum and incubate for 5 min

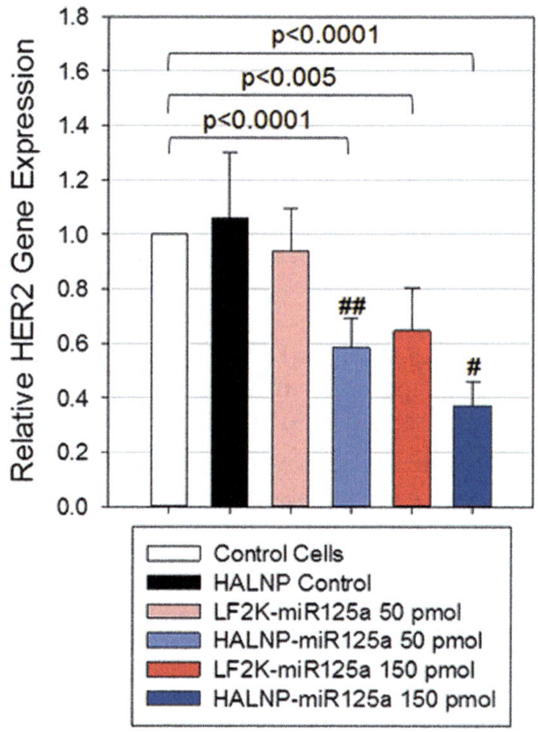

Fig. 4 Demonstration of the HALNP nanocarriers' ability to transfect cells with miR cargo and promote potent gene silencing. As a model system miR125a-5p, a miR tumor suppressor of the HER2 oncogene, was delivered to 21MT-1 HER2 positive metastatic breast cancer cells via (1) HALNPs or (2) the commercial transfection reagent Lipofectamine 2000 (LF2K) to directly compare efficacy following a 72 h transfection time (# denotes significance between LF2K and HALNP at the analogous miR125a-5p concentration; $^{\#\#}p < 0.005$, $^{\#}p < 0.05$; $n = 4$). GAPDH used as a housekeeping control. The ΔΔCt method was used to determine the change in mRNA expression. These results show that the HALNP nanocarrier is over three fold more potent than LF2K

at room temperature (Solution B). Mix Solution A and Solution B and incubate for 20 min prior to addition to cells (*see* **Note 15**).

5. Switch the seeded cells to media without serum and PS, and add the following samples types to defined wells: (a) 50 pmol HALNP-miR125a-5p as the HALNP-miR low dose, (b) 150 pmol HALNP-miR125a-5p as the HALNP-miR high dose, (c) HALNPs without miR to validate bio-inactivity of the nanocarrier, (d) 50 pmol LF2K-miR125a-5p as the low dose positive control, and (e) 150 pmol LF2K-miR125a-5p as the high dose positive control.
6. Incubate for 5 h, wash the cells once with 1× PBS, and incubate for an additional 72 h in complete media (*see* **Note 16**).
7. Extract total RNA following the standard Trizol method, synthesize cDNA (5 min 25 °C, 30 min 42 °C, 5 min 85 °C), and

run qRT-PCR with human HER2 and GAPDH (as housekeeping) primers with a 40 cycle amplification (95 °C for 10 s, 56 °C for 30 s, and 72 °C for 30 s). It is beyond the scope of the current work to provide a detailed protocol for total RNA extraction. Interested parties are directed to in-depth protocols [31].

4 Notes

1. Keep all lipids kept at −20 °C in powder form for long-term storage. PC can be stored in 100% ethanol for up to 1 week before use in MLV fabrication.
2. Scale up or down the initial lipid mass as needed. However, make sure to also scale all subsequent surface functionalization reagents as well.
3. Storing the MLV solution overnight at 4 °C allows the nanoparticles time to equilibrate and for their membranes to become more rigid, both of which help to achieve a more homogenous product post extrusion.
4. Each polycarbonate membrane can be used for about 2–3 mL of liposomal solution. However, be advised that the longer a specific membrane is utilized, the higher the chance of rupture so always check the integrity post extrusion cycle. In addition, for the smaller pore size membranes such as 200 and 80 nm, use multiple filter supports (2–3) to reduce membrane rupture.
5. Because the LNPs are neutral in charge and have high membrane curvature, they will rapidly undergo fusion. Therefore, surface functionalize the LNPs with HA as soon as possible after the extrusion process (we usually functionalize on the same day, or the next day at the latest).
6. Make sure to rehydrate the final washed HALNP sample to the volume of the initial LNP to preserve osmolarity.
7. The HALNPs are much more stable in solution than the LNPs due to their highly negative exterior charge (as seen in Table 1). Although we have validated HALNP stability for over a month at 4 °C, we try to use or lyophilize the particles within 2–3 weeks of creation.
8. The LNPs must be lyophilized to entrap cargo into the hydrophilic core upon rehydration. The lipid mass lyophilized per vial should be optimized for each individual application. Typically, 0.1–0.5 mg per vial promotes efficient cargo entrapment for in vitro experiments (>40% for dextran-based cargo, ≈25% for non-condensed nucleic acid cargo, >50% for doxorubicin) [19, 20]. Prior to lyophilization, it is a good idea to validate HA binding on the surface of the LNPs by DLS and zeta

potential analysis as described in Subheading 3.3. Dry Ice and ethanol mixture details: Break dry ice into small pieces and place into a suitable container, carefully add ethanol to cover the dry ice, and wait at least 5 min for the ethanol to cool down prior to use.

9. Wait at least 20 min for the lyophilized vial to come to room temperature before removing the cap to reduce the chance of condensation causing lipid rehydration in place of the added solution containing the therapeutic cargo of choice. This condensation effect can dramatically reduce entrapment efficiency.
10. The type of solution used for rehydration is dependent upon the cargo of choice. For nucleic acid cargo, use nuclease-free water (of buffers made with nuclease-free water). Keep in mind that certain cargoes are most stable in a particular pH or buffer type.
11. Although Method 2 allows for the quick determination of the ratio of encapsulated vs. non-encapsulated nucleic acid cargo [20, 32], the method itself does not give an actual read out for the quantity of internalized payload. Method 2 is typically used to determine the percent encapsulation, and combined with the known amount of initial cargo to indirectly determine the cargo inside the nanoparticles. Therefore, the employment of Method 2 is a valid procedure only if it is compared and agrees with Method 1 (i.e., use a standard curve to directly determine the exact amount of encapsulated cargo). We suggest using both Method 1 and Method 2 for miR encapsulation quantification, and if they agree then use Method 2 preferentially in the future.
12. Perform the entire entrapment, purification, and encapsulation efficiency procedure in the dark to reduce the chance of FITC photobleaching.
13. We have found that mixing 400 pmol of miR with 4 μL RNA binding dye ensures that all dye is complexed with miR (no free dye available). This is very important because if free dye is delivered into the cell, it will complex with any nucleic acid source and fluoresce, giving a false reading. Therefore, if all miR is complexed with dye then the fluorescence observed should only be from the delivered miR itself. Furthermore, take great care to ensure that the nucleic acid cargo chosen for analysis is the only nucleic acid source in your procedure. Please note that a nucleic acid-RNA dye saturation curve should be performed for your chosen nucleic acid type to ensure no free dye is present.
14. A 1 h time point was chosen because we have found that in 3–5 h the HALNPs rapidly escape endosomes and are homogenously distributed in the cytoplasm [20]. As a result, we chose an earlier time point to visualize the miR-dye complex still

encapsulated inside HALNPs to further ensure that the fluorescence observed is from the delivered miR and not from endogenous nucleic acid-dye interactions.

15. This procedure requires optimization for each cell type. Use these settings as a starting point, and scale/modify as necessary to achieve best results. Be sure to keep the volume between wells consistent during the transfection procedure.
16. The transfection starting time point for our studies occurs once the cells are placed into the complete medium (0 h occurs following the initial 5 h incubation in serum and PS-free medium).

Acknowledgments

We thank Dr. Vimla Band (University of Nebraska Medical Center) for kindly providing the 21MT-1 cells. We also thank Dr. Yusong Li for being able to use their labs DLS and Zeta potential machine. Lastly, we want to thank the UNL microscopy core facility for their assistance with confocal microscopy. This work was supported, in whole or in part, by P20 GM104320 (to the Nebraska Center for the Prevention of Obesity Diseases Pilot Grant to S.K.) and P20 GM113126 (to the Nebraska Center for Integrated Biomolecular Communication-Project Leader S.K.); UNL Office of Research and Development Biomedical Seed Grant (to S.K.); start up funds from University of Nebraska-Lincoln, Layman's Award, MRSEC Seed Grant, and UNL Interdisciplinary Award.

References

1. Liu Z, Sall A, Yang D (2008) MicroRNA: an emerging therapeutic target and intervention tool. Int J Mol Sci 9(6):978–999. https://doi.org/10.3390/ijms9060978
2. Cho WC (2010) MicroRNAs: potential biomarkers for cancer diagnosis, prognosis and targets for therapy. Int J Biochem Cell Biol 42(8):1273–1281. https://doi.org/10.1016/j.biocel.2009.12.014
3. Jonas S, Izaurralde E (2015) Towards a molecular understanding of microRNA-mediated gene silencing. Nat Rev Genet 16:421–433. https://doi.org/10.1038/nrg3965
4. Ha M, Kim VN (2014) Regulation of microRNA biogenesis. Nat Rev Mol Cell Biol 15(8):509–524. https://doi.org/10.1038/nrm3838
5. Sassen S, Miska EA, Caldas C (2008) MicroRNA: implications for cancer. Virchows Arch 452(1):1–10. https://doi.org/10.1007/s00428-007-0532-2
6. Wiemer EAC (2007) The role of microRNAs in cancer: no small matter. Eur J Cancer 43(10):1529–1544. https://doi.org/10.1016/j.ejca.2007.04.002
7. Mishra PK, Tyagi N, Kumar M et al (2009) MicroRNAs as a therapeutic target for cardiovascular diseases. J Cell Mol Med 13(4):778–789. https://doi.org/10.1111/j.1582-4934.2009.00744.x
8. Urbich C, Kuehbacher A, Dimmeler S (2008) Role of microRNAs in vascular diseases, inflammation, and angiogenesis. Cardiovasc Res 79(4):581–588. https://doi.org/10.1093/cvr/cvn156
9. Szabo G, Bala S (2013) MicroRNAs in liver disease. Nat Rev Gastroenterol Hepatol

10(9):542–552. https://doi.org/10.1038/nrgastro.2013.87
10. Scaria V, Hariharan M, Brahmachari SK et al (2007) microRNA: an emerging therapeutic. ChemMedChem 2(6):789–792. https://doi.org/10.1002/cmdc.200600278
11. Nana-Sinkam SP, Croce CM (2013) Clinical applications for microRNAs in cancer. Clin Pharmacol Ther 93(1):98–104. https://doi.org/10.1038/clpt.2012.192
12. Muthiah M, Park I-K, Cho CS (2013) Nanoparticle mediated delivery of therapeutic genes- focus on miRNA therapeutics. Expert Opin Drug Deliv 10(9):1259–1273
13. Zhang Y, Wang Z, Gemeinhart RA (2013) Progress in microRNA delivery. J Control Release 172(3):962–974. https://doi.org/10.1016/j.jconrel.2013.09.015
14. Torchilin VP (2010) Passive and active drug targeting: drug delivery to tumors as an example. In: Drug delivery. Springer, Berlin, pp 3–53
15. Negi LM, Talegaonkar S, Jaggi M et al (2012) Role of CD44 in tumour progression and strategies for targeting. J Drug Target 20(7):561–573
16. Eliaz RE, Szoka FC (2001) Liposome-encapsulated doxorubicin targeted to CD44 a strategy to kill CD44-overexpressing tumor cells. Cancer Res 61(6):2592–2601
17. Peer D, Margalit R (2004) Loading mitomycin C inside long circulating hyaluronan targeted nano-liposomes increases its antitumor activity in three mice tumor models. Int J Cancer 108(5):780–789. https://doi.org/10.1002/ijc.11615
18. Peer D, Park EJ, Morishita Y et al (2008) Systemic leukocyte-directed siRNA delivery revealing cyclin D1 as an anti-inflammatory target. Science 319(5863):627–630. https://doi.org/10.1126/science.1149859
19. Hayward SL, Francis DM, Sis MJ et al (2015) Ionic driven embedment of hyaluronic acid coated liposomes in polyelectrolyte multilayer films for local therapeutic delivery. Sci Rep. https://doi.org/10.1038/srep14683
20. Hayward SL, Francis DM, Kholmatov P et al (2016) Targeted delivery of MicroRNA-125a-5p by engineered lipid nanoparticles for the treatment of HER2 positive metastatic breast Cancer. J Biomed Nanotechnol. https://doi.org/10.1166/jbn.2016.2194
21. Hayward SL, Wilson CL, Kidambi S (2016) Hyaluronic acid-conjugated liposome nanoparticles for targeted delivery to CD44 overexpressing glioblastoma cells. Oncotarget 7(23):34158–34171. https://doi.org/10.18632/oncotarget.8926
22. Band V, Zajchowski D, Swisshelm K et al (1990) Tumor progression in four mammary epithelial cell lines derived from the same patient. Cancer Res 50(22):7351–7357
23. Bangham A, Hill M, Miller N (1974) Preparation and use of liposomes as models of biological membranes. In: Methods in membrane biology, vol 1. Springer, Boston, pp 1–68. https://doi.org/10.1007/978-1-4615-7422-4_1
24. Gregoriadis G (ed) (1988) Liposomes as drug carriers: recent trends and progress. John Wiley and Sons, Chichester
25. Mozafari M (2005) Liposomes an overview of manufacturing techniques. Cell Mol Biol Lett 10:711–719
26. Akbarzadeh A, Rezaei-Sadabady R, Davaran S et al (2013) Liposome: classification, preparation, and applications. Nanoscale Res Lett 8(1):102
27. Mahmood T, Yang P-C (2012) Western blot: technique, theory, and trouble shooting. N Am J Med Sci 4(9):429–434. https://doi.org/10.4103/1947-2714.100998
28. Hirano S (2012) Western blot analysis. Meth Mol Biol (Clifton, NJ) 926:87–97. https://doi.org/10.1007/978-1-62703-002-1_6
29. Engel RH, Kaklamani VG (2007) HER2-positive breast cancer: current and future treatment strategies. Drugs 67(9):1329–1341
30. Scott GK, Goga A, Bhaumik D et al (2007) Coordinate suppression of ERBB2 and ERBB3 by enforced expression of micro-RNA miR-125a or miR-125b. J Biol Chem 282(2):1479–1486. https://doi.org/10.1074/jbc.M609383200
31. Rapley R, Manning DL (1998) RNA isolation and characterization protocols, vol 86. Humana Press, New York
32. Landesman-Milo D, Goldsmith M, Leviatan Ben-Arye S et al (2013) Hyaluronan grafted lipid-based nanoparticles as RNAi carriers for cancer cells. Cancer Lett 334(2):221–227. https://doi.org/10.1016/j.canlet.2012.08.024

Chapter 9

Ultrasound and Microbubble-Mediated Blood-Brain Barrier Disruption for Targeted Delivery of Therapeutics to the Brain

Meaghan A. O'Reilly and Kullervo Hynynen

Abstract

Ultrasound and microbubble-mediated disruption of the Blood-Brain barrier is a noninvasive and targetable technique that permits the investigation of pharmacological interventions in the brain and CNS. This technique provides an alternative to direct injection of agents into the brain parenchyma or chemical disruption of the Blood-Brain barrier. Here, we detail one protocol for inducing transient Blood-Brain barrier disruption in a rodent model using a commercially available microbubble contrast agent (Definity).

Key words Focused ultrasound, Therapeutic ultrasound, Blood-brain barrier, Targeted drug delivery, Microbubble

1 Introduction

Investigation of therapeutic interventions in the brain is greatly hindered by the presence of the Blood-Brain barrier (BBB). The BBB is characterized by a reduction in both transcellular and paracellular passage of molecules from the vasculature into the brain tissue [1]. Very few therapeutic agents can pass through the intact BBB, and those that do are limited in size (<400–600 Da) and have high lipid-solubility [2]. The BBB can be disrupted globally in a whole brain hemisphere via intra-arterial injection of a hyperosmotic solution of Mannitol [3]. More targeted circumvention of the BBB can be achieved via direct injection into the brain parenchyma and convection-enhanced diffusion [4, 5], however these methods are highly invasive. Alternative strategies include design of therapeutics which can penetrate the barrier [6].

Ultrasound and microbubble-mediated BBB disruption (BBBD) is a noninvasive and targeted method to reversibly disrupt the BBB that has allowed delivery of antibodies [7–10], nanoparticles [11–13], viral vectors [14, 15], and cells [16, 17]. The ability

Rachael W. Sirianni and Bahareh Behkam (eds.), *Targeted Drug Delivery: Methods and Protocols*, Methods in Molecular Biology, vol. 1831, https://doi.org/10.1007/978-1-4939-8661-3_9, © Springer Science+Business Media, LLC, part of Springer Nature 2018

of ultrasound to impact the BBB was first reported in the 1950s [18]. However, it was almost 50 years before the addition of microbubbles to mediate the treatment allowed consistent and safe disruption to be achieved [19]. There are now over a hundred published studies on microbubble-mediated BBB disruption, from multiple different institutions. BBBD using focused ultrasound (FUS) and microbubbles (MBs) has been demonstrated in a range of animal models including mice [7, 8, 20], rats [16, 21, 22], rabbits [19, 23], pigs [24, 25], and non-human primates [26, 27].

A variety of acoustic parameters have been investigated to optimize the procedure [28–31]. Although more complex treatment schemes have been proposed which change the applied pressures to improve treatment outcome [32, 33], the majority of preclinical studies employ fixed treatment pressures throughout. Here, we describe a method for FUS-induced BBBD in a rat model. For variations on this technique we refer you to the Notes section of this chapter. The methods are divided into three major procedures: the registration of the MRI and ultrasound coordinate systems, animal preparation, and FUS delivery and outcome assessment.

2 Materials

2.1 Registration of the MRI and Ultrasound Coordinate Systems

1. Magnetic Resonance Imaging (MRI)—compatible three-axis positioning system (*see* **Note 1**).
2. Warm bath of degassed, deionized water.
3. Top-plate for water bath. The top plate should have a hole to allow the animal's head to contact the water (*see* **Note 2**).
4. MRI surface coil.
5. Spherically curved transducer or phased array operating at 0.5 MHz or other suitable operating frequencies (*see* **Notes 3** and **4**).
6. Function generator.
7. RF power amplifier.
8. Impedance matching circuit.
9. MRI scanner.
10. MRI fiducial marker plate.

2.2 Animal Preparation

1. Rats, 200–500 g (*see* **Note 5**).
2. Anesthesia machine: Isofluorane vaporizer connected to an induction chamber and a nose cone.
3. Oxygen supply.
4. Ocular lubricant ointment.
5. Betadine scrub.

6. Bridine wash.
7. Alcohol wipes.
8. 22G Angio-catheters (*see* **Note 6**).
9. Hub or 3-way stopcock.
10. Medical tape.
11. Heparinized saline: add 33 U Heparin per mL of saline.
12. Electric razor.
13. Depilatory cream.
14. Syringes, 3 and 1 mL.
15. Medical air supply (*see* **Note 7**).
16. Water-circulating heating blanket.
17. Extension tubing with nose cone sufficient to reach from the anesthetic machine to the positioning system and water bath.

2.3 Focused Ultrasound Delivery and Assessment of Outcome

1. Magnetic Resonance Imaging (MRI)—compatible three-axis positioning system.
2. Warm bath of degassed, deionized water.
3. Top-plate for water bath.
4. MRI surface coil.
5. Spherically curved transducer or phased array operating at 0.5 MHz or other suitable operating frequencies (*see* **Notes 3** and **4**).
6. Function generator.
7. RF power amplifier.
8. Impedance matching circuit.
9. MRI scanner.
10. MRI fiducial marker plate.
11. Definity microbubble contrast agent (*see* **Note 8**).
12. Gadolinium-based MRI contrast agent (*see* **Note 9**).
13. Normal saline.
14. 1 and 3 mL syringes.
15. 18G blunt-fill needles.

3 Methods

3.1 Registration of the MRI and Ultrasound Coordinate Systems

1. Place the positioning system and water bath on the bed of the MRI.
2. Place the ultrasound transducer on the arm of the positioning system within the water bath.

3. Connect the transducer to the output of the RF power amplifier via a matching network. To minimize noise, cables should be run through a grounded penetration panel.
4. Connect the function generator to the power amplifier.
5. Move the positioning arm so that the focus of the transducer is at the water surface.
6. Sonicate in continuous mode, using 0.5 W of electrical power to create a fountain on the water surface.
7. Place the fiducial marker plate over the fountain so that the ultrasound focus is aligned with the hole in the plate.
8. Turn off the function generator output.
9. With the MRI, obtain a 3-plane localizer scan and determine the location of the transducer focus in MR coordinates by measuring the location of the fiducial marker plate.

3.2 Animal Preparation

1. Place the rat in the induction chamber and anesthetize using isofluorane at 5% (*see* **Note 10**) with oxygen as the carrier gas.
2. Once the animal is anesthetized, remove from the induction chamber and continue delivery of the anesthetic at 2% via a nose cone.
3. Apply ocular lubricant ointment in each eye.
4. Use a heating blanket or heat lamp to keep the animal warm while anesthetized.
5. Clean the tail using a Betadine scrub followed by Bridine wash.
6. Wipe down the tail with alcohol (*see* **Note 11**).
7. Insert a 22G catheter into the tail vein (*see* **Notes 12** and **13**).
8. Cap the end of the catheter with a 3-way stopcock or hub, and secure the catheter to the tail using tape.
9. Flush the catheter with heparinized saline.
10. Shave the fur from the head and neck with an electric razor.
11. Apply depilatory cream to remove the remaining fur.
12. Wash the scalp with mild soap and water, being careful to completely remove any remaining depilatory cream (*see* **Note 14**).
13. Transfer the animal to the top-plate over the warm water bath. Place the animal supine, with head contacting the water bath. Use the extension tubing and nose cone to continue inhalant anesthetic.
14. Secure the animal in place using tape or other securing methods.
15. Cover the animal with the circulating water blanket to keep the animal warm.
16. Change carrier gas to medical air and continue anesthesia with isofluorane at 2% (*see* **Note 7**).

3.3 Focused Ultrasound Targeting, Delivery, and Assessment of Outcome

1. Obtain T_1-weighted and T_2-weighted scans of the animal's brain.
2. Select the target region of the brain.
3. Move the ultrasound focus to the desired target using the positioning system.
4. Set the ultrasound parameters in the function generator: burst mode, 0.23 MPa peak-negative pressure, 10 ms bursts, 1 Hz pulse repetition frequency, 120 bursts (*see* **Notes 3** and **15**).
5. Activate the microbubbles according to the manufacturer's instructions (*see* **Note 16**).
6. Using a 1 mL syringe and an 18G needle, slowly draw up a small volume of the activated bubbles.
7. Remove trapped air from the syringe by gently pulling and pushing the plunger until air pockets have moved to the top of the syringe (*see* **Note 17**).
8. Dilute the microbubbles 1:10 in normal saline by injecting 0.1 mL of microbubbles into 0.9 mL normal saline in a 1 mL syringe.
9. Mix the solution by gently inverting the syringe until the solution has a consistent appearance.
10. Inject via the tail vein any drug or agent to be delivered, followed by a 0.5 mL saline flush. Inject 0.2 mL/kg of the Definity/saline solution (0.02 mL/kg of undiluted Definity) via the tail vein and follow with a 0.5 mL saline flush.
11. Turn on the function generator output simultaneously with the microbubble injection.
12. At the end of the sonication, turn off the function generator output if this is not automatic.
13. Inject 0.2 mL/kg of MRI contrast agent (Omniscan), followed by a 0.5 mL saline flush.
14. In the MRI obtain T_1-weighted images.
15. Compare the contrast enhancement in the targeted region compared with that in a non-targeted region of the brain to confirm delivery of the contrast agent through the BBB (Fig. 1).

4 Notes

1. The positioning system can be manual or automated as long as it is MRI-compatible. If an MRI-compatible positioning system is not available then sonications can be performed outside the MRI suite and the animal can be transferred between the ultrasound platform and MRI using a frame to ensure consistent placement of the animal.

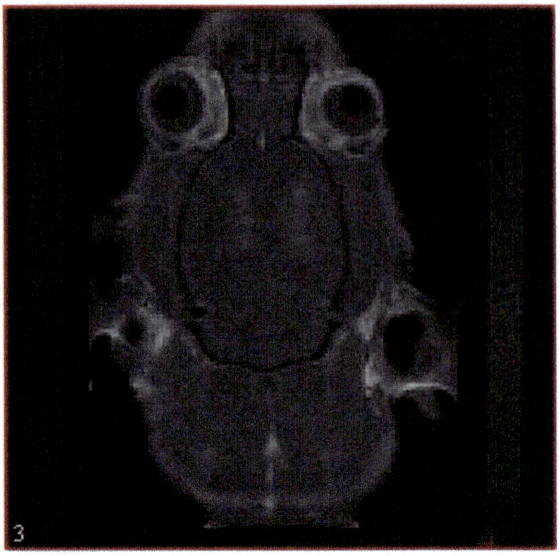

Fig. 1 T1-weighted MRI image showing disruption of the BBB in a rat brain. Six focal disruption zones form two parallel rostral/caudal lines of disruption. The ultrasound frequency in this example was 1.68 MHz

2. A film may be placed across the opening in the top plate to prevent the animal's head from falling through. In this case a small amount of ultrasound gel may be applied to the scalp to ensure good ultrasound coupling.
3. The necessary peak-negative pressures required to disrupt the BBB at different frequencies can be determined from [34].
4. Unfocused ultrasound is sometimes used when it is desirable to disrupt large regions of the brain, as for example in [35, 36].
5. For operating frequencies below 1 MHz the insertion loss of the skull can be considered a function of animal mass and in situ pressures can be determined based on the values in [37].
6. Using the largest diameter catheters and needles minimizes breakage of bubbles during injection [38]. If it is necessary to use a 24G catheter instead of a 22G catheter, extra care must be taken when injecting the microbubbles.
7. Using inhalant anesthetic results in fewer animal losses due to complications of the anesthetic. However, the use of isofluorane with oxygen as a carrier gas has been shown to reduce the effectiveness of the FUS, presumably because the use of oxygen reduces the circulation time of the bubbles [39]. We have found that using medical air as the carrier gas for the isofluorane during the treatment allows the use of inhalant anesthetic without compromising treatment efficacy.
8. Other commercial microbubble contrast agents such as SonoVue [11] or Optison [19], or custom-made bubbles [40] can also be used to disrupt the BBB.

9. Other MRI contrast agents can also be delivered. The effective area and duration of opening will be affected by the size of the contrast agent used [41].
10. The anesthetic should only be kept at 5% isofluorane for a short period of time since maintaining this level for prolonged periods may be lethal.
11. It is necessary to wipe down the tail with alcohol following the Betadine and Bridine cleaning since these washes leave a stain on the skin which makes visualization of the vein difficult.
12. To facilitate insertion of the catheter into the tail vein, the tail can be placed in warm water to open the vessel.
13. In rabbits, the ear vein may be used for catheterization.
14. It is important to remove all traces of the depilatory cream because it can cause chemical burns on the scalp.
15. These parameters are based on parameters that our group has found to be effective at disrupting the BBB. Treatment effect has been found to increase with burst length [28]. However, increasing burst length beyond 10 ms has not shown added benefit [19]. Generally, a PRF of around 1 Hz is used in order to allow sufficient time for microbubble replenishment to the treatment area [42], although one group uses a PRF of 10 Hz [40].
16. It is important to allow the Definity vial to come to room temperature before activating the microbubbles since pre-activation temperature affects the resulting bubble population [43].
17. Tapping the syringe will cause bubbles to break and may reduce the effectiveness of the treatment.

References

1. Reese T, Karnovsky MJ (1967) Fine structural localization of a blood-brain barrier to exogenous peroxidase. J Cell Biol 34(1):207–217
2. Pardridge WM (1995) Transport of small molecules through the blood-brain barrier: biology and methodology. Adv Drug Deliv Rev 15(1):5–36
3. Salahuddin TS, Johansson BB, Kalimo H, Olsson Y (1988) Structural changes in the rat brain after carotid infusions of hyperosmolar solutions. An electron microscopic study. Acta Neuropathol 77(1):5–13
4. Lidar Z, Mardor Y, Jonas T, Pfeffer R, Faibel M, Nass D, Hadani M, Ram Z (2004) Convection-enhanced delivery of paclitaxel for the treatment of recurrent malignant glioma: a phase i/ii clinical study. J Neurosurg 100(3):472–479
5. Kunwar S, Chang S, Westphal M, Vogelbaum M, Sampson J, Barnett G, Shaffrey M, Ram Z, Piepmeier J, Prados M et al (2010) Phase iii randomized trial of ced of il13-pe38qqr vs gliadel wafers for recurrent glioblastoma. Neuro-Oncology 12(8):871–881
6. Pardridge WM (2008) Re-engineering biopharmaceuticals for delivery to brain with molecular trojan horses. Bioconjug Chem 19(7):1327–1338
7. Kinoshita M, McDannold N, Jolesz FA, Hynynen K (2006) Noninvasive localized delivery of herceptin to the mouse brain by mri-guided focused ultrasound-induced blood-brain barrier disruption. Proc Natl Acad Sci U S A 103(31):11719–11723
8. Kinoshita M, McDannold N, Jolesz FA, Hynynen K (2006) Targeted delivery of antibodies through the blood-brain barrier by mri-guided focused ultrasound. Biochem Biophys Res Commun 340(4):1085–1090

9. Raymond SB, Treat LH, Dewey JD, McDannold NJ, Hynynen K, Bacskai BJ (2008) Ultrasound enhanced delivery of molecular imaging and therapeutic agents in alzheimer's disease mouse models. PLoS One 3(5):e2175
10. Jordão JF, Ayala-Grosso CA, Markham K, Huang Y, Chopra R, McLaurin J, Hynynen K, Aubert I (2010) Antibodies targeted to the brain with image-guided focused ultrasound reduces amyloid-beta plaque load in the tgcrnd8 mouse model of alzheimer's disease. PLoS One 5(5):e10549
11. Liu HL, Hua MY, Yang HW, Huang CY, Chu PC, Wu JS, Tseng IC, Wang JJ, Yen TC, Chen PY, Wei KC (2010) Magnetic resonance monitoring of focused ultrasound/magnetic nanoparticle targeting delivery of therapeutic agents to the brain. Proc Natl Acad Sci U S A 107(34):15205–15210
12. Chen PY, Liu HL, Hua MY, Yang HW, Huang CY, Chu PC, Lyu LA, Tseng IC, Feng LY, Tsai HC, Chen SM, Lu YJ, Wang JJ, Yen TC, Ma YH, Wu T, Chen JP, Chuang JI, Shin JW, Hsueh C, Wei KC (2010) Novel magnetic/ultrasound focusing system enhances nanoparticle drug delivery for glioma treatment. Neuro-Oncology 12(10):1050–1060
13. Etame AB, Diaz RJ, O'Reilly MA, Smith CA, Mainprize TG, Hynynen K, Rutka JT (2012) Enhanced delivery of gold nanoparticles with therapeutic potential into the brain using mri-guided focused ultrasound. Nanomedicine 8(7):1133–1142
14. Thévenot E, Jordão JF, O'Reilly MA, Markham K, Weng YQ, Foust KD, Kaspar BK, Hynynen K, Aubert I (2012) Targeted delivery of self-complementary adeno-associated virus serotype 9 to the brain, using magnetic resonance imaging-guided focused ultrasound. Hum Gene Ther 23(11):1144–1155
15. Alonso A, Reinz E, Leuchs B, Kleinschmidt J, Fatar M, Geers B, Lentacker I, Hennerici MG, de Smedt SC, Meairs S (2013) Focal delivery of aav2/1-transgenes into the rat brain by localized ultrasound-induced bbb opening. Mol Ther Nucleic Acids 2:e73
16. Burgess A, Ayala-Grosso CA, Ganguly M, Jordão JF, Aubert I, Hynynen K (2011) Targeted delivery of neural stem cells to the brain using mri-guided focused ultrasound to disrupt the blood-brain barrier. PLoS One 6(11):e27877
17. Alkins R, Burgess A, Ganguly M, Francia G, Kerbel R, Wels WS, Hynynen K (2013) Focused ultrasound delivers targeted immune cells to metastatic brain tumors. Cancer Res 73(6):1892–1899
18. Bakay L, Ballantine H, Hueter T, Sosa D (1956) Ultrasonically produced changes in the blood-brain barrier. AMA Arch Neurol Psychiatry 76(5):457–467
19. Hynynen K, McDannold N, Vykhodtseva N, Jolesz F (2001) Noninvasive mr imaging-guided focal opening of the blood-brain barrier in rabbits. Radiology 220(3):640–646
20. Choi JJ, Pernot M, Small SA, Konofagou EE (2007) Noninvasive, transcranial and localized opening of the blood-brain barrier using focused ultrasound in mice. Ultrasound Med Biol 33(1):95–104
21. Treat LH, McDannold N, Vykhodtseva N, Zhang Y, Tam K, Hynynen K (2007) Targeted delivery of doxorubicin to the rat brain at therapeutic levels using mri-guided focused ultrasound. Int J Cancer 121(4):901–907
22. Sheikov N, McDannold N, Sharma S, Hynynen K (2008) Effect of focused ultrasound applied with an ultrasound contrast agent on the tight junctional integrity of the brain microvascular endothelium. Ultrasound Med Biol 34(7):1093–1104
23. McDannold N, Vykhodtseva N, Hynynen K (2006) Targeted disruption of the blood-brain barrier with focused ultrasound: association with cavitation activity. Phys Med Biol 51(4):793–807
24. Xie F, Boska MD, Lof J, Uberti MG, Tsutsui JM, Porter TR (2008) Effects of transcranial ultrasound and intravenous microbubbles on blood brain barrier permeability in a large animal model. Ultrasound Med Biol 34(12):2028–2034
25. Liu HL, Chen PY, Yang HW, Wu JS, Tseng IC, Ma YJ, Huang CY, Tsai HC, Chen SM, Lu YJ, Huang CY, Hua MY, Ma YH, Yen TC, Wei KC (2011) In vivo mr quantification of superparamagnetic iron oxide nanoparticle leakage during low-frequency-ultrasound-induced blood-brain barrier opening in swine. J Magn Reson Imaging 34(6):1313–1324
26. Tung YS, Marquet F, Teichert T, Ferrera V, Konofagou E (2011) Feasibility of noninvasive cavitation-guided blood-brain barrier opening using focused ultrasound and microbubbles in nonhuman primates. Appl Phys Lett 98(16):163704
27. McDannold N, Arvanitis CD, Vykhodtseva N, Livingstone MS (2012) Temporary disruption of the blood-brain barrier by use of ultrasound and microbubbles: safety and efficacy evaluation in rhesus macaques. Cancer Res 72(14):3652–3663
28. McDannold N, Vykhodtseva N, Hynynen K (2008) Effects of acoustic parameters and

ultrasound contrast agent dose on focused-ultrasound induced blood-brain barrier disruption. Ultrasound Med Biol 34(6):930–937

29. O'Reilly MA, Waspe AC, Ganguly M, Hynynen K (2011) Focused-ultrasound disruption of the blood-brain barrier using closely-timed short pulses: influence of sonication parameters and injection rate. Ultrasound Med Biol 37(4):587–594
30. Choi JJ, Selert K, Vlachos F, Wong A, Konofagou EE (2011) Noninvasive and localized neuronal delivery using short ultrasonic pulses and microbubbles. Proc Natl Acad Sci U S A 108(40):16539–16544
31. Choi JJ, Selert K, Gao Z, Samiotaki G, Baseri B, Konofagou EE (2011) Noninvasive and localized blood-brain barrier disruption using focused ultrasound can be achieved at short pulse lengths and low pulse repetition frequencies. J Cereb Blood Flow Metab 31(2):725–737
32. O'Reilly MA, Hynynen K (2012) Blood-brain barrier: real-time feedback-controlled focused ultrasound disruption by using an acoustic emissions-based controller. Radiology 263(1):96–106
33. Arvanitis CD, Livingstone MS, Vykhodtseva N, McDannold N (2012) Controlled ultrasound-induced blood-brain barrier disruption using passive acoustic emissions monitoring. PLoS One 7(9):e45783
34. McDannold N, Vykhodtseva N, Hynynen K (2008) Blood-brain barrier disruption induced by focused ultrasound and circulating preformed microbubbles appears to be characterized by the mechanical index. Ultrasound Med Biol 34(5):834–840
35. Howles G, Bing K, Qi Y, Rosenzweig S, Nightingale K, Johnson G (2010) Contrast-enhanced in vivo magnetic resonance microscopy of the mouse brain enabled by noninvasive opening of the blood-brain barrier with ultrasound. Magn Reson Med 64(4):995–1004
36. Santin MD, Debeir T, Bridal SL, Rooney T, Dhenain M (2013) Fast in vivo imaging of amyloid plaques using μ-mri gd-staining combined with ultrasound-induced blood-brain barrier opening. NeuroImage 79:288–294
37. O'Reilly MA, Muller A, Hynynen K (2011) Ultrasound insertion loss of rat parietal bone appears to be proportional to animal mass at submegahertz frequencies. Ultrasound Med Biol 37(11):1930–1937
38. Talu E, Powell RL, Longo ML, Dayton PA (2008) Needle size and injection rate impact microbubble contrast agent population. Ultrasound Med Biol 34(7):1182–1185
39. McDannold N, Zhang Y, Vykhodtseva N (2011) Blood-brain barrier disruption and vascular damage induced by ultrasound bursts combined with microbubbles can be influenced by choice of anesthesia protocol. Ultrasound Med Biol 37(8):1259–1270
40. Choi J, Feshitan J, Baseri B, Wang S, Tung YS, Borden M, Konofagou E (2010) Microbubble-size dependence of focused ultrasound-induced bloodbrain barrier opening in mice in vivo. IEEE T Bio-Med Eng 57(1):145–154
41. Marty B, Larrat B, Landeghem MV, Robic C, Robert P, Port M, Bihan DL, Pernot M, Tanter M, Lethimonnier F, Mériaux S (2012) Dynamic study of blood-brain barrier closure after its disruption using ultrasound: a quantitative analysis. J Cereb Blood Flow Metab
42. Goertz DE, Wright C, Hynynen K (2010) Contrast agent kinetics in the rabbit brain during exposure to therapeutic ultrasound. Ultrasound Med Biol 36(6):916–924
43. Helfield BL, Huo X, Williams R, Goertz DE (2012) The effect of preactivation vial temperature on the acoustic properties of definity™. Ultrasound Med Biol 38(7):1298–1305

Chapter 10

In Vitro Validation of Targeting and Comparison to Mathematical Modeling

Jill M. Steinbach-Rankins and Michael R. Caplan

Abstract

Nanoparticle and other drug delivery platforms have demonstrated promising potential for the delivery of therapeutics or imaging agents in a specific and targeted manner. While a variety of drug delivery platforms have been applied to medicine, in vitro and in silico optimization and validation of these targeting constructs needs to be conducted to maximize in vivo delivery and efficacy. Here, we describe the mathematical and experimental models to predict and validate the transport of a peptide targeting construct through a mock tissue environment to specifically target tumor cells, relative to non-tumor cells. We provide methods to visualize and analyze fluorescence microscopy images, and also describe the methods for creating a finite element model (FEM) that validates important parameters of this experimental system. By comparing and contrasting mathematical modeling results with experimental results, important information can be imparted to the design and functionality of the targeting construct. This information will help to optimize construct design for future therapeutic delivery applications.

Key words Convection-enhanced delivery, Diffusion, Multivalent targeting, Mass transport, Finite element modeling, Cancer targeting, Peptide delivery

1 Introduction

The translation of targeted drug delivery systems from in vitro experimental systems to in vivo applications is often challenging, due to the complex factors and interactions that govern molecular transport and distribution in a given system. If in vitro validation results fail to correlate with in vivo success, this indicates that the validation test was not adequately predictive of success or failure in vivo. In fact, due to the complexity of factors involved in translating in vitro results into an in vivo delivery system, it is often difficult to discern what factors contribute to (or detract from) in vivo efficacy. Therefore, the hallmark of a successful validation tool is its predictive power to determine how the targeting construct will perform in vivo. However, given the variety of factors that can contribute to the incongruence between cell culture systems and

Rachael W. Sirianni and Bahareh Behkam (eds.), *Targeted Drug Delivery: Methods and Protocols*, Methods in Molecular Biology, vol. 1831, https://doi.org/10.1007/978-1-4939-8661-3_10, © Springer Science+Business Media, LLC, part of Springer Nature 2018

in vivo models, iterative measures are often employed to establish and optimize in vitro systems. In silico modeling, if validated with well-designed experiments, can provide a complementary method with the potential for rapid, informative, and streamlined methods to establish trends and relationships that can inform drug design and delivery.

Several experimental features are important in creating a rigorous validation system (in vitro or in silico) that will have adequate predictive power. First, the choices of target and control are critical. In vivo targets for achieving specificity of drug delivery are typically cell surface antigens or receptors. Although it is possible to use the isolated antigens/receptors themselves, the use of a whole cell displaying these antigens/receptors forces the targeting construct to bind to the antigen/receptor as it is likely to be displayed in vivo. For example, if the intracellular portions of these molecules will be inaccessible, the glycocalyx will introduce steric hindrance and charge repulsion, and the density of binding sites may affect targeting. Second, the choice of control is critical to successful validation. Use of a targeting construct without the targeting moiety (e.g., nanoparticle without ligand or antibody conjugated to the surface) is an appropriate control for verifying that that the targeting construct synthesized has functional components that have been assembled properly; however, this approach does not serve as validation to establish that targeting construct achieves the desired cell-specific targeting. A better control to validate targeting specificity is to compare binding to a cell type other than that target cell type.

Third, it is essential that the metric quantified is truly indicative of actual binding to the target site. For example, imaging is often used to quantify accumulation of targeting construct at the target site; however, many of these targeting constructs are not actually bound to the target cells. Sometimes accumulation can be seen due to ease-of-access, as in the case of the enhanced permeability and retention effect. In contrast, when performing an immunohistochemistry (IHC) assay, the cells are washed several times to remove unbound antibody or delivery vehicle before imaging. This ensures that only bound agent is visualized/detected in the imaging of the antibody-bound cells. To address these in vitro validation factors, in this chapter we demonstrate how an in vitro mock delivery system can predict targeting results analogous to in vivo conditions. More specifically, we show how constructs infused into a cell-gel matrix, representative of brain tissue, can be more accurately "targeted" using convection-enhanced delivery followed by a convective wash.

Finally, interpretation of validation results can often be challenging. The methods below detail image analysis and statistical methods that can be used to compare target to non-target regions, which provide an answer to whether preferential targeting was achieved. Often the investigator seeks additional details regarding how to optimize targeted delivery systems to achieve the largest ratio of construct on the targeted cells vs. the non-targeted cells. Due to the multitude of factors involved, a purely empirical approach to the design and development of targeted vehicles is impractical. For these purposes, mathematical modeling can be a powerful tool to vary different design parameters to predict delivery, and to understand the results obtained from in vitro experiments. The methods provided below detail how to create a finite element model that matches the important biophysics of the experimental validation procedure so that data can be compared/contrasted directly with modeling results to provide information to the investigator about the mechanisms by which targeting was achieved. In the example below, we sought to target glioblastoma cells, so selected another prevalent cell in the brain, normal human astrocytes as the non-target control.

2 In Vitro Validation

2.1 Materials

1. Targeting construct [1]: Dodecapeptides (TWYKIAFQRNRK), [3, 4] synthesized using standard solid phase synthesis, joined by poly(ethylene glycol) (PEG) to form a trivalent construct [1]. Fmoc-NH-$(PEG)_2$-COOH (20 atoms, *Nα*-Fmoc-19-amino-5-oxo-3,10,13,16-tetraoxa-6-azanonadecan-1-oic acid, Novabiochem) and 2-(1H-9-Azobenzotriazole-1-yl)-1,1,3,3-tetramethylaminium Hexafluorophosphate (HATU) in a 3:1 mixture of Dichloromethane: *N, N,*-Dimethylformamide is required to add the poly(ethylene glycol) linkers. The trivalent construct consists of three peptide sequences and two linkers (each containing three PEG molecules).
2. Normal human astrocytes (NHA).
3. Glioma cells (SF767).
4. Gel mixture: 0.3% collagen–0.3% agarose in Dulbecco's modified Eagle medium (DMEM) supplemented with 20% bovine growth serum (BGS). Stock solution of 1% collagen-1% agarose (w/v) was made in deionized (DI) water, heated until in solution, cooled until warm but still liquid, and diluted with warm 2× Dulbecco's modified Eagle medium (DMEM) supplemented with 20% bovine growth serum (BGS) to obtain a final gel concentration of 0.3% collagen–0.3% agarose.
5. Petri dishes (6 cm diameter).
6. Two metal cylinders (0.5 cm diameter) to serve as cell placeholders.
7. Syringe pump apparatus: luer lock stainless steel needle blunt tip syringe, syringe pump (compatible with 10 mL syringes),

tubing (1/4" ID Tygon works well, but any flexible tubing that fits a syringe tip and needle input will work), and xyz stage holding syringe.

8. Fluorescent microscope (inverted epifluorescence or confocal).
9. Image analysis software (Adobe Photoshop, ImageJ).

2.2 Methods

2.2.1 Setup and Creation of Mock Tissue

1. Add ~1 mg of targeting construct into 1 mL PBS. Determine the actual concentration of the trivalent construct using absorbance spectroscopy at 280 nm. Calculate the extinction coefficient based on the number of tyrosine and tryptophan residues in each construct (3 tyrosines and 3 tryptophans) [2]. This solution can be prepared in advance and flash-frozen in liquid nitrogen (stored in −80 °C), but this solution should not be stored for more than a day at 4 °C.
2. Culture NHAs and SF767 cells in separate T-75 flasks under standard culture conditions (37 °C and 5% CO_2) in DMEM supplemented with 10% BGS. Culture until the flask is confluent.
3. On the day of the experiment, add sufficient volume of Cell Dissociation Solution Non-enzymatic (Sigma) to coat the bottom of each T-75 flask (~3-5 mL). Incubate for 20 min or until cells detach from the plate (the flask may require firm rapping to promote cell detachment).
4. Place the cylindrical placeholders in a 6 cm diameter petri dish, in the locations shown in Fig. 1. The place holders should be 1.5 cm apart (center-to-center), and each cylinder edge should be 0.50 cm from the center of the petri dish.
5. Aliquot 12 mL of gel-media mixture (0.3% collagen–0.3% agarose solution prepared as described above) to Petri dish.
6. Allow the gel to cool to room temperature around the placeholders, and then remove the placeholders to create voids for the subsequent addition of the gel-cell mixture.
7. Aspirate the void spaces with a pipette to ensure the full volume is available for gel-cell allocation. Resuspend approximately 6×10^5 cells (either NHAs or SF767s) in 200 μL of 2× DMEM and then mix with 100 μL of warm 1%–1% collagen-agarose gel stock resulting in a 0.3%–0.3% collagen-agarose gel containing the desired cell density (2×10^6 cells/mL). Aliquot this cell-gel-media mixture to the appropriate location (SF767 in void to left of center, NHAs in void right of center) and allow to cool/solidify.
8. After gelation, add 2 mL of DMEM (with 10% BGS) to the top of the gel. Immediately use this apparatus for experimentation (must be used within approximately 16 h).

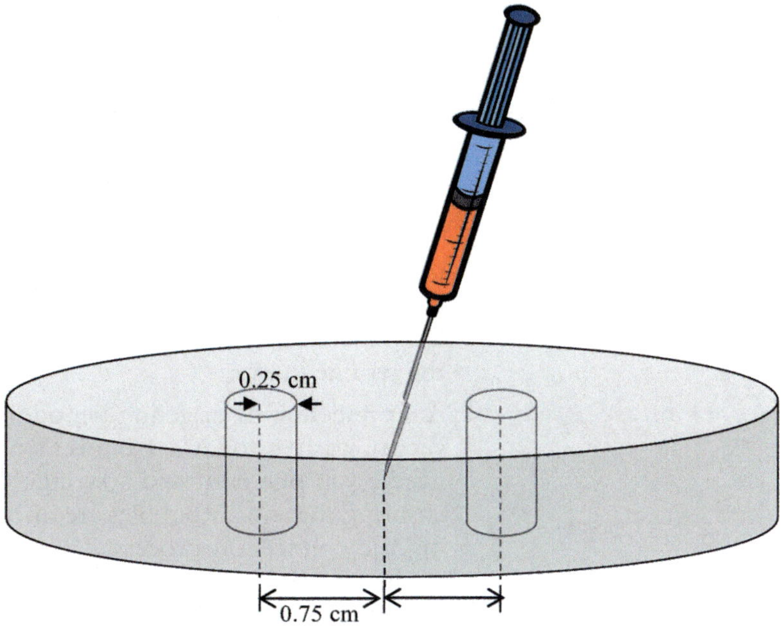

Fig. 1 Schematic of gel-cell coculture configuration

2.2.2 Convective Delivery and Convective Wash

1. Capture phase-contrast and fluorescent images of each location at this time, to serve as $t = 0$ data.
   - (a) Use phase-contrast microscopy at 20× magnification to semi-randomly select a field-of-view (FOV). The FOV should be chosen randomly but, if there are obvious abnormalities in the region (such as clumped cells, regions with fewer than expected cells, or other abnormalities to the matrix) then another FOV may need to be chosen. Capture an image of the phase-contrast view for reference. Seven to ten FOVs should be chosen for tumor, non-tumor, and acellular regions to capture representative locations in the gel, and to determine statistical significance.
   - (b) Once the FOV has been chosen by phase-contrast, switch to fluorescence imaging at 488 nm/512 nm excitation/emission (i.e., for FITC-labeled molecules) to capture a fluorescent image of the FOV.
   - (c) Select and image 7–10 FOVs for each of three regions: target region (this is the region containing SF767 cells), non-target region (this is the region containing NHA cells), and acellular region (this is another location 0.75 cm from the needle insertion point which will provide information about accumulation of targeting construct that can be attributed to mechanisms other than cell binding or internalization, such as binding to matrix).

Additionally, the acellular regions provide information about the default background levels of auto-fluorescence in the gel.

2. Insert the blunt tip needle in the center of the dish, midway between the SF767 and NHA regions (*see* Fig. 1 for dimensions).
3. Inject 50 μL of a 50 μM targeting construct solution (here, trivalent peptide) through the needle. Care must be taken not to jostle the syringe/needle when performing this injection. This injection is done as a bolus injection—not infused with the syringe pump.
4. After injection of targeting peptide construct, begin the convective wash as follows. Connect small diameter tubing to the needle (on one end) and a syringe (on the other end), while ensuring that no air bubbles are introduced to the needle during the connection process. Fill the syringe with cell culture media containing no targeting construct. Place the syringe in the syringe pump, with the pump calibrated to deliver 5.0 μL/min. Run the syringe pump for the remainder of the experiment except when noted otherwise.
5. If the experiment is run overnight, or for more than 4 h, cover the petri dish in parafilm or foil with a small slit in the parafilm to allow some of the fluid build-up to evaporate. Typical infusion times are approximately 12–16 h at 5.0 μL/min. Infusion times were established based on the time needed to convect fluid without construct past the cellular regions within the gel. Calculation of different infusion rates and infusion durations can be performed by comparing the volume of gel including radii up to and including the gel containing cells (1 cm radius includes all of the cells; therefore, $V \approx 1.35\ cm^3$ assuming a gel height of approximately 0.43 cm—which should result from pouring 12 mL of agar solution in a 6 cm petri dish) with the rate of infusion (5.0 μL/min will infuse 1.35 cm^3 after 270 min = 4.5 h). To see the full effect of a convective wash, infusion duration should be approximately 3 times this calculated infusion time.

2.2.3 Imaging

Acquire images of several locations in the mock tissue at several time points. Recommended time points are 0, 1, 2, 4, and 13.5 h after initiating the convective wash; however, additional or extended time points may be included.

1. Imaging with the needle in place is generally preferred. If the microscope does not permit this, use the motorized stage to remove the needle, then capture images. After imaging, replace the needle using the motorized stage, and restart the convective wash as described above.

2. When imaging, begin by using phase-contrast microscopy at 20× magnification to semi-randomly select a field-of-view (FOV). The FOV should be chosen randomly but, if there are obvious abnormalities in the region (such as clumped cells, regions with fewer than expected cells, or other abnormalities to the matrix) then another FOV may need to be chosen. Capture an image of the phase-contrast view for reference. Seven to ten FOVs should be chosen for tumor, non-tumor, and acellular regions to capture representative locations in the gel, and to determine statistical significance.
3. Once the FOV has been chosen by phase-contrast, switch to fluorescence imaging at 488 nm/512 nm excitation/emission (i.e., for FITC-labeled molecules) to capture a fluorescent image of the FOV.
4. Select and image 7–10 FOVs for each of three regions:
   (a) Target region: this is the region containing SF767 cells.
   (b) Non-target region: this is the region containing NHA cells.
   (c) Acellular region: this is another location 0.75 cm from the needle insertion point which will provide information about accumulation of targeting construct that can be attributed to mechanisms other than cell binding or internalization, such as binding to matrix. Additionally, the acellular regions provide information about the default background levels of auto-fluorescence in the gel.
5. Ensure that there are similar numbers of cells in NHA and SF767 FOVs by inspection of the phase-contrast images. If there are not similar numbers of cells, the experiment may still provide meaningful results; however, the following factors should be considered. If the concentration of construct is depleted substantially by the cells (i.e., most of the construct binds to cells), this can result in lesser binding per cell in the region with greater cell density. Conversely, in regions of lesser cells, more binding per cell may occur, or construct may be less physically hindered to perfuse greater distances in the gel matrix. While observations may be made, another gel-cell mock tissue should be selected at the beginning of the experiment. Statistical problems in analysis (Subheading 2.2.4) may arise due to large differences in the number of cells analyzed in one region vs. the other, one of these is that there may be unequal variance.
6. Repeat **step 4** until data for all desired time points have been collected. *See* Subheading 2.2.2, **step 5** for the method to calculate the appropriate infusion time, τ. Recommended time points for data collection are 0, 1, 0.5τ, τ, and 3τ.

2.2.4 Data Analysis and Statistics

1. For a given FOV in the phase-contrast image, select at least 10 cells for analysis, prior to fluorescence visualization to avoid bias). Using image analysis software (e.g., Adobe Photoshop or NIH Image J), select one of the cells in the fluorescent image by drawing an outline around its perimeter. Use the software to calculate the average intensity of fluorescence across all pixels in that cell. Record that value. Repeat for all of the cells chosen in that FOV.
2. Repeat **step 1** for each FOV imaged (7–10 cell-containing FOVs per cell region per time point).
3. Select an acellular region as a background control. In this image, choose approximate areas similar in size to a cell from the phase-contrast image (avoiding regions with obvious abnormalities). Abnormalities often appear as very bright spots, and are likely due to aggregation of construct or some other locale of dense matrix in which construct has accumulated. Analyze the selected acellular FOV regions as described for the cellular regions, instead outlining the perimeter of the chosen region that is similar in size to a cell.
4. To analyze the data by time point, bin the data into a histogram (fluorescence vs. count) so that bins are sized to allow the number of cells/regions in each bin at a reasonable number (bins near the peak should be well above 1 but there should be 5–10 bins with counts >1). If the reader is unfamiliar with selecting appropriate data bins, please see: https://support.microsoft.com/en-us/help/214269/how-to-use-the-histogram-tool-in-excel. Plot a histogram for the SF767 region, another for the NHA region, and a third for the acellular region. Visually analyze these histograms to compare/contrast binding of the targeting construct to the cells and/or matrix. An ideal result will show a normal distribution for both regions with the SF767 peak at greater fluorescence than the NHA peak. Any deviations from this should be noted. Statistical comparison can be performed with a non-parametric test such as a Chi-squared test.
5. Using each cell outlined at an "independent" measurement, calculate the mean and standard deviation (and/or 95% confidence interval) of the data for the SF767, NHA, and acellular regions. Use a Student's t-test ($p < 0.05$) to compare the data from the SF767 and NHA regions. If the p-value is less than 0.05 and the mean of the SF767 region is greater than the mean of the NHA region, you can conclude that the targeting construct preferentially targets the SF767 cells at that time point. Perform an ANOVA with all three populations to ensure that the SF767 cells are also different from the acellular region. [Note: Using each cell outlined as an independent measure-

ment is not acceptable under strict interpretation of statistical methods. To publish these data, you will need to repeat this entire experiment three (or more) times, use the means (mean of SF767 region, mean of NHA region) of the single experiment as the "independent" measurement, and perform a t-test upon those measurements to ensure the difference is reproducible and robust.]

2.3 Notes

1. To study the biophysics of binding in the absence of endocytosis, construct internalization by the cells can be minimized by conducting the experiments at 4 °C. In this work, cell binding and internalization were not differentiated. A more in-depth approach would be needed to semi-quantitatively or quantitatively assess cell internalization. Therefore, the described measurements account for cellular association (both binding and internalization).
2. In these experiments, we have used a trivalent, biomacromolecular construct targeted to the $\alpha_6\beta_1$-integrin via a dodecapeptide ligand derived from laminin (TWYKIAFQRNRK) [3, 4]. Detailed protocols for the synthesis of the construct are published by Rosca et al. [1, 5]. Briefly, the trivalent construct, consisting of three peptide sequences and two linkers (each containing three PEG molecules), is synthesized using standard solid-phase peptide synthesis. The three dodecapeptides (TWYKIAFQRNRK) are connected by two linkers which are each constructed of three units of Fmoc-NH-$(PEG)_2$-COOH (20 atoms, *Nα*-Fmoc-19-amino-5-oxo-3,10,13,16-tetraoxa-6-azanonadecan-1-oic acid, Novabiochem) to form a peptide-linker-peptide-linker-peptide structure. At the N-terminus, a molecule of fluorescein isothiocyanate (FITC, Anaspec #20151) is added according to the manufacturer's protocol. The constructs are cleaved from the resin, purified using standard protocols, and verified by matrix assisted laser desorption ionization—time of flight mass spectroscopy (MALDI-TOF-MS).
3. NHA and SF767 cells are human cells so Biosafety Level 2 (BSL2) precautions should be used at all times.
4. An inverted epifluorescence microscope is acceptable; however, confocal microscopy provides clearer depictions of individual cells if available. For the fluorophores used in these experiments, a FITC filter (488 nm/512 nm, excitation/emission), digital camera (e.g., SPOT-RT3), and real-time imaging software (Diagnostic Imaging, Inc.) were used.
5. A 0.3% collagen–0.3% agarose gel provides a relevant brain tissue mimic by providing comparable matrix porosity and mechanical properties. Due to the anchorage and extracellular

matrix (e.g., collagen I) dependence of NHA and SF767 cells, agar alone is inadequate and may result in cell death.

6. Non-enzymatic dissociation of cells from the cell culture flask is necessary to maintain the structure and functionality of the cell surface antigens/receptors being targeted.
7. The 0.3% collagen–0.3% agarose gel-cell solution must be made before the collagen-agarose stock mixture begins to solidify. Once the serum has been added, subsequent reheating to maintain liquidity, may inactivate serum for cell maintenance. When cooling this mixture, care must be taken to cool at room temperature. Inserting the petri dish in the freezer or refrigerator, to accelerate cooling, for greater than 1–3 min, will result in a harder edge consistency between tumor and non-tumor regions.
8. The 3 tyrosines and 3 tryptophans in this peptide construct are used to calculate the extinction coefficient for absorbance spectroscopy (280 nm), and determine the concentration prior to infusion.
9. It is essential that the needle be inserted exactly vertically, because any slant to the tip will create a region around the needle that is mechanically disrupted. Any disruption to the gel-cell matrix may promote fluid convection or backflow through the needle insertion path rather than through the collagen-agarose gel. We recommend the use of a motorized stage to ensure both slow and steady insertion pressure and vertical needle insertion. The needle should also be primed with peptide solution to remove air bubbles, prior to vertical insertion in the gel.
10. A flow rate of 5 μL/min was chosen because it is the maximum clinically viable infusion rate for convection-enhanced delivery to the brain, due to the necessity of avoiding edema and backflow up the catheter insertion path [6, 7]. However, a range of flow rates spanning 0.5–5 μL/min may be used to evaluate convection-enhanced delivery as desired.
11. Immediately after the initial bolus injection, very little construct is likely to be observed bound to cells, as construct will likely be contained primarily at the center of the gel (corresponding to the injection site). For the infusion conditions described here, a typical progression of fluorescence signal follows. At the 1 h time-point, the fluorescence intensity observed in the background is likely to be high for both the SF767s and NHAs due to unbound construct at the site of these cells. After approximately 2 h of wash, background fluorescence will likely decrease slightly and, if targeting is successful, SF767 cells are

likely to be distinguishable from background. After 4 h, trivalent constructs are likely to remain bound to SF767 cells and lower background fluorescence will lead to greater contrast between cells and background. After 13.5 h, the intensity of trivalent construct bound to SF767s will likely decrease, but the intensity of background fluorescence will likely decrease more rapidly, enhancing the contrast between cells and background.

12. The concentration of the initial bolus of targeting construct must be chosen carefully, based on the avidity of the targeting construct for its target cell receptor. Recent research in the development of drug targeting constructs for cancer therapeutics has focused on increasing the avidity of the targeting constructs for target cells [1, 5, 8–12]. The results in our previous papers suggested that increased avidity was not sufficient to achieve specific targeting in cell monolayers [1]. We showed that a low level of specificity was achieved when high construct concentrations (10 μM) were added, and that enhanced specificity (due to multivalency) was only achieved when the construct concentration was less than the affinity of the receptor-ligand bond (robust intensity and specificity were observed at 0.625 μM, compared to the construct's avidity of 4.3 μM).

    However, in the case described here, which incorporates convective transport, the bolus needs to exceed the concentration indicated by the avidity, so that the construct binds to the cells, but also remains at detectable levels after the convective wash removes unbound construct from the region. The remaining bound concentration (less than the construct-receptor avidity) will provide specificity between the target and non-target cells. Therefore, 3D cell-gel experiments will require a higher concentration of construct than 2D-binding assays. A range of concentrations greater than those observed to attain binding specificity in 2D culture should be chosen to conduct preliminary assays with, prior to choosing a final concentration for infusion. In this arrangement, we found using an injected concentration of approximately 10× avidity to be optimal. The avidity of the trivalent construct for SF767 cells is approximately 4.3 μM [5], and we found an injection concentration of 50 μM to be optimal.

13. Dispose of material from the experiment following your institution's waste disposal procedures. For experiments using the human cells described in this protocol, follow BSL2 disposal procedures. The construct contains FITC and so may be considered hazardous waste.

3 Comparison to Mathematical Modeling

3.1 Materials

COMSOL Multiphysics was used to simulate the experimental system based on mass transport and binding equations found in [13]. We recommend COMSOL Multiphysics with the Chemical Reaction Engineering Module be installed on a PC having RAM (≥16GB) to accelerate simulations. Also, a capable video card is important to visualize 3D simulations. Most standard PCs should be sufficient to run the simulations described here.

3.2 Methods

The simulation program solves Darcy's Law and mass transport equations to determine the fluid velocities and spatiotemporal targeting construct concentrations. Table 1 enumerates the equations used: where P is the local pressure, v is the local velocity of the fluid, K is the permeability of the gel, C_0 is the concentration of unbound construct, C_1 is the concentration of construct bound by one ligand, C_2 is the concentration of construct bound by two ligands, C_3 is the concentration of construct bound by three ligands, D_{eff} is the effective diffusion coefficient of construct through the gel, k_f and k_r are the association/dissociation constants of the ligand/antibody to the receptor/antigen, V_R is the binding enhancement factor (accounting for increased effective concentration once one ligand/antigen is bound), and R is the density of available receptors/antigens at the particular location (target cells, non-target cells, or acellular matrix). Rationale for the parameter settings chosen can be found in Stukel, Heys, and Caplan [14] or are discussed in Subheading 3.3.

Table 1
Equations for finite element simulations [14]

Trivalent	Peptide/antibody (monovalent)
$\nabla^2 P = 0$ & $\vec{v} = K\nabla P$	$\nabla^2 P = 0$ & $\vec{v} = K\nabla P$
$\frac{\partial C_0}{\partial t} = D_{\text{eff}}\nabla^2 C_0 - \vec{v}\cdot\nabla C_0 - 3k_f R C_0 + k_r C_1$	$\frac{\partial C_0}{\partial t} = D_{\text{eff}}\nabla^2 C_0 - \vec{v}\cdot\nabla C_0 - 3k_f R C_0 + k_r C_1$
$\frac{\partial C_1}{\partial t} = 3k_f R C_0 - k_r C_1 - 2k_f V_R R C_1 + 2k_r C_2$	$\frac{\partial C_1}{\partial t} = 3k_f R C_0 - k_r C_1$
$\frac{\partial C_2}{\partial t} = 2k_f V_R R C_1 - 2k_r C_2 - k_f V_R R C_2 + 3k_r C_3$	
$\frac{\partial C_3}{\partial t} = k_f V_R R C_2 - 3k_r C_3$	
$R = R_{\text{initial}} - C_1 - 2C_2 - 3C_3$	$R = R_{\text{initial}} - C_1$

1. Open the COMSOL program, choose 2D simulation, and in the Chemical Reaction Engineering Module choose "Mass Transport > Convection and Diffusion > Transient Analysis" as the model type. Click "Multiphysics" in the panel to the right, click "Add." With the same model type chosen, change the "Dependent variable" name to "c1," and click "Add." Repeat twice more with "Dependent variable" names "c2" and "c3" respectively. This will yield 4 convection and diffusion models in total, to model a trivalent targeting construct. Next, choose "Momentum Transport > Porous Media Flow > Darcy's Law > Steady State Analysis" and click "Add". Set the first "Convection and Diffusion" model (chcd) as the "ruling application module." Click "OK" to establish these arrangements.
2. In Draw > Draw Mode, create a circle with the center at (0,0) and a radius of 0.03 m (COMSOL usually defaults to using meters as units of length, but double-check this when you enter your parameter values below). Create another circle centered at (−0.0075,0) with radius of 0.00125 m. Copy and paste this circle, when prompted by COMSOL for a displacement, enter (0.015,0) to place the center of the pasted circle at (0.0075,0). Create one more circle with center at (0,0) with radius of 0.0005 m.
3. In Physics > Subdomain Settings, click on "Darcy's Law" in the left-hand menu bar, then (while holding down the control key) click on all of the subdomains. Set the density (ρ) to 1000 kg/m^3, the hydraulic permeability (K) to 1×10^{-15} m^2 (type as "1e-15"), and the fluid viscosity (η) to 1×10^{-3} Pa·s. Click "Apply." Then click only on the small circle centered at (0,0) which represents the injection needle. Uncheck the box that says "Active in this Domain." Click "Apply."
4. Still in Physics > Subdomain Settings, click on the first "Convection and Diffusion" model in the left-hand menu bar, then click on the "target" subdomain (0.025 m diameter circle at (−0.0075,0)). Set the isotropic diffusion coefficient (D_{eff}) to 6×10^{-10} m^2/s. Set the x-direction velocity to "u_chdl," and set the y-direction velocity to "v_chdl." In the field for "R," type "-3*kf*Rtarget*c + kr*c1." Click "Apply."
5. Repeat **step 4** for the "non-target" subdomain by clicking on the non-target subdomain (0.025 m diameter circle at (0.0075,0)) and setting its parameters identically except that the reaction field (R) will read "-3*kf*Rnon*c + kr*c1."
6. Repeat **step 4** for the "acellular" subdomain by clicking on the large circle (radius 0.03 m) at a point not inside either of the other subdomains, and set its parameters identically except that the reaction field (R) will read "0."

7. Still in Physics > Subdomain settings, click only on the small circle centered at (0,0) which represents the injection needle. Uncheck the box that says "Active in this Domain."
8. Still in Physics > Subdomain Settings, click on the second "Convection and Diffusion" model in the left-hand menu bar, then click on the "target" subdomain. Set the Diffusion coefficient to "0" (a targeting construct does not diffuse once it is bound to the cell). Also make sure the x-direction and y-direction velocities are set to "0." In the reaction field (R), type "3*kf*Rtarget*c – kr*c1 – 2*kf*Vr*Rtarget*c1 + 2*kr *c2". Click "Apply."
9. Repeat **step 8** for the "non-target" subdomain and set its parameters identically except that the reaction field (R) will read "3*kf*Rnon*c – kr*c1 – 2*kf*Vr*Rnon*c1 + 2*kr*c2."
10. Nothing needs to be done for the acellular gel subdomain because its parameters are already set appropriately for the other convection and diffusion models. Set the injection needle to Inactive for the 2nd, 3rd, and 4th convection/diffusion models.
11. Still in Physics > Subdomain Settings, click on the third "Convection and Diffusion" model in the left-hand menu bar, then click on the "target" subdomain. Set the Diffusion coefficient to "0" and make sure the x-direction and y-direction velocities are set to "0." In the reaction field (R), type "2*kf* Vr*Rtarget*c1 – 2*kr*c2 – kf*Vr*Rtarget*c2 + 3*kr*c3." Repeat this for the "non-target" subdomain and set its parameters identically except that the reaction field (R) will read "2* kf*Vr*Rnon*c1 – 2*kr*c2 – kf*Vr*Rnon*c2 + 3*kr*c3".
12. Still in Physics > Subdomain Settings, click on the fourth "Convection and Diffusion" model in the left-hand menu bar, then click on the "target" subdomain. Set the Diffusion coefficient to "0" and make sure the x-direction and y-direction velocities are set to "0." In the reaction field (R), type "kf*Vr*Rtarget*c2 – 3*kr*c3." Repeat this for the "non-target" subdomain and set its parameters identically except that the reaction field (R) will read "kf*Vr*Rnon*c2 – 3*kr*c3."
13. In Physics > Boundary Settings, click on "Darcy's Law" in the left-hand menu bar, then (while holding down the control key) click on all of the arcs defining the largest circle. Set the boundary condition type to "Pressure" and set to atmospheric pressure (101325 Pa). Deselect these boundaries. Then select all of the arcs defining the smallest circle (representing the injection needle). Set the boundary condition type to "inflow/outflow" and set to 1×10^{-5} m/s.
14. In Physics > Boundary Settings, click on the first "Convection and Diffusion" model in the left-hand menu bar, then select all of the arcs defining the largest circle. Set the boundary condition type to "Insulated/Symmetry." Deselect these boundaries.

Then select all of the arcs defining the smallest circle (representing the injection needle). Set the boundary condition type to "concentration" and set to "(0.05–0.05 * flc1hs(t-0.0063,0.001))". *See* Subheading 3.3, **steps 1** and **2** below for explanation of this boundary condition.

15. The boundary settings for the 2nd, 3rd, and 4th "Convection and Diffusion" models should be set to "Insulated/Symmetry" at both boundaries which is likely to be the default.

16. In Options > Constants, define the following parameters:
    (a) Rtargetinitial = 6.25×10^{-7} mol/m^3 (this has units of concentration because there are a defined number of cells in this volume, and each cell has a known number of receptors). This value represents the concentration of receptors on target tumor cells.
    (b) Rnoninitial = 2.19×10^{-7} mol/m^3. This value represents the concentration of receptors on non-target non-cancerous cells.
    (c) kf = 8.0 (mol/m^3)$^{-1}$ s^{-1}. This represents the association rate of a ligand to its receptor.
    (d) kr = 0.03424 s^{-1}. This represents the dissociation rate of a ligand from the receptor.
    (e) Vr = 1×10^6. This represents the volume enhancement factor which accounts for the fact that a construct bound by at least one receptor is held in close proximity to the cell surface, giving it enhanced likelihood of contacting another receptor.

17. In Options > Expressions > Global Expressions, define the following parameters:
    (a) Rtarget = Rtargetinitial – (c1 + 2*c2 + 3*c3). This represents the number of target receptors still available for binding to a ligand.
    (b) Rnon = Rnoninitial – (c1 + 2*c2 + 3*c3). This represents the number of non-target receptors available for binding to a ligand.
    (c) c_total = c + c1 + c2 + c3. This represents the total concentration of constructs in a location.
    (d) c_bound = c1 + c2 + c3. This represents the concentration of bound ligands.

18. Click the toolbar button to "Initialize Mesh." The elements may not be fine/small enough to provide appropriate data. If so, click the toolbar button for "Refine Mesh."

19. In Solver Parameters, make sure that the "Darcy's Law" solver is set to "Stationary" to provide a steady state solution to the Darcy's Law equation. All four of the "Convection and Diffusion" models should be set to "Transient." Set the duration

of the simulation to run from 0 s to 48,600 s (t = 0 to t = 13.5 h) with time steps of 600 s by typing "range(0,600,48600)" into the "Times" box (600 s is the length of time between data output, the step size for simulation is set elsewhere). Click on the "Time Stepping" tab, set the initial time step to 0.0001 s, and set the maximum step size to 5 s. The other Solver Parameters will likely work at their default settings.

20. Save the simulation prior to running the simulation (always important, but particularly so when initiating a long and memory-intensive simulation). Click the toolbar button to "Solve" the simulation. When the simulation is complete, save again.
21. In Post Processing > Plot Parameters, click on the "General" tab, choose the "solution time" that you wish to analyze, and check the boxes for plot types "Surface" and "Geometry Edges." Click on the "Surface" tab, and type "c_total" into the "Expression" box, then click "OK." This will provide a plot of total concentration (bound plus unbound) at each location in the gel at the chosen time point.
22. In Post Processing > Plot Parameters, click on the "Animate" tab, highlight all time points, then click "Start Animation." This will show a time course of the surface plots from **step 20** over all time points in the simulation.

3.3 Notes

1. When running, view the Progress on the "Log" tab. Monitor the "stepsize," "Tfail," and "Nfail" columns. Tfail is a tolerance fail and does not necessarily mean that there is a problem, but frequent tolerance failures will decrease step size and may indicate that your solution will not be as precise as it should be. If Nfail occurs more than a few times, this likely indicates a problem with the solution; thus, you should try to determine why the Nfails are occurring and attempt to change the simulation to avoid those. Tfail and even a few Nfail errors are likely to occur near t = 0.0063 in this simulation when the injection is switched from including targeting construct to injection of only buffer without targeting construct. The function for that boundary condition, "(0.05–0.05 * flc1hs(t-0.0063,0.001))," ramps the concentration of targeting construct down over several milliseconds rather than making an abrupt transition. This makes the solution less stiff, and minimizes the likelihood of Tfail or Nfail errors. If Tfail or Nfail errors occur in your simulations, consider changes like this to make the numerical solution less stiff.
2. The FEM is designed to have the same geometric configuration as the experimental setup. Also, many of the parameters are fixed at experimentally determined values. Tumor and non-tumor sub-regions were assigned 6.25×10^{-7} and 2.19×10^{-7} mol of

receptors per cubic meter (corresponding to approximately 37,600 and 13,210 receptors per cell respectively—values based on experimental measurement by fluorescence activated cell sorting) [1]. Boundary condition at the syringe was set to 50 μM for 0.0063 s (to simulate the injection of 50 μL) and then set to 0 μM for the remainder of the simulation, with velocity from the needle set to 1×10^{-5} m/s. Association (k_f) and dissociation (k_r) rates were set to 8.0 $(\mathrm{mol/m^3})^{-1}\ \mathrm{s^{-1}}$ and 0.03424 $\mathrm{s^{-1}}$ respectively (matching experimentally measured affinity, k_r/k_f) [1]; V_R was set to 1×10^6. The diffusion coefficient $D_{eff} = 6 \times 10^{-10}\ \mathrm{m^2/s}$, density $\rho = 1000\ \mathrm{kg/m^3}$, hydraulic permeability $K = 1 \times 10^{-15}\ \mathrm{m^2}$, and fluid viscosity $\eta = 1 \times 10^{-3}$ Pa·s complete the parameter set. The only parameters not experimentally verified are k_f (association rate) and K (permeability). The model is insensitive to the value of permeability because the boundary condition is a flow rate and the fluid is incompressible. The association rate is held constant for all construct types and the value is consistent with other peptide ligands for receptors measured by surface plasmon resonance [15]. Thus, the only parameter that might be considered fitted is V_R, although information about the reasonability of 1×10^6 has been published [1]. Setting as many as possible of these parameters to known values allows comparison between model and experiment to yield more informative conclusions. One parameter value not included, although implicitly included as $f = 1$, is the filtration coefficient. This value will be 1 if the construct velocity equals the fluid velocity, but can be less than 1 if the matrix retards convection of the construct. For the biomacromolecular constructs modeled here, $f = 1$ is likely to be a reasonable approximation; however, this can be easily adjusted by changing the x-direction and y-direction velocities to "f*u_chdl" and "f*v_chdl" respectively.

3. Running this finite element simulation provides the results shown in Fig. 2 for the trivalent peptide construct (Fig. 2a–d), monovalent peptide (Fig. 2e–h), and fluorescently labeled antibody (Fig. 2i–l). Equations for peptide and antibody simulations are shown in Table 1; the dissociation rate (k_r) for the antibody was changed to $8.0 \times 10^{-7}\ \mathrm{s^{-1}}$. Although there is substantial binding of all three types of constructs to the SF767 cells at early time points (Figs. 2a/b, 2e/f, 2i/j: left cell region), the very high background concentration obscures the concentration difference between the SF767 and NHA regions (right cell region in same Figures). After 4 h of convective wash (Fig. 2c, g, k), the bolus of injected construct moves beyond the cell regions and becomes diluted as convection and diffusion spread the bolus over a longer distance (radii). The model accurately predicts that the concentration of trivalent construct remaining on the SF767s (~0.07 μM) is

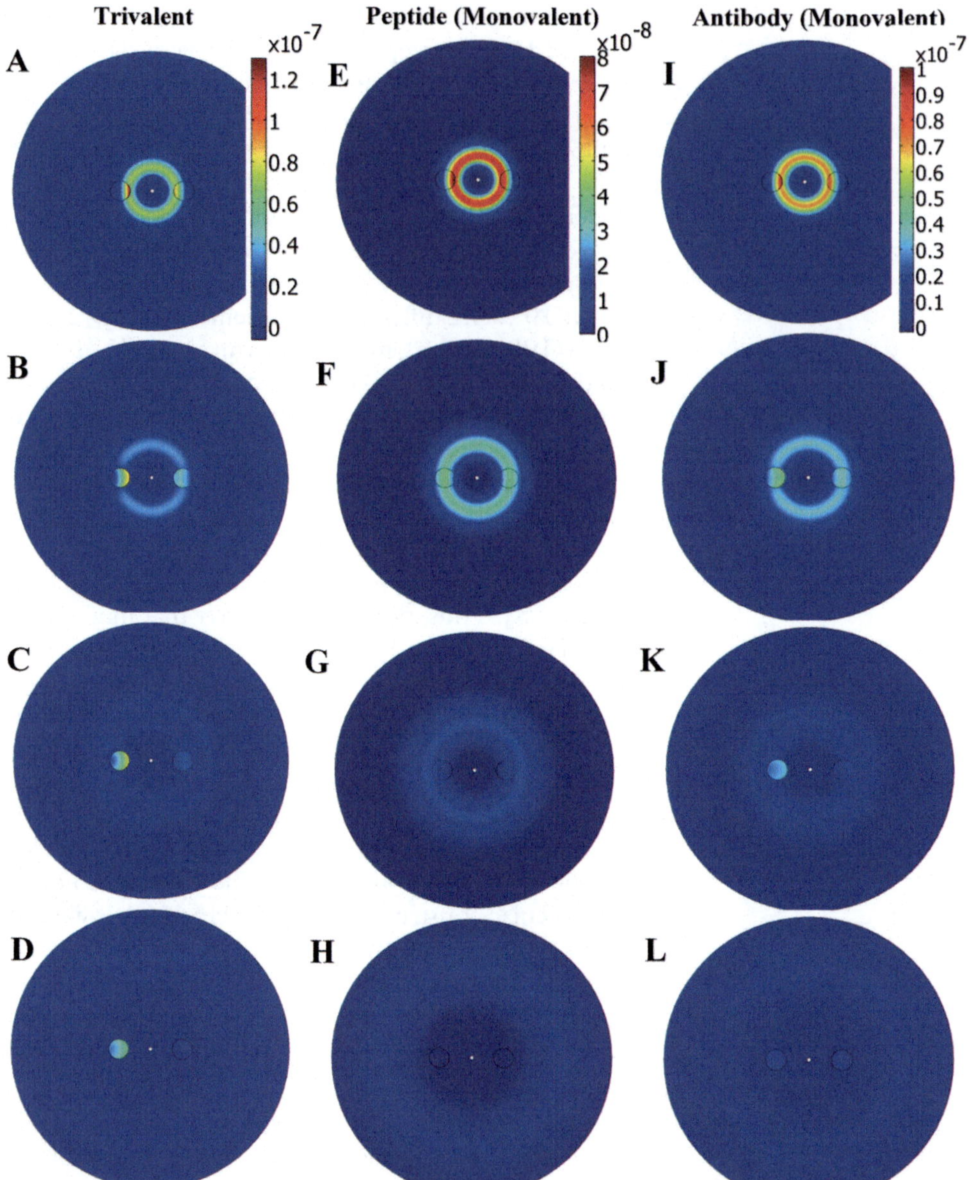

Fig. 2 Mathematical modeling results of construct concentration vs. location as a function of time. Circular sub-regions to the left and right of the injection site represent SF767 and NHA regions respectively. Modeling results after 1 h (**a**, **e**, **i**), 2 h (**b**, **f**, **j**), 4 h (**c**, **g**, **k**), and 13.5 h (**d**, **h**, **l**) of convective wash are shown for injection of a trivalent peptide construct (**a**–**d**), monovalent peptide (**e**–**h**), and antibody for comparison (**i**–**l**). Color maps show concentration in molarity (M)

significantly greater than that remaining on the NHAs (~0.02 μM). As the wash continues to 13.5 h (Fig. 2d), the concentration of trivalent construct decreases in both regions (~0.04 and 0.01 μM respectively), but the contrast is greater due to the transport of the bolus past the cell regions and dilution by convection and diffusion.

4. These predictions can be compared to the fluorescent images of SF767s and NHAs collected experimentally as described above (example images provided in Fig. 3). If the concentration of each fluorescently labeled targeting construct is known, the experimental fluorescent intensity can be quantitatively compared with the model results. However, exact values should be cautiously compared, due to a variety of factors that may affect the accuracy of this method. Instead, data trends observed between the SF767 and NHA or acellular regions may be compared more readily.
   (a) As an example, the model data predict that, after 4 h, the concentration of trivalent construct remaining on the SF767s (~0.07 μM) is approximately 3.5 times greater than the concentration remaining on the NHAs (~0.02 μM). The experimental data can be analyzed to determine if the fluorescence intensity in the SF767 region is approximately 3.5 times the fluorescence intensity in the NHA region.
   (b) After 13.5 h, the model predicts that the construct concentration in both the SF767 and NHA regions will decrease. Moreover, the concentration in the acellular region will decrease more rapidly, thus increasing contrast. The c_total ratios of the SF767 or NHA regions, relative to the acellular, can be calculated and compared to experimental results.
5. Substantial differences between modeling and experimental results may indicate that the model is not accurately capturing one or more important aspects of the biophysics. For example, cellular uptake (internalization) of the targeting construct can lead to accumulation in the cell. This phenomenon is not modeled in the above protocol, but the reaction term of the SF767 and NHA subdomains can be modified to simulate cellular uptake. Modeling is usually most informative when such mismatch between modeling and experimental results forces additional biophysical phenomena to be considered to achieve approximate agreement.

Acknowledgments

The authors thank our funding sources: NIH (R01 CA097360, R21 NS051310), Arizona Biomedical Research Commission contract #0606 and our collaborators Robert J. Gillies (Moffitt Cancer Institute, University of South Florida), Michael Berens

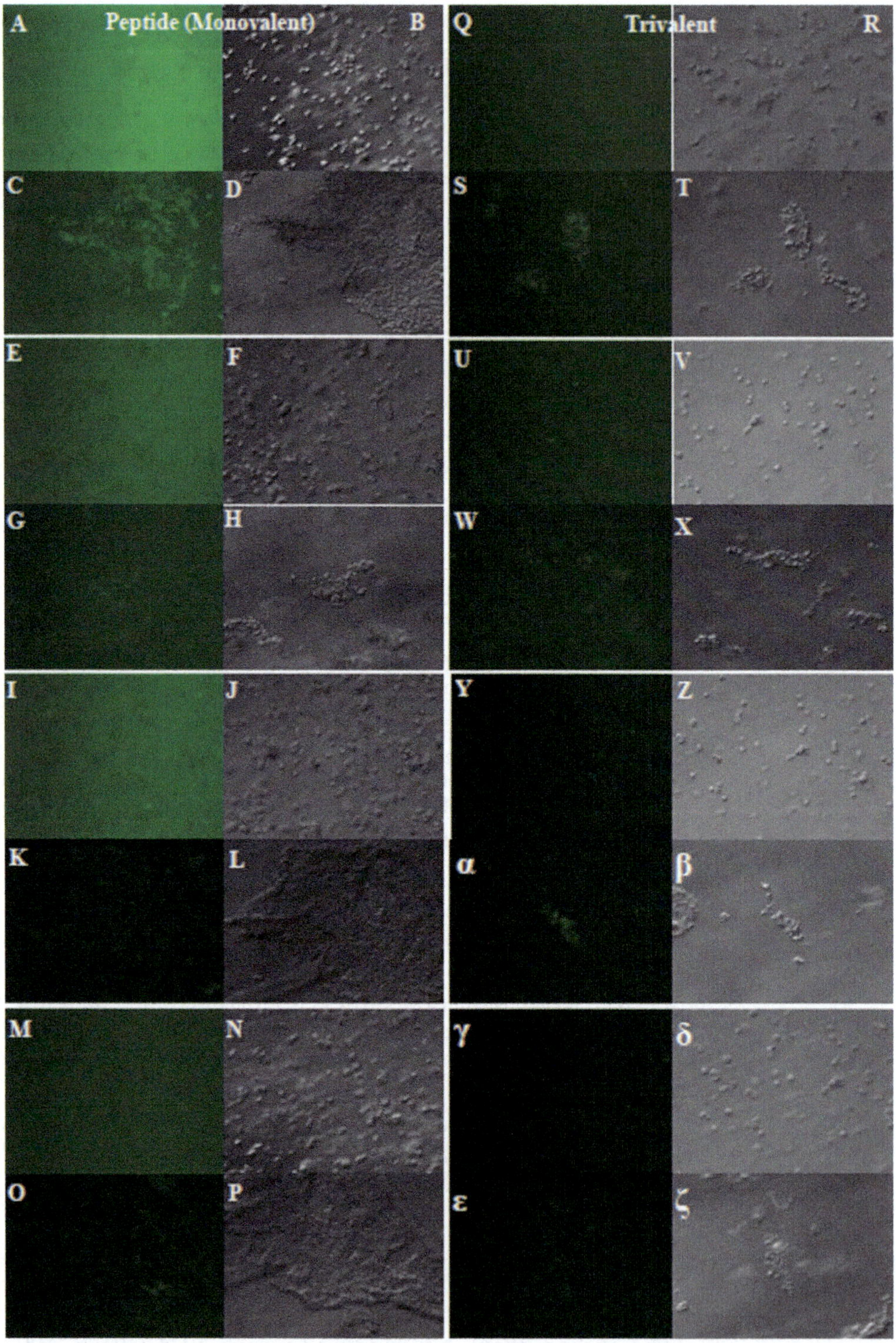

Fig. 3 Representative epifluorescent microscopy images of peptide (**a**–**p**) and trivalent construct (**q**-**ζ**) near SF767 and NHA cells after 1 h (**a**–**d**, **q**–**t**), 2 h (**e**–**h**, **u**–**x**), 4 h (**i**–**l**, **y**-**β**), and 13.5 h (**m**–**p**, **γ**-**ζ**) of convective wash. Epifluorescence of FITC-labeled constructs (1st and 3rd columns) and phase contrast (2nd and 4th columns) images are depicted. Images of NHA cell region: a/b, e/f, i/j, m/n, q/r, u/v, y/z, γ/δ. Images of SF767 cell region: c/d, g/h, k/l, o/p, s/t, w/x, α/β, ε/ζ

(Translational Genomic Institute), Josef Vagner (University of Arizona), and Heather Maynard (UCLA). Recognition is given to Dr. Michael Berens, Dr. Dominique Hoelzinger, and Dr. Tim Demuth for assistance with obtaining and validating cell lines. We thank Dr. Christine Pauken for assisting with the imaging. We also thank Dr. Dan Brune and John Lopez for their generous assistance and advice with the construct synthesis.

References

1. Rosca EV, Gillies RJ, Caplan MR (2009) Glioblastoma targeting via Integrins is concentration dependent. Biotechnol Bioeng 104(2):408–417
2. ThermoScientific. Tech Tip #6 Extinction Coefficients: A guide to understanding extinction coefficients, with emphasis on spectrophotometric determination of protein concentration (TR0006.4). 2006; https://tools.thermofisher.com/content/sfs/brochures/TR0006-Extinction-coefficients.pdf.
3. Nakahara H, Nomizu M, Akiyama SK, Yamada Y, Yeh Y, Chen WT (1996) A mechanism for regulation of melanoma invasion. Ligation of alpha6beta1 integrin by laminin G peptides. J Biol Chem 271(44):27221–27224
4. Nomizu M, Kuratomi Y, Malinda KM, Song SY, Miyoshi K, Otaka A, Powell SK, Hoffman MP, Kleinman HK, Yamada Y (1998) Cell binding sequences in mouse laminin alpha1 chain. J Biol Chem 273(49):32491–32499
5. Rosca EV, Stukel JM, Gillies RJ, Vagner J, Caplan MR (2007) Specificity and mobility of biomacromolecular, multivalent constructs for cellular targeting. Biomacromolecules 8(12):3830–3835
6. Morrison PF, Chen MY, Chadwick RS, Lonser RR, Oldfield EH (1999) Focal delivery during direct infusion to brain: role of flow rate, catheter diameter, and tissue mechanics. Am J Phys 277(4 Pt 2):R1218–R1229
7. Raghavan R, Brady ML, Rodriguez-Ponce MI, Hartlep A, Pedain C, Sampson JH (2006) Convection-enhanced delivery of therapeutics for brain disease, and its optimization. Neurosurg Focus 20(4):E12
8. Gao X, Yang L, Petros JA, Marshall FF, Simons JW, Nie S (2005) In vivo molecular and cellular imaging with quantum dots. Curr Opin Biotechnol 16(1):63–72
9. Handl HL, Vagner J, Han H, Mash E, Hruby VJ, Gillies RJ (2004) Hitting multiple targets with multimeric ligands. Expert Opin Ther Targets 8(6):565–586
10. Kioi M, Husain SR, Croteau D, Kunwar S, Puri RK (2006) Convection-enhanced delivery of interleukin-13 receptor-directed cytotoxin for malignant glioma therapy. Technol Cancer Res Treat 5(3):239–250
11. Lowery AR, Gobin AM, Day ES, Halas NJ, West JL (2006) Immunonanoshells for targeted photothermal ablation of tumor cells. Int J Nanomedicine 1(2):149–154
12. Michalet X, Pinaud FF, Bentolila LA, Tsay JM, Doose S, Li JJ, Sundaresan G, Wu AM, Gambhir SS, Weiss S (2005) Quantum dots for live cells, in vivo imaging, and diagnostics. Science 307(5709):538–544
13. Stukel JM, Parks J, Caplan MR, Helms Tillery SI (2008) Temporal and spatial control of neural effects following Intracerebral microinfusion. J Drug Target 16(3):198–205
14. Stukel JM, Heys JJ, Caplan MR (2008) Optimizing delivery of multivalent targeting constructs for detection of secondary tumors. Ann Biomed Eng 36(7):1291–1304
15. Jovanovic J, Takagi J, Choulier L, Abrescia NGA, Stuart DI, van der Merwe PA, Mardon HJ, Handford PA (2007) aVb6 is a novel receptor for human Fibrillin-1. J Biol Chem 282(9):6743–6751

Part III

Measuring Delivery and Efficacy

Chapter 11

Enzyme-Linked Immunosorbent Assay to Quantify Targeting Molecules on Nanoparticles

Rachel S. Riley, Jilian R. Melamed, and Emily S. Day

Abstract

Molecular targeting presents a promising means of improving the specificity of cancer therapeutics, increasing accumulation at the cancer site and limiting off-target effects. These targeting schemes can be applied to nanoparticle-based treatments to further enhance their anticancer efficacy. Here, we describe methods to conjugate antibodies to silica-gold nanoshells and to quantify the resulting antibody content on the nanoparticles using a solution-based enzyme-linked immunosorbent assay (ELISA). Although we will be using anti-EGFR (epidermal growth factor receptor) antibodies conjugated to gold-silica nanoshells as a model system, this method is adaptable to quantify a range of targeting antibodies and proteins on various types of nanoparticles.

Key words ELISA, Nanoparticles, Molecular targeting, Antibodies, Cancer nanotechnology

1 Introduction

Over the last several decades, nanoparticles have emerged as promising agents for cancer therapy. They have proven effective as agents for drug and gene delivery [1, 2], biomarker detection [3], image contrast enhancement [4], and tumor ablation via hyperthermia [5–7]. Several first-generation nanoparticles are currently in clinical use or in clinical trials [8, 9]. However, many of these therapies are limited by poor specificity for diseased tissue and rapid clearance from circulation. Incorporating molecular targeting ligands into nanoparticle systems can overcome these limitations.

Targeted nanoparticle systems for cancer therapies can utilize either passive or active targeting. In passive targeting, nanoparticles exploit the leaky vasculature characteristic of tumors to extravasate into the tumor bed; once within the tumor, the nanoparticles are retained due to the poorly organized lymphatic system. This

Rachel S. Riley and Jilian R. Melamed contributed equally to this chapter.

Rachael W. Sirianni and Bahareh Behkam (eds.), *Targeted Drug Delivery: Methods and Protocols*, Methods in Molecular Biology, vol. 1831, https://doi.org/10.1007/978-1-4939-8661-3_11, © Springer Science+Business Media, LLC, part of Springer Nature 2018

phenomenon, which allows nanoparticles to accumulate within cancerous lesions, is known as the enhanced permeability and retention effect [10]. However, passive targeting is limited by a lack of specificity for the disease site versus normal tissue, producing off-target effects associated with conventional therapies. Furthermore, passively targeted particles often fail to accumulate at therapeutic concentrations at the disease site [11]. These limitations can be overcome through active targeting.

Actively targeted nanoparticles are coated with bioactive ligands such as antibodies, peptides, aptamers, or proteins that can be recognized by cancer cells. This allows the nanoparticles to select for cancerous cells over normal cells, reducing off-target effects. Importantly, active targeting greatly enhances cellular uptake of nanoparticles, which is essential for both drug and gene delivery [12]. Antibody targeting has also been shown to improve the efficacy of photothermal tumor ablation [13–17]. A number of antibody-based anticancer therapeutics are already in clinical use [18], further indicating the clinical utility of antibody-targeted nanoparticles. Peptides and proteins have also been explored as a means of nanoparticle targeting; for example, nanoparticles have been conjugated to RGD or VEGF (vascular endothelial growth factor) to promote binding to tumor vasculature [6, 19]. Overall, there is substantial evidence in the literature to support continued development of molecular-targeting strategies for nanoparticle-based therapeutics. For these strategies to succeed, researchers must precisely characterize their systems, including quantification of targeting molecules present on nanoparticle surfaces.

Several methods currently exist to characterize antibody loading on nanoparticles, many of which rely on fluorescent labels conjugated to the antibody [20, 21]. However, these methods are limited in that the fluorescent label may interfere with antibody-binding affinity, which in turn affects characterization precision and targeting efficacy. For example, the fluorophores may be quenched due to close proximity to each other and the nanoparticle surface, resulting in inaccurate measures of loading. Here, we present a solution-based ELISA to directly quantify antibody loading on nanoparticles without the use of fluorescent labels. Briefly, a heterobifunctional poly(ethylene) glycol (PEG) chain is used to provide a link between the antibody and the nanoparticle surface. This PEG molecule contains an N-hydroxysuccinimide (NHS) group at one end that acts as a leaving group to allow the primary amines on targeting agents to react with the PEG molecules. At the other end of the PEG molecule is an orthopyridyl disulfide (OPSS) ligand that facilitates covalent attachment to the nanoparticle surface via a gold-sulfur bond. First, the antibody is PEGylated, and then the entire PEG-antibody conjugate is attached to the nanoparticle surface, as demonstrated in Fig. 1. ELISA characterization is performed after conjugation. This method differs from traditional ELISA methods in that antigens are

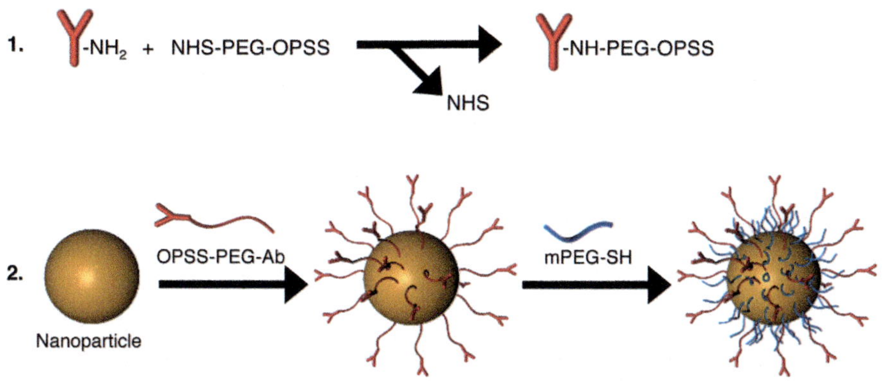

Fig. 1 Antibody conjugation to nanoparticles with a gold surface can be achieved using orthopyridyl disulfide-poly(ethylene glycol)-N-hydroxysuccinimide (OPSS-PEG-NHS) as a linker. First, the antibody reacts with OPSS-PEG-NHS to form a stable amide bond between the PEG and primary amines on the antibody. The OPSS-PEG-Antibody conjugate and mPEG-SH are then bound to the nanoparticles through gold-sulfur bonding mediated by the disulfide or thiol terminus, respectively

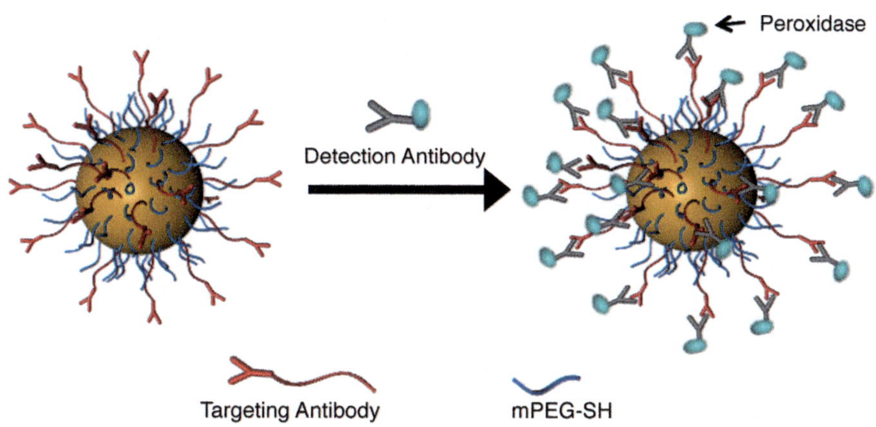

Fig. 2 To quantify targeting antibodies on nanoparticles, a secondary detection antibody is added to the solution. This detection antibody, which binds the primary targeting antibody, is conjugated to horseradish peroxidase to enable colormetric detection and quantification of the primary antibody

not used to capture the primary antibody, as the primary antibody has already been attached to the nanoparticle surface. Secondary antibodies are added directly to the nanoparticle sample, followed by the addition of a color-producing substrate (Figs. 2 and 3). It is important to note that the concentration of nanoparticles in the sample must also be measured in order to accurately quantify the number of antibodies per nanoparticle.

In this protocol, we conjugate mouse-anti-human EGFR to 150 nm diameter silica core/gold shell nanoshells and detect the anti-EGFR with horseradish peroxidase (HRP)-conjugated goat anti-mouse IgG. These selections are meant to serve as model molecules and nanoparticles; the protocols we describe are adaptable to other antibodies and proteins (Fig. 4). For example, we have

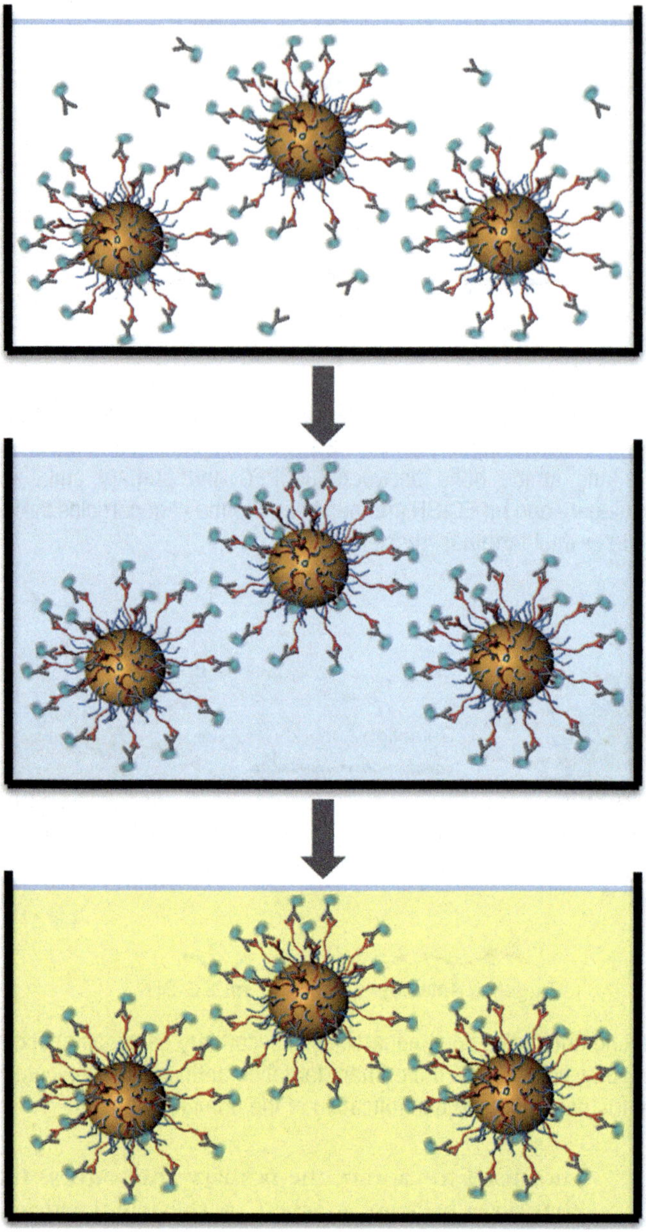

Fig. 3 Steps of the quantification assay. Detection antibodies (gray) that bind targeting antibodies (red) on the nanoparticle surface are added to the solution. Unbound detection antibodies are then removed by centrifugation. Finally, a color changing substrate that reacts with the horseradish peroxidase (blue) on the detection antibodies is added, followed by a stop solution, to produce a color change that enables quantification of the targeting antibodies

previously reported conjugation and quantification of anti-HER2 (human epidermal growth factor receptor 2) antibodies, anti-Frizzled7 antibodies, or VEGF molecules on nanoshells, nanorods, and gold-gold sulfide nanoparticles by this method [6, 13, 16, 17, 22]. Importantly, the concentrations used in this protocol should be optimized for specific antibodies, nanoparticles, and applications.

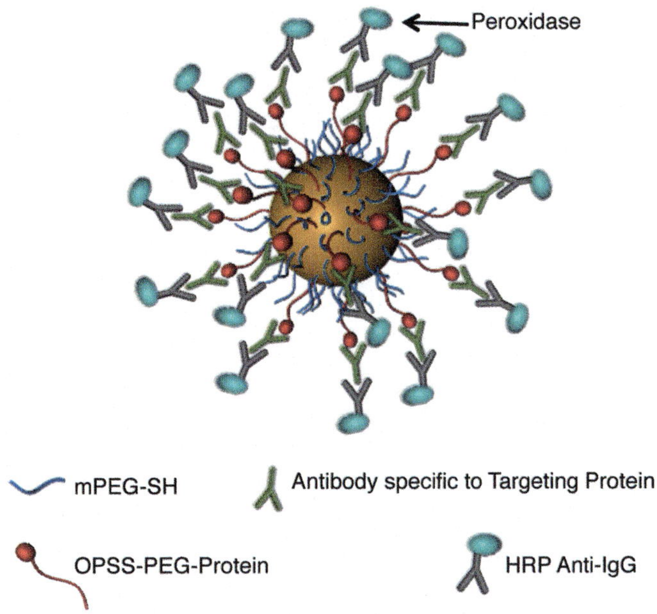

Fig. 4 This method can be modified to detect many types of targeting molecules. For example, if the nanoparticle is coated with a PEG-conjugated protein (red), then a primary antibody specific to that protein (green) is added. Following a centrifugation step to remove unbound antibodies, a secondary horseradish peroxidase-conjugated detection antibody (gray and blue) is added to the sample. The remaining steps of the procedure are performed as described in the methods

2 Materials

Prepare all solutions using ultrapure water unless otherwise noted, and store at appropriate temperatures as indicated below.

2.1 OPSS-PEG-Anti-EGFR (OPSS-PEG-Antibody) Preparation

1. 100 mM sodium bicarbonate solution (pH 8.5, MW 84 g/mol)): Combine 210 mg sodium bicarbonate and 25 mL ultrapure water. Store at room temperature.
2. OPSS-PEG-NHS at desired molecular weight (*see* **Note 1**): Store at −80 °C under argon.
3. Mouse anti-human EGFR antibody (suspended in amine-free buffer): This is referred to as the targeting antibody and concentration is dependent on the chosen targeting antibody. Store at −20 °C for long term, or 4 °C for short term, or in accordance with manufacturer recommendations. Avoid repeated freeze-thaw cycles.

2.2 Antibody-Conjugation to Nanoshells

1. Prepared nanoshells: Place 10 mL nanoshell solution into microcentrifuge tubes in 1 mL batches. Centrifuge for 5 min at 2000 × *g*. Aspirate the supernatant and resuspend in ultrapure water to an optical density (OD) of 1.5.

2. 1 mM mPEG-SH (methoxy PEG thiol) at desired molecular weight (*see* **Note 2**): Store mPEG-SH as a lyophilized powder under argon at −80 °C. Prepare fresh 1 mM solution in ultrapure water for each use.
3. OPSS-PEG-Anti-EGFR (OPSS-PEG-Antibody): prepare as described in the Methods (Subheading 3.1).

2.3 Solution-Based ELISA

1. 1× PBS (phosphate-buffered saline): Store at room temperature.
2. 2 M Sulfuric Acid: Make a large stock solution by slowly adding 12.5 mL 18 M sulfuric acid (MW 98.08 g/mol) to 100 mL ultrapure water. Use caution when handling acids. Store at room temperature.
3. HRP-conjugated goat anti-mouse IgG: This is referred to as the detection antibody. Prepare as described in Subheading 3.3.
4. 3% BSA in PBS: Weigh 600 mg BSA (bovine serum albumin) and combine with 20 mL PBS. Vortex until completely dissolved. Store at 4 °C.
5. Phosphate Citrate Buffer: Combine one phosphate citrate buffer capsule with 100 mL H_2O and vortex thoroughly. Make fresh immediately prior to use.
6. TMB substrate: Combine 2 TMB (3,3′,5,5′-tetramthylbenzidine) tablets with 20 mL fresh phosphate citrate buffer and vortex thoroughly to dissolve tablets. Make fresh immediately prior to use.
7. OPSS-PEG-Anti-EGFR (OPSS-PEG-Antibody)-conjugated nanoshells: Prepare as described in the Methods (Subheading 3.2).

3 Methods

3.1 Prepare OPSS-PEG-Anti-EGFR (OPSS-PEG-Antibody)

Perform this procedure on ice.

1. Suspend targeting antibody in buffer recommended by the manufacturer to desired concentration. The recommendation for mouse anti-human EGFR (for this protocol) is 1 mg/mL in 1× PBS.
2. Thaw OPSS-PEG-NHS on ice. Dilute the OPSS-PEG-NHS in sodium bicarbonate buffer (*see* **Note 3)** to a concentration such that the solution (in Subheading 3.1, **step 3**) will be at 1 part PEG to 9 parts antibody following addition of the antibody. At this time, the molar ratio of PEG to antibody will be 2:1. Once the PEG is in buffer, proceed quickly to the next step.
3. Add 1 part PEG to every 9 parts antibody solution (for example, 12 μL OPSS-PEG-NHS plus 100 μL targeting antibody) (*see* **Note 4**). Allow the reaction to proceed 2–8 h at 4 °C.

4. Either use OPSS-PEG-Antibody immediately for conjugation to nanoparticles or aliquot and store at −80 °C (*see* **Note 5**).

3.2 Attach OPSS-PEG-Anti-EGFR (OPSS-PEG-Antibody) to Nanoshells

1. If frozen, thaw previously prepared OPSS-PEG-Anti-EGFR on ice.
2. Resuspend nanoshells to OD 1.5 in ultrapure water, if obtained at a concentration other than this. Label two 15 mL conical tubes (*see* **Note 6**), for Treatments 1 and 2, respectively, representing the antibody-conjugated nanoshells (treatment group) and nanoshells containing only PEG (control group). For Treatment 1, place 5 mL nanoshells into the tube, followed by the addition of 4 μL OPSS-PEG-Anti-EGFR (*see* **Note 7**). For Treatment 2, add 5 mL nanoshells only at OD 1.5. Vortex both samples and gently rock at 4 °C for 4 h.
3. Backfill both treatment solutions with 5 μM mPEG-SH by adding 25 μL of 1 mM mPEG-SH for every 5 mL of nanoshells at OD 1.5. Allow reaction to rock gently at 4 °C overnight (*see* **Note 8**).
4. After overnight conjugation, centrifuge samples in 1 mL batches one time at 2000 × *g* for 5 min (*see* **Note 9**). Resuspend in milli-Q water to 1.5 mL total volume for each of the two treatments. This will remove any unbound PEG and antibody molecules. Equalize OD across groups by diluting as necessary.

3.3 Incubation with Detection Antibody

1. Pre-coat six microcentrifuge tubes with 1 mL 3% BSA in PBS (PBSA) for 30 min at room temperature, then remove the PBSA (*see* **Note 10**). Place 450 μL of Treatment 1 into each of three tubes, and place 450 μL of Treatment 2 into each of three tubes.
2. Prepare detection antibody at 100 μg/mL in PBSA and add 50 μL to each of the six tubes. Vortex and allow to react for 1 h at room temperature. Store the antibody on ice for the remainder of the assay (*see* **Note 11**). Figure 2 displays a schematic of detection antibodies binding to targeting antibodies on a nanoparticle surface.
3. Centrifuge all samples at 2000 × *g* for 5 min, remove the supernatant, and resuspend in 3% PBSA. Repeat 2–3 times. After each spin, be sure to add the exact volume of PBSA that was taken out (*see* **Note 12**). The purpose of this step is to remove from the solution any detection antibodies that are not bound specifically to the targeting antibodies on the nanoparticle surface. This step is depicted visually in Fig. 3.
4. Remove 100 μL of each sample and place into six new tubes. These will be used to quantify targeting antibodies bound to nanoshells. Place another 200 μL of each sample into six disposable UV-vis cuvettes for later nanoshell quantification (*see* **Note 13**).

5. Centrifuge the remaining 200 μL in the original six sample tubes and place 100 μL of the supernatant into another set of six new tubes (*see* **Note 14**). These samples will serve as a control for any background signal.

3.4 Preliminary Enzyme Assay

The preliminary assay is used to determine the optimal sample dilution that will provide the best reading.

1. For the preliminary assay, use the A batches (1-A-, 1-A+, 2-A-, 2-A+). Remove 50 μL of each of the four samples and place each into a tube with 450 μL PBS. This is the first dilution. Continue dilutions for all four A samples for 10X, 100X, and 1000X dilutions in PBS (*see* **Note 15**). Once diluted, transfer 70 μL of each dilution into a separate tube (*see* **Note 16**).
2. Make fresh phosphate citrate buffer by mixing 1 tablet with 100 mL H_2O and vortex until completely dissolved. The buffer must be used within 30 min.
3. Make TMB solution by mixing 2 TMB tablets with 20 mL of the fresh phosphate citrate buffer. Add 700 μL TMB solution to each tube containing 70 μL of each dilution (from **step 1**) and develop in the dark for 15 min (*see* **Note 17**). After the waiting period, the solution will appear blue.
4. To stop the reaction, add 200 μL of 2 M sulfuric acid to each tube. Centrifuge at 500 × *g* for 5 min to remove any large aggregates and transfer 850 μL of the supernatant to UV-vis cuvettes, labeled appropriately (*see* **Note 18**). After adding the stop solution, the color will change to yellow (Fig. 3). Note that Fig. 3 does not display all of the transfer and centrifugation steps leading up to this point in order to maintain visual simplicity.
5. Measure A^{450} of each dilution cuvette and note the dilution that provides a reading between 0.5–1 for the "+" samples (*see* **Note 19**).

3.5 Performing True Enzyme Assay

1. Use the optimal dilution determined by the preliminary assay to prepare samples B and C of each of the four treatments by repeating Subheading 3.4 (*see* **Note 20**), as outlined below.
2. Prepare the detection antibody standard curve solutions. Dilute the detection antibody stock previously prepared (Subheading 3.3, **step 2**) over the following range, and continue diluting 2× until there are 10 standard dilutions to form the standard curve:
   (a) 10 μL HRP-AM +9.99 mL 1× PBS.
   (b) 500 μL of dilution 1 + 500 μL 1× PBS.
   (c) 500 μL of dilution 2 + 500 μL 1× PBS.
   (d) Continue 2× dilutions.

3. In microcentrifuge tubes, add 70 μL of each diluted sample and all standard samples (*see* **Note 16**).
4. Prepare a fresh TMB solution by combining two TMB tablets and 20 mL of fresh phosphate-citrate buffer (Subheading 3.4, **steps 2** and **3**).
5. Measure A^{450} for B and C samples by repeating Subheading 3.4, **steps 4** and **5**.
6. Calculate original detection antibody concentration in each treatment group.

3.6 Quantification of Nanoshells and Bound Antibodies

1. Add 300 μL ultrapure water to the cuvettes containing nanoshells from Subheading 3.3, **step 4**. Mix cuvette contents well (*see* **Note 21**) and measure the peak nanoshell absorbance.
2. Determine the original and final nanoshell concentration in each sample using the measured absorbance and known extinction coefficient (*see* **Note 22**).
3. Subtract the two sample groups (+ and −) and calculate the concentration of antibody present in the solution by comparison against the standard curve of the detection antibody. Divide the antibody present in each sample by the number of nanoshells present in each sample to quantify the number of targeting molecules bound per nanoshell. If it is desirable to report loading in terms of surface coverage, calculate the surface area of the nanoparticles. Using this data, divide the antibody content by the total nanoshell area, which gives the final amount of antibody bound to the nanoshells in pmol/cm^2.

4 Notes

1. Typical OPSS-PEG-NHS molecular weight is 2000 Da. However, this can be adjusted from 2000 to 5000 Da, depending on the specific nanoparticle design.
2. Typical mPEG-SH molecular weight is 5000 Da. This can be modified for the specific application. Recommended molecular weight is within the 2000–10,000 Da range.
3. Sodium Bicarbonate with pH 8.5 is used because the higher pH accelerates the reaction. Make sure final pH is 8.5–9.0, because the antibody is most likely stored at pH 7.0. Make sure OPSS-PEG-NHS is completely thawed and at room temperature prior to opening the bottle. If the vial is still cold, condensation may accumulate which will degrade the PEG. OPSS-PEG-NHS is a PEG derivative used to modify materials via thiol groups. Once suspended in buffer, the NHS groups have a short half-life, so work as quickly as possible.

4. One part PEG to every nine parts antibody is ideal but depends on antibody stock concentration. It may be helpful to add the PEG solution to the antibody in a drop-wise fashion.
5. PEGylated targeting molecules may be dialyzed at this point to purify the sample, if desired.
6. If samples are sticking to the sides of the conical tubes, use glass scintillation vials during conjugation instead of plastic conical tubes.
7. For this step, use 4 μL OPSS-PEG-Anti-EGFR per 5 mL of OD 1.5 nanoshells. This represents adding 1500 antibody molecules per nanoshell. Note that excess PEGylated targeting molecules are used in the reaction since less than 100% of the molecules will attach to the nanoparticle surface. This ratio may need to be altered if different volumes or concentrations of materials are being used than described in this protocol, or if the nanoparticle size or shape is different. For example, we typically add only 150 antibodies per nanoparticle in conjugation reactions for 35 nm diameter nanoparticles.
8. To make the mPEG-SH solution, weigh 5 kDa mPEG-SH carefully by weighing the PEG storage vial before and after PEG is removed, in addition to weighing the PEG in the vial in which it will be diluted. The recommended final PEG concentration in the nanoparticle solution is 5 μM, but a range of 2.5–10 μM has been used satisfactorily. It may be necessary to adjust the volume of PEG added for different concentrations and/or types of nanoparticles.
9. Centrifugation times may need to be adjusted, but it is recommended not to exceed 2500 × *g* speeds. When working with small volumes, samples can be purified by centrifugation. For larger volumes, it may be easier/faster to purify by transflow filtration.
10. Pre-coating tubes with PBSA is not necessary, but is a cautionary step to prevent particles from sticking to the sides of the tubes. Ensure that the pre-coated tubes are dry before proceeding. If preferred, scintillation vials may be used. It is recommended to label microcentrifuge tubes by letter and number (i.e., 1–A, 1–B, 1–C, 2–A, 2–B, 2–C).
11. To prepare the detection antibody (HRP-AM; HRP goat anti-mouse IgG) at 100 μg/mL in PBSA from a 1 mg/mL antibody stock, combine 360 μL PBSA with 40 μL stock. If the assay yields high background, allow the reaction to proceed for 8 h at 4C rather than 1 h at room temperature. The 100 μg/mL antibody solution will be required later, so ensure that it is kept on ice or at 4 °C.
12. The centrifugation details should be adjusted to form a pellet accordingly. It is recommended to aspirate 350 μL of the

supernatant after each spin and add in exactly 350 μL PBSA prior to the next spin.

13. The tubes should be labeled 1–A+, 1–B+, 1–C+, 2–A+, 2-B+, 2–C+.
14. The tubes should be labeled 1–A–, 1–B–, 1–C–, 2–A–, 2–B–, 2–C–. Keep all tubes until the assay is completed. Later, HRP quantification on the + and – samples will be performed by subtracting their respective HRP content. By doing this, background noise will be eliminated and you can determine the quantity of HRP present on the nanoparticles.
15. The first standard dilution is diluted 10× with 50 μL sample and 450 μL PBS. The next dilution (100×) will have 50 μL of the first dilution plus 450 μL PBS; repeat to create a 1000× dilution. To avoid confusion, tubes should be labeled 1A–10, 1A–100, 1A–1000, 1A + 10, 1A + 100, 1A + 1000.
16. The 70 μL of each dilution is used for the reaction. Tubes should be labeled 1A–10*, 1A-100*, etc. accordingly.
17. It is important to add the TMB solution to samples in the same order that sulfuric acid will be added after the 15 min reaction time so that the reaction time for all tubes is equivalent. After adding TMB solution, place the samples in the dark for the 15 min development.
18. By centrifuging for 5 min at 500 × *g*, any clumps will pellet. This is not a necessary step, but is precautionary to improve reading accuracy.
19. Ideally, the A^{450} will be between 0.5 and 1 for all the "+" samples and the reading for the "–" samples will be quite low. Usually, the 100× dilution is best.
20. This is the same procedure as Subheading 3.4, **steps 1–4**, but for B and C samples of both treatment groups. It is recommended to label these according to Treatment, +/–, and B and C. For example, 1B–100, 1B + 100, 2B–100, 2B + 100, and the same for C samples.
21. Do not vortex the cuvette samples, as this will create bubbles that will interfere with the absorbance measurements. Instead, gently pipette the sample. Measure the absorbance from 1100 to 400 nm.
22. Beer's Law states that $A = \varepsilon cl$ where A is the nanoparticle absorbance at its peak resonance wavelength as measured by a spectrophotometer, ε is the extinction coefficient, c is the concentration of the nanoparticles, and l is the path length of the sample. The extinction coefficient for nanoshells depends on their exact core diameter and shell thickness, as discussed by Erickson and Tunnell [23]. As readers adapt this protocol to other nanoparticle types, they should confirm the extinction coefficient of their material

and calculate the nanoparticle concentration according to Beer's law. For nanoshells, an optical density of 1 corresponds to approximately 3×10^9 nanoshells/mL.

References

1. Jensen SA, Day ES, Ko CH, Hurley LA, Luciano JP, Kouri FM, Merkel TJ, Luthi AJ, Patel PC, Cutler JI, Daniel WL, Scott AW, Rotz MW, Meade TJ, Giljohann DA, Mirkin CA, Stegh AH (2013) Spherical nucleic acid nanoparticle conjugates as an RNAi-based therapy for glioblastoma. Sci Transl Med 5(209):209ra152 *equal contribution
2. Deng ZJ, Morton SW, Ben-Akiva E, Dreaden EC, Shopsowitz KE, Hammond PT (2013) Layer-by-layer nanoparticles for systemic codelivery of an anticancer drug and siRNA for potential triple-negative breast cancer treatment. ACS Nano 7(11):9571–9584
3. Zheng D, Seferos DS, Giljohann DA, Patel PC, Mirkin CA (2009) Aptamer nano-flares for molecular detection in living cells. Nano Lett 9(9):3258–3261
4. Kircher MF, de la Zerda A, Jokerst JV, Zavaleta CL, Kempen PJ, Mittra E, Pitter K, Huang R, Campos C, Habte F, Sinclair R, Brennan CW, Mellinghoff IK, Holland EC, Gambhir SS (2012) A brain tumor molecular imaging strategy using a new triple-modality MRI-photoacoustic-Raman nanoparticle. Nat Med 18(5):829–835
5. Hirsch LR, Stafford RJ, Bankson JA, Sershen SR, Rivera B, Price RE, Hazle JD, Halas NJ, West JL (2003) Nanoshell-mediated near-infrared thermal therapy of tumors under magnetic resonance guidance. Proc Natl Acad Sci U S A 100(23):13549–13554
6. Day ES, Zhang L, Thompson PA, Zawaski JA, Kaffes CC, Gaber MW, Blaney SM, West JL (2012) Vascular-targeted photothermal therapy of an orthotopic murine glioma model. Nanomedicine (Lond) 7(8):1133–1148
7. Day ES, Thompson PA, Zhang L, Lewinski NA, Ahmed N, Drezek RA, Blaney SM, West JL (2011) Nanoshell-mediated photothermal therapy improves survival in a murine glioma model. J Neuro-Oncol 104(1):55–63
8. Schütz CA, Juillerat-Jeanneret L, Mueller H, Lynch I, Riediker M (2013) Therapeutic nanoparticles in clinics and under clinical evaluation. Nanomedicine (Lond) 8(3):449–467
9. Zhang L, Gu FX, Chan JM, Wang AZ, Langer RS, Farokhzad OC (2008) Nanoparticles in medicine: therapeutic applications and developments. Clin Pharmacol Ther 83(5):761–769
10. Matsumura Y, Maeda H (1986) A new concept for macromolecular therapeutics in cancer chemotherapy: mechanism of tumoritropic accumulation of proteins and the antitumor agent smancs. Cancer Res 46(12 Part 1):6387–6392
11. Huynh NT, Roger E, Lautram N, Benoît J-P, Passirani C (2010) The rise and rise of stealth nanocarriers for cancer therapy: passive versus active targeting. Nanomedicine (Lond) 5(9):1415–1433
12. Byrne JD, Betancourt T, Brannon-Peppas L (2008) Active targeting schemes for nanoparticle systems in cancer therapeutics. Adv Drug Deliv Rev 60(15):1615–1626
13. Day ES, Bickford LR, Slater JH, Riggall NS, Drezek RA, West JL (2010) Antibody-conjugated gold-gold sulfide nanoparticles as multifunctional agents for imaging and therapy of breast cancer. Int J Nanomedicine 5:445–454
14. El-Sayed IH, Huang X, El-Sayed MA (2006) Selective laser photo-thermal therapy of epithelial carcinoma using anti-EGFR antibody conjugated gold nanoparticles. Cancer Lett 239(1):129–135
15. Loo C, Lowery A, Halas N, West J, Drezek R (2005) Immunotargeted nanoshells for integrated cancer imaging and therapy. Nano Lett 5(4):709–711
16. Lowery AR, Gobin AM, Day ES, Halas NJ, West JL (2006) Immunonanoshells for targeted photothermal ablation of tumor cells. Int J Nanomedicine 1(2):149–154
17. Steichen SD, Caldorera-Moore M, Peppas NA (2013) A review of current nanoparticle and targeting moieties for the delivery of cancer therapeutics. Eur J Pharm Sci 48(3):416–427
18. Rostro-Kohanloo BC, Bickford LR, Payne CM, Day ES, Anderson LJE, Zhong M, Lee S, Mayer KM, Zal T, Adam L, Dinney CPN, Drezek RA, West JL, Hafner JH (2009) The stabilization and targeting of surfactant-synthesized gold nanorods. Nanotechnology 20(43):434005
19. Pasqualini R, Koivenuen E, Ruoslahti E (1997) Alpha v integrins as receptors for tumor targeting by circulating ligands. Nat Biotechnol 15(6):542–546
20. Kumar S, Aaron J, Sokolov K (2008) Directional conjugation of antibodies to nanoparticles for synthesis of multiplexed optical contrast agents with both delivery and targeting moieties. Nat Protoc 3(2):314–320

21. Kocbek P, Obermajer N, Cegnar M, Kos J, Kristl J (2007) Targeting cancer cells using PLGA nanoparticles surface modified with monoclonal antibody. J Control Release 120(1-2):18–26
22. Riley RS, Day ES (2017) Frizzled7 antibody-functionalized nanoshells enable multivalent binding for Wnt signaling inhibition in triple negative breast cancer cells. Small 13(26): 1700544
23. Erickson TA, Tunnell JW (2010) Gold nanoshells in biomedical applications. In: Kumar SSRC (ed) Nanotechnologies for the life sciences, vol 3. Wiley, Weinheim, pp 1–44

Chapter 12

Tunable Collagen Microfluidic Platform to Study Nanoparticle Transport in the Tumor Microenvironment

Matthew R. DeWitt and M. Nichole Rylander

Abstract

This chapter describes the motivation and protocol for creating a perfused 3D microfluidic in vitro platform representative of the tumor microenvironment to study nanoparticle transport. The cylindrical vascularized tumor platform described consists of a central endothelialized microchannel surrounded by a collagen hydrogel matrix containing cancer cells. This system can be employed to investigate key nanoparticle transport events in the tumor such as extravasation, diffusion within the extracellular matrix, and nanoparticle uptake. This easily manufactured tumor platform can be used for novel nanoparticle refinement focused on optimizing nanoparticle features such as size, shape, and functionalization method. This can yield ideal nanoparticles with properties that facilitate increased transport within the tumor microenvironment, leading to more effective nanoparticle-based treatments for cancer including nanoparticle-based drug delivery systems.

Key words Tumor engineering, Microfluidics, Nanoparticle transport, Tumor microenvironment, Drug delivery

1 Introduction

The ultimate goal of nanoparticle-based cancer therapy is to deliver a sufficient concentration of particles to a targeted tumor site, resulting in high treatment efficacy with minimal systemic toxicity [1]. Nanoparticles have shown promise in enhancing localized delivery of drug payloads at effective concentrations to achieve therapeutic benefit, highlighting their potential as drug-delivery systems [2, 3]. Nanoparticles have also been utilized as antennas to direct external energy sources to deliver therapeutic heat to ablate tumors from within [4–7]. The Oncological application of nanoparticles is based on harnessing the unique pathophysiology of tumors to result in passive nanoparticle targeting and customizing features of nanoparticles to develop active targeting strategies that enhance specificity of particles to the tumor [1]. Novel nanomedicines made of a variety of materials are currently studied

Rachael W. Sirianni and Bahareh Behkam (eds.), *Targeted Drug Delivery: Methods and Protocols*, Methods in Molecular Biology, vol. 1831, https://doi.org/10.1007/978-1-4939-8661-3_12, © Springer Science+Business Media, LLC, part of Springer Nature 2018

including polymers [8, 9], magnetic materials [10, 11], gold [12–15], and a wide range of carbon nanoparticles [6, 16–18]. Rigorous and established preclinical models are needed to optimize these novel particles in the early stages of research and development, which will lead to improved therapeutic efficacy and functionality in future cancer treatments.

The efficacy of nanoparticle-based tumor therapies relies on the ability of the particles to make their way from a systemic delivery to targeted tumor cells [19]. Along this path, particles encounter a variety of different barriers to transport that regulate the ultimate particle concentration at their targeted site. The pro-angiogenic environment of the tumor, which is hypothesized to occur as the result of a rapidly growing vascular bed that feeds the expanding tumor, is known to result in a leaky vasculature, leading to localized transvascular nanoparticle transport [20]. The leakiness and lack of a functioning lymphatic bed leads to the well-known enhanced permeability and retention (EPR) effect [21, 22]. This phenomenon results in passive targeting for accumulation of particles <400 nm into the tumor [23, 24]. Tumors were shown to have an order of magnitude larger endothelial pore size than healthy tissue, which corresponded to selective nanoparticle extravasation [25]. Nanoparticle transvascular transport is an important first step in nanoparticle tumor transport and can be modeled as a flux across a semi-permeable membrane down a pressure gradient and diffusion down a concentration gradient, which allows for coupling of experimental and in silico models [26]. Increasing nanoparticle extravasation at the tumor site should be studied in the early stages of nanoparticle formulations to develop more targeted and less toxic treatments [27].

After translocation across the tumor capillaries nanoparticles must travel through the tumor interstitium to the targeted tumor cells. In many cases, the tumor interstitium is known to be predominantly composed of collagen and other elastic fibers along with a matrix of extracellular biomacromolecules that together form an extracellular matrix (ECM) [28]. Additionally, the high interstitial pressure often present in the tumor microenvironment can serve as an added hindrance to NP transport due to the lack of a driving pressure gradient from the vasculature to the lymphatic bed [29]. Previous research has shown even with elimination of pressure gradients, penetration of macromolecules is hindered in the tumor interstitium resulting in nanoparticle transport exclusively by diffusion as particles larger than approximately 5 nm are known to undergo mass transport by diffusion once inside the tumor [30–32]. The properties of nanoparticles including shape, size, surface charge, and solubility have been shown to affect their interaction with the ECM and can ultimately influence their mass transport [33, 34]. Thus, novel nanoparticle therapies should be studied in a controlled environment before costly animal models are utilized as shown in Fig. 1a to determine nanoparticle extravasation and diffusion in the tumor.

Specific uptake of nanotherapeutics is another significant consideration when designing nanoparticles to achieve maximum therapeutic efficacy with minimal toxicity [35]. It has been found that nanoparticle shape and size can play important roles in the process of internalization and therefore must be considered for optimization [36]. Current work has utilized tools such as flow activated cell sorting (FACS) and confocal imaging to study the dynamics of cellular uptake of nanoparticles [37]. However, many of these studies are accomplished in 2D cell culture models and therefore

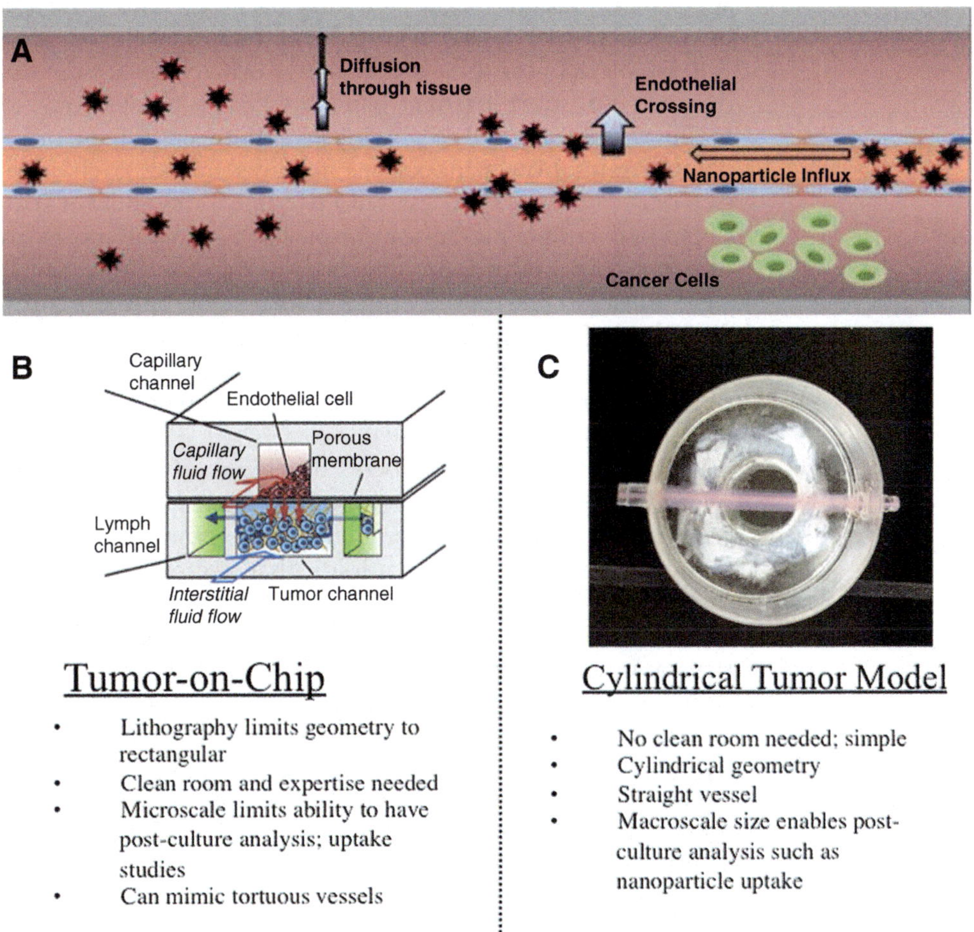

Fig. 1 In vitro modeling of the tumor microenvironment for nanoparticle transport studies. (**a**) Depiction of key transport barriers in the tumor microenvironment including extravasation of nanoparticles across a leaky endothelium, and diffusion in the ECM. (**b**) Tumor-on-chip platforms used to study nanoparticle transport and its key features [53]. (**c**) Image of cylindrical tumor platform described in this protocol with a central microvessel filled with fluorescent nanoparticles

may not accurately model the uptake process. Internalization or uptake of particles represents the last transport barrier nanoparticles must overcome in order to achieve therapeutic efficacy, and the role of uptake in the treatment process cannot be overlooked. While there is a broad research field focused on optimizing nanoparticle features for increased circulation or extravasation, these factors may compound other transport processes and therefore should be studied in parallel with particle uptake [38].

Many novel therapeutic and diagnostic nanoparticles have been developed and optimized utilizing in vitro studies; however, there has been relatively minimal success in their in vivo translation. These static in vitro models do not mimic transport processes that nanoparticles encounter in the tumor microenvironment and are primarily used to understand how particle features affect uptake by affecting their interaction with cell membrane by endocytosis. Animal models can provide a framework for understanding the dynamic transport barriers nanoparticles face, but they can be highly variable and fail to provide an easily accessible platform that demonstrates how nanoparticle features impact each individual step of the transport process. Additionally, the significant cost associated with animal models can be prohibitive in parametric analysis of nanoparticle feature optimization for increased efficacy [39]. In vitro 3D cultures such as multicellular spheroids can provide a functional platform for studying particle penetration into avascular regions of tumors, but they do not recreate the transport boundary of extravasation and do not necessarily contain the physiologic fluid flow seen in tumors [40].

The integration of protocols developed in tissue engineering, microfluidics, and cancer biology has spurred the field of tumor engineering [41–43]. Tumor engineering is the creation of biomimetic microfluidic-based scaffolds that recreate the native 3D tumor microenvironment within a highly controllable cell culture system predominantly utilizing collagen or a mixture of proteins that make up the tumor ECM [44]. These systems have primarily been utilized and developed to study key events in tumor progression such as angiogenesis, to access drug efficacy, and evaluate novel therapies [45–48]. Conventional polydimethylsiloxane (PDMS) microfluidic platforms allow for precise control of chemical and nutrient gradients within a micro-scale system and can permit the study of cellular migration and remodeling of ECM during tumor progression [49]. Additionally, these in vitro systems have been designed to enable high-resolution visualization of cell events in tumor progression such as angiogenesis, tumor hypoxia, and metastasis in real time in a non-destructive manner [50, 51].

Recently, groups have begun to utilize tumor engineering to study nanoparticle transport. Ng et al. have developed PDMS-Matrigel microfluidic devices to study nanoparticle penetration in a 3D matrix under varied pressure gradients and fluid flows, highlighting the importance of convective flow and showing the steric hindrance from ECM components on nanoparticle transport [52]. However, this model does not include an endothelial barrier, which is an important transport barrier that should be considered when optimizing nanoparticles to increase aggregation in the tumor. More recently, Kwak et al. have developed a tumor-microenvironment-on-chip platform to simulate transport of particles and were able to show the size-dependent transport of nanoparticles within a tumor microenvironment that has physiologic flow. Their platform is shown in Fig. 1b where lithographic techniques are used to create endothelial and lymphatic vessels with a central area containing a bulk collagen hydrogel to study nanoparticle transport [53]. However, the PDMS-based platform utilized does not contain a sufficient quantity of cells to allow for Fluorescence-activated cell sorting (FACS) determining uptake of particles by cells within the system and therefore cannot be used to draw conclusions on nanoparticle properties that affect uptake in a 3D microenvironment. Additionally, the lithography techniques used to create these platforms cannot produce a cylindrical vessel, which is important for flow profile estimation and for simplifying in silico modeling of transport to a 1D axisymmetric system. Finally, the need for a cleanroom to create these PDMS-based platforms can be prohibitive for researchers.

Here, we present a protocol for a high-throughput 3D microfluidic engineered tumor platform that recreates the tumor microenvironment through the incorporation of a cylindrical endothelialized microchannel within a collagen 3D matrix containing human cancer cells in order to study nanoparticle transport as shown in Fig. 1c. The optically clear platform allows for high imaging resolution without the need for a cleanroom microlithography and the size of the platform allows for post-culture recovery and analysis. This is the first use of a cylindrical model of the tumor microenvironment containing an endothelialized microvessel to measure nanoparticle transport at the tissue and cellular level, and a comparison of this system Fig. 1c with tumor-on-a-chip platforms is seen in Fig. 1b. The system can be utilized to quantify transvascular transport and transport within the ECM using particles delivered via the central microchannel. A fluorescence microscope can be used to track intensity of particle translocation from the central vessel to the collagen ECM matrix containing cancer cells over time. Lastly, this system can be used to study the last step of nanoparticle transport in tumors, cellular uptake as the system enables post-culture analysis. Ultimately, novel 3D cell culture models such as the one described in this protocol should be used during development stages of nanoparticle design. The use of these models will allow for optimization of particles based on predicted in vivo transport barriers, and lessening of the disparity between in vitro and in vivo efficacy.

2 Materials

The materials and cell culture procedures are specified according to the cells utilized in this study. Please prepare all cell solutions according to cell source guidelines. Prepare and store all reagents at room temperature (unless indicated otherwise). Follow all waste disposal protocols especially concerning nanoparticle-generated waste.

2.1 Construction of Tumor Platform and Endothelial Cell Preconditioning

1. 35 mm glass bottom petri dish with 10–14 mm glass diameter.
2. Fluorinated Ethylene Propylene (FEP) tubing 1/4″ ID × 3/8″ OD.
3. Silicone 1/16″ ID × 1/8 OD″ tubing.
4. 60 mL Syringes with luer connection.
5. Programmable Syringe Pump.
6. 70% Ethanol in DI water.
7. Female and Male luer ×1/16″ barb adapter.
8. 22G 2″n and 0.5″ blunt needles.
9. AEF Filter serving as bubble trap such as Pall Supor AEF Filter.
10. Endothelial cell culture media. Store at 4 °C.
11. Cancer cell culture media (DMEM with 10% FBS, 1% Pen-Strep). Store at 4 °C.
12. 0.5% Trypsin/EDTA. Store at 4 °C.
13. 500 mL Erlenmeyer flask with 3-way stopper.
14. 1% polyethyleneimine (PEI) in dH_2O. Store at 4 °C.
15. 0.1% glutaraldehyde in dH_2O. Store at 4 °C.
16. 3 Syringes, 3 mL capacity.
17. 18G Needle.
18. Metal spatula for mixing in tubes.
19. MDA-MB-231; ATCC.
20. Telomerase Immortalized Microvascular Endothelial Cells (TIME) stably transfected to produce GFP; ATCC.
21. Polydimethylsiloxane (PDMS).

2.2 Nanoparticle Imaging and Post Culture Analysis

1. Fluorescent polystyrene nanoparticles, 50 nm. Store at 4 °C.
2. Microscope with environmental chamber capable of temperature and CO_2 control.
3. Phosphate-Buffered Saline (PBS). Store at 4 °C.
4. ImageJ (NIH) or other image-processing software.
5. Collagenase Type 3- Filtered. Store at 4 °C.
6. Flow Activated Cell Sorter.
7. 2–5 mL Round-Bottom Polystyrene Tubes.

3 Methods

Carry out all procedures at room temperature in a sterilized environment such as a biological safety cabinet unless otherwise stated.

3.1 Platform and Accessory Preparation and Sterilization

1. Cut silicone tubing for input (~ 0.2 m) bubble trap (~0.05 m), and output (~0.15 m), as seen in Fig. 2a.
2. Arrange fluid flow lines including in line bubble trap as seen in Fig. 2a.
3. Autoclave all tubing, syringes, and needles.
4. Sterilize all valves and connectors by submerging them in 70% ethanol under ultraviolet light in a biosafety cabinet for 1 h; allow drying overnight in sterile environment.
5. Clean petri dishes with 70% ethanol, ensuring imaging glass is clean and secure.
6. Cut FEP tubing slightly longer than the petri dish (+0.5 cm) and clean FEP tubing and PDMS needle guides in 70% ethanol and UV for 1 h; allow drying overnight (*see* **Note 1**).

3.2 Experimental System Setup

1. Plasma treat the cut FEP tubing held in a petri dish without PDMS needle guides for 4 min to enable collagen attachment to surface through surface activation in air plasma under vacuum on high utilizing plasma cleaner such as Harrick Plasma PDC-32G.
2. Insert PDMS needle guides and use soldering iron to heat shrink FEP tubing around needle guides until firmly secure, as seen in Fig. 2b.
3. Use a 3 mL syringe with a 22G needle to inject 1% polyethyleneimine in dH_2O into FEP tubing capped with PDMS needle guides and incubate at 37 °C for 15 min.
4. Vacuum PEI solution out of system and inject sterile 0.1% glutaraldehyde in dH_2O into FEP tubing; incubate at 37 °C for 30 min.
5. Carefully remove glutaraldehyde and wash (2×) with dH_2O at room temperature, removing residual glutaraldehyde and ensuring a dry surface by forcing water out with empty syringe all within a biological safety cabinet. The surface is now treated, has active carboxyl groups to interact with collagen, and is ready to be filled.
6. During surface treatment of FEP make sure to wipe down incubators and syringe pump with 70% ethanol to ensure sterile environment for 72 h preconditioning.
7. Place sterile syringes, stoppers, tubing, and valves in biological safety hood.

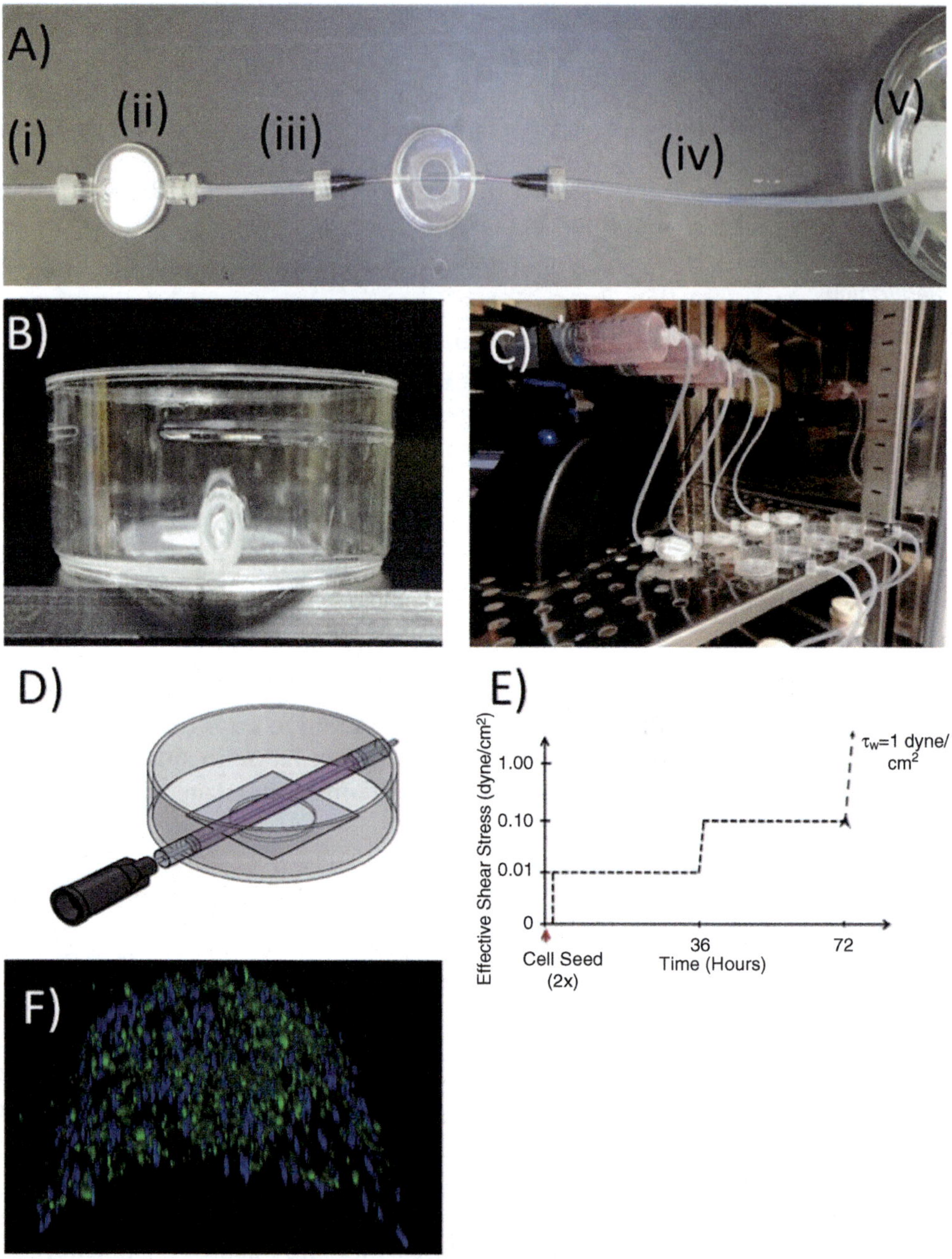

Fig. 2 Protocol for forming and conditioning 3D cylindrical tumor model. (**a**) Flow setup with (i) input line connected to Syringe on Syringe pump, (ii) bubble trap, (iii) 2 in. line to connect the platform input, (iv) output line connected to output of platform, and (v) collection flask. (**b**) Side image of platform showing central hole in PDMS needle guides used to direct and hold 22G needles (**c**) Image of setup showing ability to have multiple platforms in-line (**d**) Depiction of collagen hydrogel polymerization with 22G needle in place to form central cylindrical microvessel (**e**) 72 h Preconditioning flow profile where flow rates are adjusted to achieve plotted wall shear stress in central vessel. (**f**) Fluorescent image of confluent and aligned endothelium on central microvessel after 72 h flow protocol

8. Connect tubing to syringes and fill syringe with media using the tubing submerged in media, and prime syringes to remove air and visible bubbles.
9. Attach male luer barb adapter to end of media tubing as seen in Fig. 2a i.
10. Prepare collection reservoirs by attaching 3-hole stopper on Erlenmeyer flask and insert tubing into the flask. Attach a male luer barb adapter to the end of tubing, then attach 22G needle to male luer barb and place in incubator as seen in Fig. 2a iv (*see* **Note 2**).
11. Secure syringes on syringe pump, maintaining the sterility of tubing and syringes while placing pump with loaded syringes into an incubator. Set up the tubing and syringes in parallel as seen in Fig. 2c to enable high throughput.

3.3 Collagen Hydrogel Microchannel Fabrication

Prepare all collagen solutions 72 h in advance of tumor platform creation. Store all resulting solutions at 4 °C unless otherwise noted.

1. Prepare collagen stock solution by dissolving rat tail tendons in 10 mM HCl (pH 2.0) overnight at 4 °C.
2. Following centrifugation at 30,000 × *g* for 30 min, the monomerized collagen supernatant should be collected and lyophilized for long-term storage.
3. Making a working stock solution of collagen in 10 mM HCL (pH 2.0), the working stock solution should be 2× the final concentration of collagen in the microfluidic platform (4–20 mg/mL).
4. Immediately after experimental flow setup, place collagen stock solution, NaOH, 10× DMEM,1× DMEM and supplies on ice.
5. The collagen hydrogel is prepared by mixing a collagen stock solution (2× final concentration) with 10% 10× DMEM, sufficient 1 N NaOH to neutralize the HCl, supplemented with DMEM.
6. Use a spatula for an evenly mixed solution without bubbles. If a coculture setup with tumor cells within the matrix is desired, mix a final concentration of 1×10^6 cells/mL cancer cells into neutralizing buffer before adding the collagen, and mix on ice (*see* **Note 3**).
7. Swiftly use 1 mL syringe with 18G needle to pull up neutralized collagen and switch needle with 22G needle.
8. Carefully inject the neutralized collagen solution into the treated FEP tubing through the PDMS needle guide (*see* **Note 4**).

9. Insert a 2 in 22G needle into platform concentrically using the PDMS needle guides to create central void or vessel as seen in Fig. 2d (*see* **Note 5**).
10. Incubate platform containing collagen and 2 in 2G needle at 37 °C for 20–25 min allowing the collagen to gel around the needle (*see* **Note 6**).
11. Gently remove the 22G needle, creating the central microchannel void within the collagen hydrogel.

3.4 Endothelial Seeding and Flow Preconditioning

A 3-day graded shear stress or flow rate protocol previously developed should be utilized in order to maintain endothelial integrity and establish a confluent monolayer of endothelial cells within the central vessel [54]. The 72 h preconditioning scheme is described below and a final flow rate that results in a wall shear stress of 1 dyne/cm^2 should be reached for a total of 6 h after the 72 h preconditioning in order to align endothelial cells according to the previously published literature and shown in Fig. 2e [55]. If tumor-endothelial cell coculture is used, we have previously shown an increase in permeability in coculture compared to endothelial monoculture occurs due to pro-angiogenic crosstalk between endothelial and cancer cells, highlighting the systems capability to accurately model a leaky tumor microenvironment [55].

1. Start trypsinizing endothelial cells during collagen incubation utilizing 0.05% Tyrpsin EDTA.
2. Prepare a 20 × 10^6 cells/mL solution in culture medium by spinning cells at 120 × *g* for 5 min and suspending cells in an appropriate volume of cell culture medium.
3. Use a 20 μL pipette to inject 20 μL of the endothelial cell suspension into microchannel.
4. Rotate complete platform 90° around central vessel axis every 30 s (4×), 1 min (4×), 2 min (8×), for a total 22 min to ensure even distribution of endothelial cells along the central vessel.
5. Carefully repeat **steps 3** and **4** for a total of 2 cell solution injections to ensure complete endothelialization.
6. Attach input tubing along with an in-line bubble trap as seen in Fig. 2e. Prime the input line with syringe pump, allowing the media to flow through bubble trap.
7. Apply 72 h graded preconditioning graded fluid flow introduction protocol as shown in Fig. 2e in order to align and elongate endothelial cells within the central microvessel. Additionally, this flow enables ample tumor - endothelial signaling that promotes an in vivo like leaky tumor vasculature [41]. Specifically, initially flow will be ramped to 0.01 dynes/cm^2 over 1 h and held constant at 0.01 dynes/cm^2 for 36 h. Afterwards, the flow

will be ramped to 0.1 dynes/cm^2 over one hour and likewise held for an additional 36 h. Finally, after approximately 72 h, the flow is ramped to 1 dynes/cm^2 and can be used for permeability studies.

8. Collect media from reservoirs after 48 h. Use 22 μm filter to sterilize and reuse media as necessary.
9. Continue flow at 1 dynes/cm^2 for 72 h followed by 6 h of increased flow with a wall shear stress of 1 dyne/cm^2 before experimentation (*see* **Note 7**).

3.5 Imaging of Nanoparticle Transport

This section will describe how to dynamically and nondestructively image nanoparticle transport in the 3D tumor platform after it has undergone 78 h of endothelial preconditioning. Data from this system can be utilized to compare extravasation time constants, diffusion constants, and penetration of nanoparticles into the tumor space. The data can be used to quantitatively compare transport for different nanoparticles of similar or varying properties to elucidate the effects of particle parameters on overall transport efficacy or the 1D data can be utilized easily for in silico models.

1. Set the microscope incubated chamber to 37 °C with 0.5% CO2 atmosphere.
2. Measure nanoparticles for desired concentration using a microbalance and resuspend in 20 mL of endothelial cell culture media (*see* **Note 8**).
3. Sonicate cell culture media containing fluorescent nanoparticles for 30 min to disassociate aggregates (*see* **Note 9**).
4. Place the platform in microscope stage (*see* **Note 10**).
5. Add 37 °C dH_2O to petri dish holder as seen in Fig. 3a, using a small amount of vacuum grease where FEP tubes meet petri dish to avoid water leakage. The water acts both as a temperature regulator and to match refractive indices of the platform to enable high-resolution imaging.
6. Place a 20 mL syringe of nanoparticle media on syringe pump. Prime the tubing and connect a 22G needle using male luer adapter and connect 22G needle at output of platform as seen in Fig. 3a.
7. Use fluorescently tagged endothelial cells or brightfield imaging to locate endothelial vessel in the collagen hydrogel, set the focus of the microscope.
8. Take background image of vessel (make sure there are no fluorescent particles in the media).
9. Connect the input flow needle that is connected to a syringe containing nanoparticle solution on syringe pump to the input needle guide. Connect output tubing to nanoparticle waste collection and start flow.

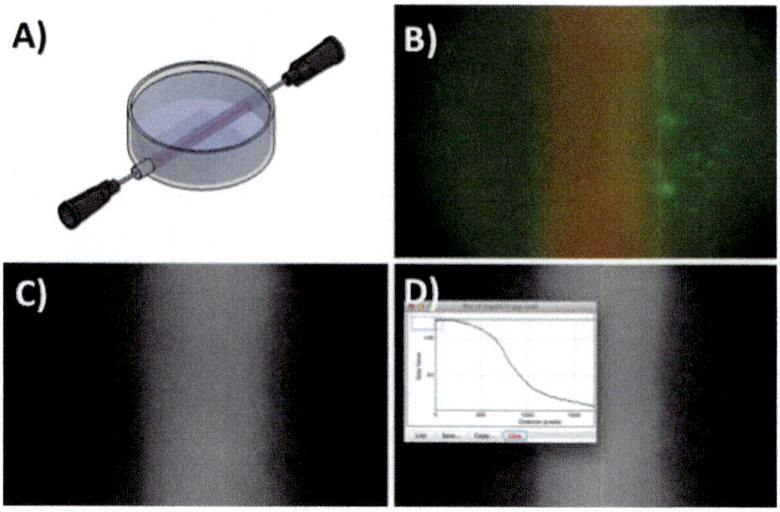

Fig. 3 Nanoparticle Transport Imaging and Analysis. (**a**) Depiction of platform with heated water to enable high-resolution imaging with steady temperature with input and output needle. (**b**) Example image at early time point showing red nanoparticles contained within vessel and green cancer cells in the matrix. (**c**) Gray scale image produced for comparison showing location of nanoparticles. (**d**) image analysis to create radial distribution

10. Capture an initial image as seen in Fig. 3b where nanoparticles are located completely within microvessel and the vessel is aligned in the middle of the image. Find the z-axis where vessel is at widest (center of vessel).
11. Wait 5 min and capture another image, acquiring an image every 5 min for the next 6–12 h, creating a time-lapse of the same location in the vessel keeping same exposure time for each image.
12. Collect nanoparticle waste from output line.

3.6 Image Analysis for Nanoparticle Transport

Imaging nanoparticle transport within the system allows for understanding the dynamic process of extravasation including accumulation around the endothelial wall and diffusion into the collagen matrix over time. By performing image analysis on a time-lapse series, a better understanding of the timing of nanoparticle transport can be accomplished. Data collected in this manner can be used to understand how these properties affect extravasation and diffusion to optimize these features to result in increased transport.

1. Take time-lapse image set for each experiment and import into ImageJ or other image processing software.
2. Separate color layers if multiple fluorescence wavelengths are used, selecting for signal corresponding to nanoparticles and transform data to grey scale as seen in Fig. 3c (*see* **Note 11**).

3. Find the middle of central microvessel using measuring tools.
4. Plot the average pixel intensity from the center of the vessel to the edge of image. Export the now radial data as seen in Fig. 3d.
5. Average the left and right half of the vessel to get an average radial distribution of nanoparticles for each time point. Plot data at different time points to show translocation of particles across endothelial wall and diffusion throughout the matrix. An example of 50 nm polystyrene fluorescent particles data is shown in Fig. 4a-d, highlighting the value of quantitative data that could be used to refine nanoparticles to optimize their transport based on different particle properties such as size, shape, and surface charge.

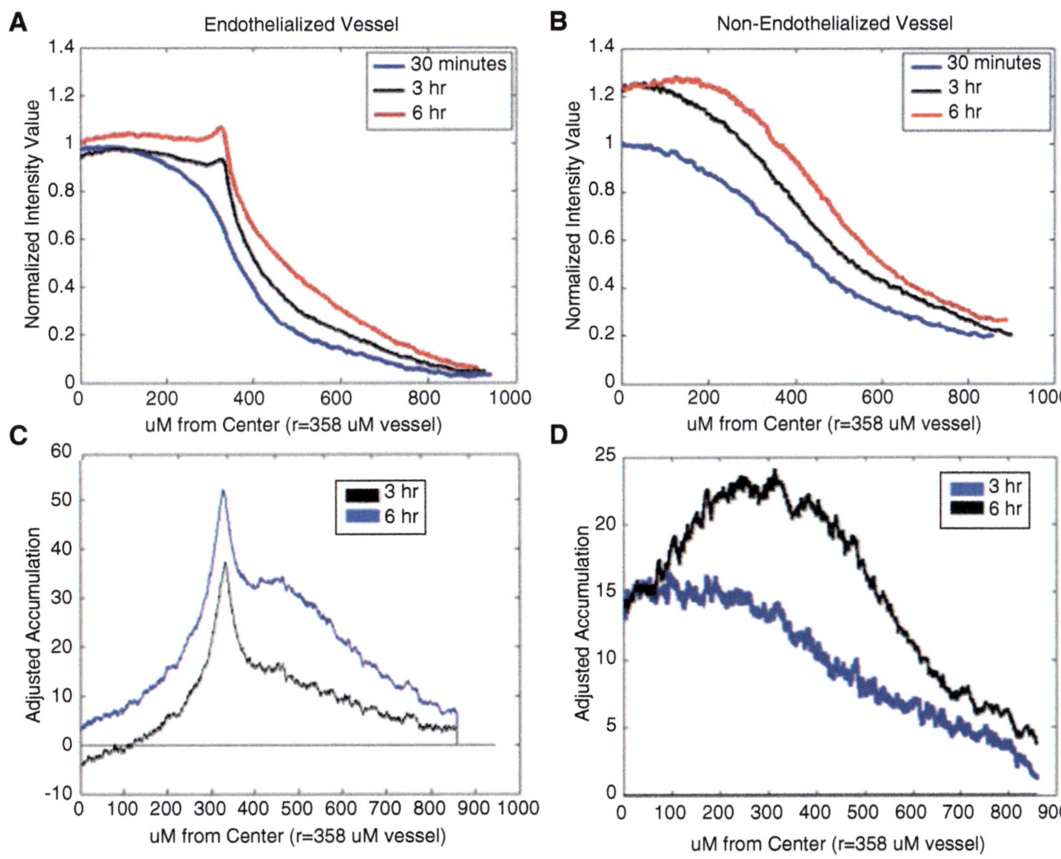

Fig. 4 Example of normalized radial transport data in platform. (**a**) Radial distribution of relative fluorescence for 50 nm polystyrene nanoparticles in a coculture platform at different time-points over 6 h. (**b**) Radial data for non-endothelialized channel. (**c** and **d**) Difference in intensity in 6 h and 3 h and 30 min, showing accumulation of particles near endothelial wall as the characteristic peaks seen at ~350 micron from vessel center and diffusion of particles in collagen matrix for both endothelialized and non-endothelialized platforms

In this specific case a coculture setup Fig. 4a is compared to a tumor only setup Fig. 4b in which endothelialization of the vessel does not occur. The results seen in Fig. 4c and d show the importance of the barrier function of the endothelialized channel and highlight the importance of including an endothelium in an in vitro tumor platform through the differences in accumulation at wall and level of nanoparticle extravasation.

3.7 Nanoparticle Uptake Analysis

While great strides are being made to highlight the usefulness of tumor-on-chip platforms for studying nanoparticle transport, the microscale of many of these systems limits their ability to perform post-culture analysis due to the quantity of cells required for these assays. Recovery and isolation of a sufficient quantity of cells in a macroscale platform exposed to nanoparticles allows for analysis and conclusion of nanoparticle uptake. The protocol described below allows for post-culture analysis of nanoparticle uptake by tumor and endothelial cells in the tumor platform allowing simultaneous extravasation and diffusion live imaging studies to more fully understand nanoparticle transport in the tumor microenvironment.

1. After nanoparticles are flowed through the system for sufficient time (1–6 h), remove all nanoparticle media and tubing and replace with clean, sterilized tubing connected to PBS at 37C in a syringe on a syringe pump. Wash samples with perfused PBS for 1 h to wash all uninternalized nanoparticles.
2. To recover and isolate cells from the device, remove all tubing and use tweezers to remove PDMS needle guides.
3. Gently push collagen hydrogel with blunt needle into a cell culture well containing a metalloprotease dispase solution in PBS at 50 caseionolytic units per mL. Incubate together at 37 °C with 5% CO_2 for 3 h for complete collagen dissolution without harm to the cells.
4. Add EDTA in PBS solution (5 mM) to halt collagen degradation and add fresh cell culture media. Centrifuge at 150 × *g* for 5 min.
5. Wash cell suspension 2× with ice-cold PBS, centrifuging at 120 × *g* for 5 min between each wash.
6. Resuspend cells in 200 μL PBS placed on ice in a 5 mL round-bottom polystyrene tube until analysis with flow cytometer.
7. Use side scattering vs. forward scattering on flow cytometer to differentiate between cell debris and live cells.
8. To separate endothelial and tumor cells, endothelial cells were utilized that stably produce green fluorescent protein (GFP) and cancer (MDA-MB-231-ATCC) cells, which have no fluo-

rescence signature, were used. It is only necessary to have one fluorescent cell type and for the emission of those cells to be different than the chosen nanoparticle fluorophore.

9. Uptake of red (ex/em 660/680 nm) particles was assessed using a flow cytometer.
10. A plot of nanoparticle fluorescence as a function of cell fluorescence can then be created as seen in Fig. 5 a-c for 1, 3, and12 h respectively where the top two quadrants are nanoparticle positive cells and the right two quadrants are green endothelial cells.
11. Take control groups with no nanoparticle exposure for each cell type.

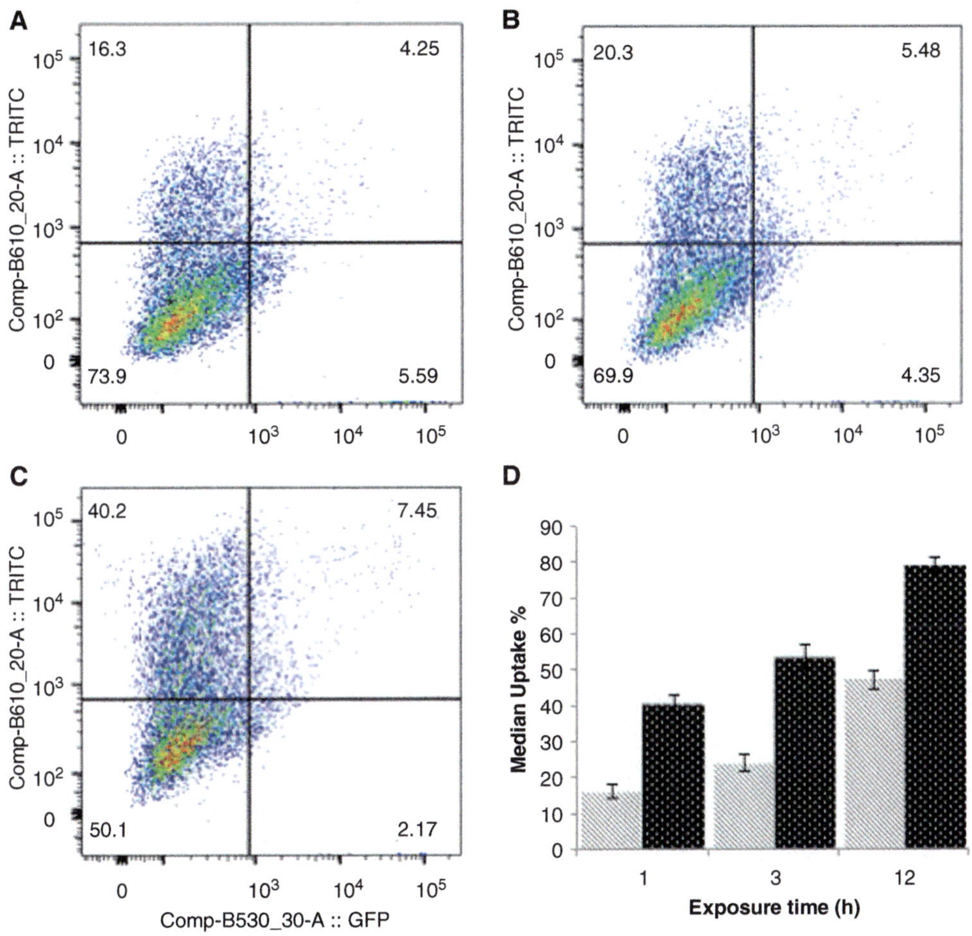

Fig. 5 FACS data for nanoparticle uptake in platform. Highlighting platforms ability to get sufficient quantity of cells for post-culture analysis. (**a**–**c**) Following 1, 3, 12 h exposure to nanoparticle flow in central vessel representative data showing gating employed for cell type(x-axis) and nanoparticle uptake (y-axis). (**d**) Uptake % of cancer and endothelial cells over the 12 h experiment, showing a statistically significant increase ($p < 0.01$) in uptake over time by both cancer (gray) and endothelial cells (black)

12. Employ gating to first separate cell type based on fluorescence (green-endothelial negative—cancer).
13. Utilizing nanoparticle negative groups and each cell type to separate based on particle uptake (y-axis).
14. Median Uptake % can be plotted as seen in Fig. 5d where % uptake is defined by gating determined from controls. Uptake by non-fluorescent cancer cells can be distinguished from free NPs and debris through forward and side scattering (*see* **Note 12**).

In this case the data highlights the capability of the system to show increased uptake of particles over time. Since ultimately many nanoparticles must be uptaken by cells, these experiments can impart important quantitative information on this last step of nanoparticle transport so that optimization of particle features that result in higher uptake can be accomplished in parallel with dynamic extravasation and diffusion imaging which is nondestructive.

4 Notes

1. It is important that the holes in the petri dish that hold FEP tubing are as close to the OD size of the FEP tubing as possible to ensure a tight seal and to prevent leakage with the addition of water. To make sliding of the FEP into the petri dish easier, the front end of FEP tubing can be cut at an angle. PDMS guides should be just long enough to be able to heat shrink FEP around it and hold a 22G needle during flow. The PDMS guides should be created using the FEP tubing. The tube should be filled completely with PDMS and polymerized around a 22G needle. The needle is removed after polymerization and the long cylinder should be cut into short (3–5 mm) PDMS guide caps.
2. For the collection of endothelial media previously flowed through the system the flask must be sealed. Parafilm can be used over the stopper to ensure a closed system where outflow media from the tumor platform enters the flask via tubing going through stopper.
3. An appropriate collagen concentration should be chosen to result in a sturdy platform. At least a final 5 mg/mL collagen solution has been used for reproducible collagen platforms with a robust matrix.
4. Make sure collagen completely fills FEP tubing, from one PDMS guide to the other. Any holes at the ends will result in collagen collapse and leaks.
5. We have previously published on the ability to select collagen polymerization parameters to result in tunable collagen hydro-

gels with desired pore size and stiffness. Specific collagen polymerization parameters and collagen concentrations should be chosen to best model the specific tissue properties based on work previously published by our group [56].

6. Collagen Polymerization time should not exceed 25 min to ensure viability of cancer cells in the matrix. The 22G needle does not need to be treated but should be sterile.
7. A final flow resulting in a shear stress of 1 dyne/cm^2 for 6 h results in a leaky coculture setup that nanoparticles up to 200 nm can extravasate [55]. Increased flow rates (10 dynes/cm^2) will result in tighter endothelial barrier and can be varied to result in changes in permeability. Endothelial media will provide nutrients for endothelial cells and cancer cells through diffusion into the hydrogel.
8. Nanoparticle concentration for different fluorescent nanoparticles depends on the intensity of the fluorophore. Concentration of nanoparticles should be chosen to result in adequate signal to noise ratio with minimal concentration of particles and ensuring colloidal stability of particles. A sensitivity analysis should be performed to find optimized nanoparticle concentration for imaging.
9. Leave the lid off of the sonicator to reduce heat that could possibly confound results.
10. A petri dish holder insert compatible with the microscope stage used can be utilized. Alternatively, a plate adapter can be cut that fits to the size of a well plate stage insert with a whole cut to the size of the petri dish and needles in place as shown in Fig. 3a.
11. Select a wavelength for particle fluorescence in red or blue as collagen hydrogels can be highly autofluorescent in green wavelengths, which can confound results.
12. The data presented in Fig. 5 is gated so that the left two quadrants are green negative tumor cells and to the right are green positive endothelial cells. Positive and negative for cell uptake can be gated using cell populations with no particle exposure.

Acknowledgments

Funding for this work was provided by the National Science Foundation Early CAREER Award CBET 0955072 and 0933571, the National Institutes of Health Grant R211R21CA158454-01A1. A special thanks to Rhys J Michna for his help in solidworks depictions of the 3D platform.

References

1. Cho K, Wang X, Nie S, Chen ZG, Shin DM (2008) Therapeutic nanoparticles for drug delivery in cancer. Clin Cancer Res 14:1310–1316
2. Singh R, Lillard JW Jr (2009) Nanoparticle-based targeted drug delivery. Exp Mol Pathol 86:215–223
3. Stover TC, Kim YS, Lowe TL, Kester M (2008) Thermoresponsive and biodegradable linear-dendritic nanoparticles for targeted and sustained release of a pro-apoptotic drug. Biomaterials 29:359–369
4. Whitney J, DeWitt M, Whited BM, Carswell W, Simon A et al (2013) 3D viability imaging of tumor phantoms treated with single-walled carbon nanohorns and photothermal therapy. Nanotechnology 24:275102
5. Carpin LB, Bickford LR, Agollah G, Yu TK, Schiff R et al (2011) Immunoconjugated gold nanoshell-mediated photothermal ablation of trastuzumab-resistant breast cancer cells. Breast Cancer Res Treat 125:27–34
6. Burke A, Ding X, Singh R, Kraft RA, Levi-Polyachenko N et al (2009) Long-term survival following a single treatment of kidney tumors with multiwalled carbon nanotubes and near-infrared radiation. Proc Natl Acad Sci U S A 106:12897–12902
7. Hood RL, Carswell WF, Rodgers A, Kosoglu MA, Rylander MN et al (2013) Spatially controlled photothermal heating of bladder tissue through single-walled carbon nanohorns delivered with a fiberoptic microneedle device. Lasers Med Sci 28:1143–1150
8. Kumari A, Yadav SK, Yadav SC (2010) Biodegradable polymeric nanoparticles based drug delivery systems. Colloids Surf B Biointerfaces 75:1–18
9. Owens DE 3rd, Peppas NA (2006) Opsonization, biodistribution, and pharmacokinetics of polymeric nanoparticles. Int J Pharm 307:93–102
10. McBain SC, Yiu HH, Dobson J (2008) Magnetic nanoparticles for gene and drug delivery. Int J Nanomedicine 3:169–180
11. Giustini AJ, Petryk AA, Cassim SM, Tate JA, Baker I et al (2010) Magnetic nanoparticle hyperthermia in Cancer treatment. Nano Life 1:01n02
12. Kennedy LC, Bickford LR, Lewinski NA, Coughlin AJ, Hu Y et al (2011) A new era for cancer treatment: gold-nanoparticle-mediated thermal therapies. Small 7:169–183
13. O'Neal DP, Hirsch LR, Halas NJ, Payne JD, West JL (2004) Photo-thermal tumor ablation in mice using near infrared-absorbing nanoparticles. Cancer Lett 209:171–176
14. Loo C, Lowery A, Halas N, West J, Drezek R (2005) Immunotargeted nanoshells for integrated cancer imaging and therapy. Nano Lett 5:709–711
15. Qin Z, Bischof JC (2012) Thermophysical and biological responses of gold nanoparticle laser heating. Chem Soc Rev 41:1191–1217
16. Pekkanen AM, DeWitt MR, Rylander MN (2014) Nanoparticle enhanced optical imaging and phototherapy of cancer. J Biomed Nanotechnol 10:1677–1712
17. Whitney JR, Sarkar S, Zhang J, Do T, Young T et al (2011) Single walled carbon nanohorns as photothermal cancer agents. Lasers Surg Med 43:43–51
18. DeWitt MR, Pekkanen AM, Robertson J, Rylander CG, Nichole Rylander M (2014) Influence of hyperthermia on efficacy and uptake of carbon nanohorn-cisplatin conjugates. J Biomech Eng 136:021003
19. Jain RK (1987) Transport of molecules across tumor vasculature. Cancer Metastasis Rev 6:559–593
20. Nagy JA, Chang SH, Shih SC, Dvorak AM, Dvorak HF (2010) Heterogeneity of the tumor vasculature. Semin Thromb Hemost 36:321–331
21. Maeda H, Wu J, Sawa T, Matsumura Y, Hori K (2000) Tumor vascular permeability and the EPR effect in macromolecular therapeutics: a review. J Control Release 65:271–284
22. Hansen AE, Petersen AL, Henriksen JR, Boerresen B, Rasmussen P et al (2015) Positron emission tomography based elucidation of the enhanced permeability and retention effect in dogs with Cancer using Copper-64 liposomes. ACS Nano 9:6985–6995
23. Hobbs SK, Monsky WL, Yuan F, Roberts WG, Griffith L et al (1998) Regulation of transport pathways in tumor vessels: role of tumor type and microenvironment. Proc Natl Acad Sci U S A 95:4607–4612
24. Hashizume H, Baluk P, Morikawa S, McLean JW, Thurston G et al (2000) Openings between defective endothelial cells explain tumor vessel leakiness. Am J Pathol 156:1363–1380
25. Yuan F, Dellian M, Fukumura D, Leunig M, Berk DA et al (1995) Vascular permeability in a human tumor xenograft: molecular size dependence and cutoff size. Cancer Res 55:3752–3756
26. Kedem O, Katchalsky A (1958) Thermodynamic analysis of the permeability

of biological membranes to non-electrolytes. Biochim Biophys Acta 27:229–246
27. Jain RK, Stylianopoulos T (2010) Delivering nanomedicine to solid tumors. Nat Rev Clin Oncol 7:653–664
28. Jain RK (1987) Transport of molecules in the tumor interstitium: a review. Cancer Res 47:3039–3051
29. Goel S, Duda DG, Xu L, Munn LL, Boucher Y et al (2011) Normalization of the vasculature for treatment of cancer and other diseases. Physiol Rev 91:1071–1121
30. Baxter LT, Jain RK (1991) Transport of fluid and macromolecules in tumors. III. Role of binding and metabolism. Microvasc Res 41:5–23
31. Baxter LT, Jain RK (1989) Transport of fluid and macromolecules in tumors. I. Role of interstitial pressure and convection. Microvasc Res 37:77–104
32. Flessner MF, Choi J, Credit K, Deverkadra R, Henderson K (2005) Resistance of tumor interstitial pressure to the penetration of intraperitoneally delivered antibodies into metastatic ovarian tumors. Clin Cancer Res 11:3117–3125
33. Adriani G, de Tullio MD, Ferrari M, Hussain F, Pascazio G et al (2012) The preferential targeting of the diseased microvasculature by disk-like particles. Biomaterials 33:5504–5513
34. Decuzzi P, Godin B, Tanaka T, Lee SY, Chiappini C et al (2010) Size and shape effects in the biodistribution of intravascularly injected particles. J Control Release 141:320–327
35. Barua S, Mitragotri S (2014) Challenges associated with penetration of nanoparticles across cell and tissue barriers: a review of current status and future prospects. Nano Today 9:223–243
36. Chithrani BD, Ghazani AA, Chan WC (2006) Determining the size and shape dependence of gold nanoparticle uptake into mammalian cells. Nano Lett 6:662–668
37. Iversen TG, Skotland T, Sandvig K (2011) Endocytosis and intracellular transport of nanoparticles: present knowledge and need for future studies. Nano Today 6:176–185
38. Lazarovits J, Chen YY, Sykes EA, Chan WC (2015) Nanoparticle-blood interactions: the implications on solid tumour targeting. Chem Commun (Camb) 51:2756–2767
39. Stirland DL, Nichols JW, Miura S, Bae YH (2013) Mind the gap: a survey of how cancer drug carriers are susceptible to the gap between research and practice. J Control Release 172:1045–1064
40. Gao Y, Li M, Chen B, Shen Z, Guo P et al (2013) Predictive models of diffusive nanoparticle transport in 3-dimensional tumor cell spheroids. AAPS J 15:816–831
41. Buchanan C, Rylander MN (2013) Microfluidic culture models to study the hydrodynamics of tumor progression and therapeutic response. Biotechnol Bioeng 110:2063–2072
42. Szot CS, Buchanan CF, Freeman JW, Rylander MN (2011) 3D in vitro bioengineered tumors based on collagen I hydrogels. Biomaterials 32:7905–7912
43. Griffith LG, Swartz MA (2006) Capturing complex 3D tissue physiology in vitro. Nat Rev Mol Cell Biol 7:211–224
44. Ghajar CM, Bissell MJ (2010) Tumor engineering: the other face of tissue engineering. Tissue Eng Part A 16:2153–2156
45. Cross VL, Zheng Y, Won Choi N, Verbridge SS, Sutermaster BA et al (2010) Dense type I collagen matrices that support cellular remodeling and microfabrication for studies of tumor angiogenesis and vasculogenesis in vitro. Biomaterials 31:8596–8607
46. Esch MB, King TL, Shuler ML (2011) The role of body-on-a-chip devices in drug and toxicity studies. Annu Rev Biomed Eng 13:55–72
47. Verbridge SS, Chandler EM, Fischbach C (2010) Tissue-engineered three-dimensional tumor models to study tumor angiogenesis. Tissue Eng Part A 16:2147–2152
48. Sano MB, Arena CB, Bittleman KR, DeWitt MR, Cho HJ et al (2015) Bursts of bipolar microsecond pulses inhibit tumor growth. Sci Rep 5:14999
49. Farahat WA, Wood LB, Zervantonakis IK, Schor A, Ong S et al (2012) Ensemble analysis of angiogenic growth in three-dimensional microfluidic cell cultures. PLoS One 7:e37333
50. Sung KE, Yang N, Pehlke C, Keely PJ, Eliceiri KW et al (2011) Transition to invasion in breast cancer: a microfluidic in vitro model enables examination of spatial and temporal effects. Integr Biol (Camb) 3:439–450
51. DelNero P, Song YH, Fischbach C (2013) Microengineered tumor models: insights & opportunities from a physical sciences-oncology perspective. Biomed Microdevices 15:583–593
52. Ng CP, Pun SH (2008) A perfusable 3D cell-matrix tissue culture chamber for in situ evaluation of nanoparticle vehicle penetration and transport. Biotechnol Bioeng 99:1490–1501
53. Kwak B, Ozcelikkale A, Shin CS, Park K, Han B (2014) Simulation of complex transport of nanoparticles around a tumor using tumor-microenvironment-on-chip. J Control Release 194:157–167
54. Buchanan CF, Voigt EE, Szot CS, Freeman JW, Vlachos PP et al (2014) Three-dimensional

microfluidic collagen hydrogels for investigating flow-mediated tumor-endothelial signaling and vascular organization. Tissue Eng Part C Methods 20:64–75

55. Buchanan CF, Verbridge SS, Vlachos PP, Rylander MN (2014) Flow shear stress regulates endothelial barrier function and expression of angiogenic factors in a 3D microfluidic tumor vascular model. Cell Adhes Migr 8:517–524

56. Antoine EE, Vlachos PP, Rylander MN (2015) Tunable collagen I hydrogels for engineered physiological tissue micro-environments. PLoS One 10:e0122500

Chapter 13

Utilizing the Lung as a Model to Study Nanoparticle-Based Drug Delivery Systems

Dylan K. McDaniel, Veronica M. Ringel-Scaia, Sheryl L. Coutermarsh-Ott, and Irving C. Allen

Abstract

Intranasal administration is a highly effective route for drug delivery and biodistribution studies. Indeed, this route of delivery has become the method of choice to distribute diverse pharmacological agents both locally and systemically. In the majority of preclinical animal models and in human patients, intranasal administration is the preferred method to deliver therapeutic agents to the airways and lungs. However, issues with drug stability and controlled release in the respiratory tract are common problems with many therapeutic agents. Nanoparticle delivery via intranasal administration has tremendous potential to circumvent these common issues. Over the past 30 years nanoparticles have gained increased interest as therapeutic delivery vehicles and as tools for improved bioimaging. Integral to the success of nanoparticles in drug delivery and biodistribution is the utilization of mouse models to characterize therapeutic strategies under physiologically relevant in situ conditions. Here, we describe a model of nanoparticle administration to the lungs utilizing intranasal administration and discuss a variety of highly useful techniques to evaluate nanoparticle up-take, biodistribution, and immune response. While these protocols have been optimized for intranasal administration of common fluorescently labeled nanoparticles, they can be applied to any nanoparticle or drug delivery system of interest targeting the lungs and airways.

Key words Biodistribution, Intranasal administration, Inflammation, Airway, Flow cytometry

1 Introduction

Intranasal administration has long been utilized as a route for the delivery of topical or local acting agents because it offers easy access to large mucosal surfaces and large porous endothelial membranes [1, 2]. In addition, interest centers on the intranasal route of administration for the purpose of delivering agents systemically [3], to the brain [4], and most relevant to the methodology presented here—to the lungs [5]. Pulmonary delivery of therapeutics is highly relevant, both clinically and physiologically, as the lungs are able to absorb agents for both local delivery and systemic release. In addition, the lungs have a high surface area and exhibit relatively limited enzymatic activity enabling stable and controlled deposition of therapeutics in the air spaces. The intranasal

Rachael W. Sirianni and Bahareh Behkam (eds.), *Targeted Drug Delivery: Methods and Protocols*, Methods in Molecular Biology, vol. 1831, https://doi.org/10.1007/978-1-4939-8661-3_13, © Springer Science+Business Media, LLC, part of Springer Nature 2018

route yields unusual pharmacokinetics related to variations in absorption and distribution that are based on the properties of the agent administered, and specifically the ability of the agent to cross the mucosal barrier [6]. In order to enhance the bioavailability of intranasally administered therapeutics, one highly efficient modification is to couple the drug of interest to the payload of a nanoparticle-based delivery platform.

Nanoparticles represent an increasingly explored method for enhanced delivery of therapeutics [7]. Particles on the nanoscale exhibit unique properties, such as increased surface area-to-volume ratio and reduced immunostimulatory properties that make them superior to other comparable therapeutic delivery methods for applications in the lungs [8]. These unique properties allow for improved bioavailability, biodistribution, and controlled release of therapeutics. Indeed, several different formulations of novel nanoparticles have demonstrated these features in preclinical murine models [9–11].

Here, we describe a highly efficient method of intranasal administration of nanoparticle-based agents in mice. Unique to this protocol, we provide details that facilitate succinct and efficient evaluation of resultant biodistribution in the lung following nanoparticle exposure, which is made possible by the addition of a fluorophore or fluorescent protein coupled to the nanoparticle and subsequent evaluation with flow cytometry. We also outline procedures to allow biodistribution assessments on lung tissue sections prepared for histopathology and methods to robustly evaluate the host immune response following nanoparticle administration (*see* **Note 1**). This model is highly flexible and can be readily modified to evaluate any type of nanoscale drug delivery platform, coupled with a diverse range of fluorescent markers. Likewise, this protocol is ideal to evaluate nanoparticle-based therapeutic delivery in conjunction with any preclinical mouse model of airway or lung disease, including pneumonia, asthma, chronic obstructive pulmonary disease (COPD), or cancer.

2 Materials

2.1 Mice

1. Adult, 6–12 week-old male or female mice (*see* **Note 2**).

Mice should be acclimated to the housing facility for at least 5 days prior to the beginning of the experiment (*see* **Note 3**).

2.2 Reagents and Solutions

1. Isoflurane.
2. Sterile, 1× PBS.
3. Trypan blue.
4. Diff-Quik stains.

5. 10× Buffered formalin.
6. Permount.
7. Hoechst Nuclear Stain (10 μg/mL) (*see* **Note 4**).
8. Deionized (DI) water.
9. Sterile 10× PBS.

2.3 Materials and Equipment for Nanoparticle Administration

1. Scale with weighing container.
2. Anesthesia machine.
3. 20–200 μL pipette tips.
4. 20–200 μL pipetter.
5. Nanoparticles in PBS.

2.4 Materials and Equipment for Necropsy

1. CO_2 Tank and euthanasia chamber.
2. Mouse necropsy tools: 1 pair of large blunt scissors; 1 pair of straight forceps; 1 pair of blunt 90° angled forceps; 1 pair of sharp 90° angled scissors; 1 pair of slightly curved blunt scissors.
3. 1.5 mL microcentrifuge tubes.
4. Microcentrifuge.
5. 10 mL Syringes (with 27 gauge needles).
6. 1 mL Syringes (without needles).
7. 15 mL conical tubes.
8. Tracheal Cannula (*see* **Note 5**) (Harvard Apparatus, MA, USA).
9. 4–0, Silk Surgical Suture.
10. Refrigerated bench top centrifuge (with rotor to accommodate 15 mL conical tubes).
11. Hemacytometer.
12. Microscope (10× and 20× objectives).
13. Cytospin centrifuge.
14. Microscope Slides.
15. Coverslips.
16. 10 mL syringe with a 6 inch piece of medical tubing fitted at the hub and stopcock.
17. 50 mL conical tubes.

2.5 Materials and Equipment for Evaluation of Nanoparticle Immunogenicity

Murine IL-6 ELISA kit.

2.6 Materials and Equipment for Evaluation of Nanoparticle Distribution

Nanoparticles with fluorescent marker.

Flow Cytometer/ImageStream.

3 Methods

3.1 Preparation of Nanoparticles for Intranasal Administration

1. Prepare nanoparticle solution at a concentration of 1 mg/mL in PBS using aseptic techniques (*see* **Note 6**).

3.2 Nanoparticle Lung Inoculation Using Intranasal Administration

1. Record initial body weights.
2. Anesthetize mice in an induction chamber using isoflurane (*see* **Note 7**).
3. Withdraw 25 μL of nanoparticle solution into a pipetter.
4. When fully anesthetized (*see* **Note 8**), scruff mouse and angle head such that the liquid will easily slide down the nostril into the airway (Fig. 1).
5. Slowly dispense 25 μL of fluorophore-loaded nanoparticles into one nostril, allowing the animal to slowly aspirate the liquid through normal breathing (*see* **Note 9**).
6. Maintain the animal in an upright position for 15–30 s to allow full aspiration and dispersal of the liquid.

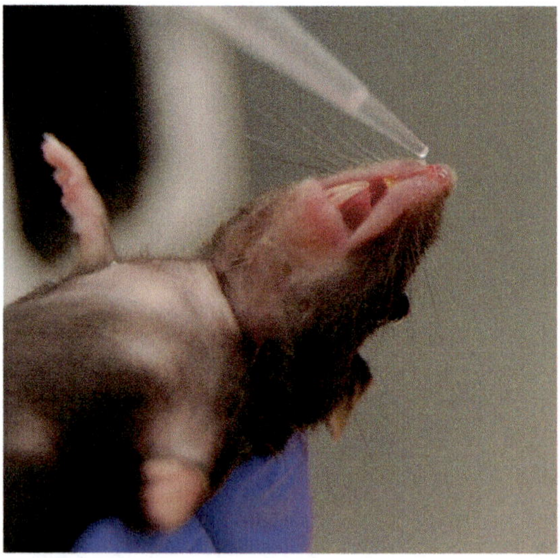

Fig. 1 *Intranasal Administration.* This image illustrates the proper mouse handling technique for intranasal administration

3.3 Cell and Tissue Collection to Evaluate Immune Response and Nanoparticle Distribution in the Lung

1. Euthanize mouse via CO_2 24 h after nanoparticle administration. Ensure proper euthanasia by checking toe pinch reflex.
2. Immediately following euthanasia, whole blood should be acquired by cardiac puncture (*see* **Note 10**). The blood should be aliquoted into 1.5 mL centrifuge tubes and allowed to settle for 30 min prior to centrifugation.
3. Use blunt scissors to incise and dissect the skin away from the mouse in such a way that will allow adequate visualization and access to the thoracic and abdominal organs later in the procedure. Remove the large salivary glands overlying the throat.
4. Incise the peritoneum to fully expose the abdominal organs. Gently move the freely moveable intestinal tract to the side to expose either the right or the left kidney. Transect the large renal vessels entering the kidney at the hilus (indent). This will allow for drainage of fluid administered during perfusion.
5. Make a small incision in the diaphragm being especially careful not to puncture the lungs. The lungs are pale/white and can often be seen through the diaphragm. They are tightly abutted to the diaphragm due to negative thoracic pressure, however, you can often visualize a small window where they are not so intimately associated. Once the incision is made, the negative pressure will be released and the lungs and heart will retract. At this point, you should be able to visualize and access the heart. If not, use the blunt end of your scissors to widen the incision.
6. Using a 27-gauge needle on a 10 mL syringe, slowly and evenly infuse 3–5 mL 1× PBS into the heart. This whole body perfusion is performed to clear the vessels of the lungs (and other organs) of excessive erythrocytes. Excessive erythrocytes can potentially interfere with cytokine analysis, as well as, visualization of changes in the lungs via histopathology assessments. During the perfusion, you should visualize blood-tinged fluid exiting the body from the severed renal vessels. This fluid should become clearer as the perfusion progresses. If the chest cavity fills with fluid, slowly back your needle out as you may have punctured through the heart.
7. Once the perfusion is complete, the thoracic organs can then be exposed. Using the blunt end of your scissors, incise the remainder of the diaphragm. Slowly and carefully transect the rib cage as close to the body as possible, but without cutting any lung tissue. If enough of the rib cage is not removed, this may negatively impact your formalin perfusion. Using the blunt end of your scissors, cut away the collar bone being careful to avoid cutting the trachea. At this point, you should have good visualization of the trachea. If there are excessive amounts of soft, white tissue at the thoracic inlet (thymus)

impairing this visualization, this can carefully be trimmed away at this time.

8. Using the 90° angled sharp scissors, make a small incision into the trachea approximately 1–3 rings beneath the larynx. Make sure to only extend the incision halfway across the dorsal portion of the trachea; do not completely sever the trachea.
9. Carefully insert the tracheal cannula into the incision.
10. Secure the cannula in place with one, proximal, securely tightened suture. Do this by threading a single piece of silk suture underneath the trachea and using an instrument tie to encircle the cannulated portion of the trachea. Place a second ligature distal to the first such that it is surrounding the trachea, but not including the cannula. This should be loosely secured so that it can be tightened following formalin infusion.
11. The next steps will involve infusion of 1× PBS through the cannula into the lungs to acquire bronchoalveolar lavage fluid (BALF). Make sure to have three 1 mL syringes each filled with 1 mL of 1× PBS ready. These should have no air bubbles as this can interfere with infusion/recovery. Take the first of the three syringes and gently attach it to the tracheal cannula. Steadily infuse 0.9 mL of the 1× PBS into the lungs. As you infuse the PBS, the lungs should steadily inflate with no evidence of fluid leakage. After infusing 0.9 mL, the fluid should then be steadily and smoothly removed into the same syringe with gentle, but continuous traction on the plunger. The recovered BALF should then be placed into a labeled 15 mL conical tube on ice. This process should then be repeated with the remaining two 1 mL syringes; however, in these instances, the entire 1 mL of PBS should be infused.
12. Record the total BALF amount recovered.
13. The next steps are set forth to optimize formalin perfusion of the lungs and, thus, histopathologic visualization (*see* **Note 11**). Fill a 10 mL syringe (without needle or plunger) with 10× buffered formalin and attach medical tubing. Make sure the tubing is filled with formalin and there are no air bubbles. Firmly attach the end of the medical tubing to the tracheal cannula. Open the stop cock and allow formalin to fill the lungs via gravity inflation. Once again, the lungs should steadily inflate with no evidence of fluid leakage (*see* **Note 12**). Once the lungs are fully inflated, tighten the second ligature around the trachea (making sure NOT to include the cannula) in order to secure the formalin. Close the stopcock and remove the medical tubing from the cannula.
14. Carefully transect the trachea below the tip of the cannula but above your second (tightened) ligature. Grasp the excess suture with your forceps and carefully retract the lungs from

the body. Carefully cut all attachments to the body with your curved scissors making sure not to cut the lungs. The final attachments of the lung to the body (caudal vena cava, esophagus, and aorta) can be transected immediately above the diaphragm.

15. Place the lungs in individually labeled 50 mL conical tubes filled with ~25 mL formalin and allow to fix for at least 24 h at room temperature before paraffin embedding.
16. Properly dispose of the remainder of the animal carcass.

3.4 Sample Analysis

Cytokine Analysis Using ELISA

1. For the analysis of systemic cytokines in the serum, allow blood samples to settle and coagulate for ~30 min after collection. Spin coagulated samples in a microcentrifuge at maximum speed (~16,200 × *g*) for 5 min. Gently remove the tubes from the microcentrifuge. Each tube should now contain two visible layers. The serum resides in the clear, slightly yellowish top layer. Carefully remove this layer (making sure not to aspirate the bottom layer composed of coagulated red and white blood cells) and place it in a new, appropriately labeled 1.5 mL centrifuge tube. These can then be stored at −80 °C for future analysis. Due to low volumes, serum samples can be run at half volumes in ELISA assays. Additionally, serum samples can be diluted 1:3–1:5 to spare additional volume.
2. Cell-free BALF can also be used for cytokine analysis. Place BALF samples (after recovered volumes have been recorded) into a centrifuge and spin at 200 × *g* for 5 min at 4 °C. Upon removing the 15 mL conical tubes from the centrifuge, a small cell pellet may or may not be visible at the bottom of the tube. Being careful not to aspirate/disturb the cell pellet, remove the supernatant and place into 1.5 mL microcentrifuge tubes. These cell-free supernatants can be stored at −80° C.
3. For use in ELISA, cell-free BALF can be used neat or diluted 1:5 in assay diluent.

Lysing Red Blood Cells in BALF

4. Following removal of the cell-free supernatants, cell pellets recovered from BALF need to be resuspended. Additionally, there may be blood contamination as a result of BALF recovery. This can potentially affect cell counts and/or differential analysis and so this resuspension procedure is designed to also include red blood cell lysis. For each sample, resuspend the cell pellet in 900 μL of DI water followed immediately by 100 μL of 10× PBS. Samples should be processed one at a time. Allowing cells to incubate with DI water alone for an extended period may lead to lysis of the cells of interest (i.e., leukocytes) (*see* **Note 13**).

5. Remove 800 μL for flow cytometry. The following steps are performed using the remaining 200 μL of BALF.
6. Determine BALF cellularity using Trypan blue and a hemacytometer.

Differential Staining for Cell Counts

7. To determine cell differentials, aliquot 150–200 μL of the BALF cells into a cytospin slide holder and funnel correctly fitted with a labeled microscope slide. Spin at 100 × *g* for 5 min in an appropriate cytospin/centrifuge. Allow slides to air dry overnight before staining (e.g., with Diff-Quik).
8. Stain slides with an appropriate differential stain and according to the manufacturer's directions. Allow the slides to air dry overnight and then coverslip using permount. Evaluate the slides using a microscope equipped with a 20× and 40× objective (*see* **Note 14**).

Histopathology Analysis

9. Formalin-fixed samples can be prepared for histopathologic evaluation. After ≥24 h of formalin fixation, the whole inflated lungs should be ventrally orientated and embedded in paraffin. The resultant blocks should be cut to expose the main conducting airway. Increased scoring accuracy can be achieved by orientating the lungs in the same position and cut to the same depth. Five micron serial sections of the lungs should be cut and stained with Hemotoxylin and Eosin (H&E). Additional sections can be cut and prepared for in situ hybridization using standard protocols.

3.5 Utilization of Flow Cytometry to Assess Nanoparticle Uptake

1. Add Hoechst to the remaining 800 μL of BALF (*see* **step 5** in Subheading 3.4) at a concentration of 10 μg/mL. The Hoechst staining will allow for the visualization of the nucleus. Target cells can also be counterstained with antibodies targeting specific cell populations to allow for more robust downstream data analysis following the suppliers recommended protocols.
2. Incubate in the dark at room temperature for 15 min.
3. Spin at 600 × *g* for 5 min and resuspend in 20 μL of sterile PBS in a 1.5 mL tube (*see* **Note 15**).
4. Set gates appropriately (i.e., single cells, cell specific markers, etc.) and load the samples into the flow cytometer (*see* **Note 16**).
5. In order to quantify nanoparticle uptake, fluorophore-loaded nanoparticles can be detected inside the cells by the flow cytometer. This can be done by changing the gates so that the single cells containing the fluorophore and those without will be counted separately.

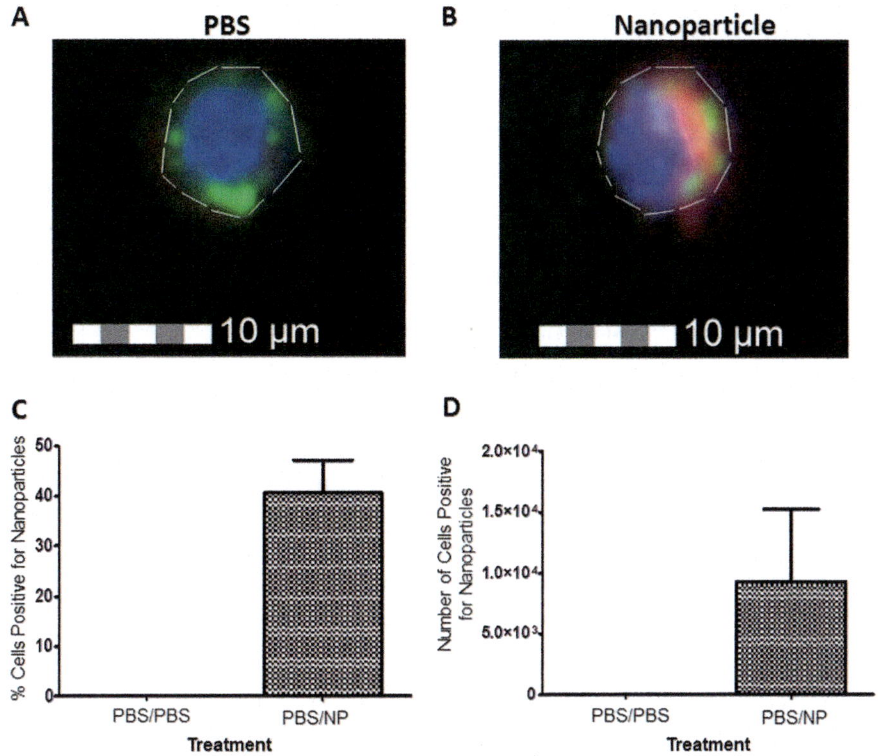

Fig. 2 *Analysis and Visualization of Cellular Uptake of Fluorescently Labeled Nanoparticles Using Flow Cytometry.* (**a**) Sample images of cells from the lungs of mice treated with PBS and (**b**) fluorescently labeled PEO-PDLLA nanoparticles. These images were taken using Amnis ImageStream and three individual fluorescent images were overlayed: green (autofluorescence of the cell), blue (DNA labeled with Hoechst dye), and red (TIPS pentacene). (**c**) Percentage of cells positive for TIPS pentacene-loaded nanoparticles using flow cytometry. (**d**) The number of cells positive for nanoparticle uptake. This number was obtained by multiplying the percentage of cells positive for nanoparticles (shown in **a**) by the number of cells calculated using Trypan blue exclusion, described in the protocol

6. This information can be used to determine the percentage of cells positive for nanoparticles by calculating the percentage of cells gated for the fluorophore as well as analyzing the mean fluorescence intensity of a given sample (Fig. 2c) (*see* **Note 17**).
7. Cells can be imaged using ImageStream and analyzed using the manufacturer's software or utilizing routine fluorescence microscopy (Fig. 2a, b).
8. Single color images can be overlayed to give a single image containing all colors of interest (i.e., cells, nucleus and nanoparticles) (Fig. 2a, b) (*see* **Note 18**).

4 Notes

1. Using our methods, the host immune response following nanoparticle treatment can be robustly evaluated in the lungs. For example, our methods are ideal for soluble mediators, such as cytokines, as well as histopathology. We recommended evaluating pro-inflammatory cytokines such as IL-6, IL-1β and TNF. Using histopathology, the infiltration of leukocytes can be observed in the air spaces to determine the extent of an inflammatory response in the lung.
2. We have successfully used 6–12 week-old C57BL/6 mice in this assay. However, the protocol can be applied to any mouse strain of interest.
3. All studies should be conducted in accordance with the institutional animal care and use guidelines and in accordance with the prevailing national regulations.
4. This protocol was optimized using Hoechst 33342 (Excitation/ Emission bound to DNA: 350/461 nm).
5. We recommend using specialized, commercially available tracheal cannulas. However, 16-gauge needles can be used if necessary. In our experience, these are most useful when the sharp tips are ground down and blunted.
6. This protocol has been successfully performed using polyethylene glycol (PEG), poly(lactic-co-glycolic acid) (PLGA), and polyethylene oxide-poly-DL-lactic acid (PEO-PDLLA) nanoparticles. We do not anticipate any problems when utilizing nanoparticles of other compositions.
7. The use of inhalant anesthetics (in this case, isoflurane) can potentially lead to some confounding effects when evaluating lung physiology. These can be minimized by limiting the animal's exposure to the inhalant as much as possible and by utilizing appropriate control animals.
8. Mouse is fully anesthetized when it reaches the surgical plane of anesthesia. Specifically, the mouse should be unconscious and will not respond to external stimuli.
9. Add nanoparticles to one nostril at time; taking care to avoid getting liquid in the cleft.
10. Cardiac puncture should be performed using a 1 mL syringe with 27-gauge needle attached. There are multiple acceptable ways to acquire whole blood from the heart. However, we choose to do so prior to making any incisions. Following confirmation of euthanasia, pin the mouse to a surgical board. Spray the animal with 70% ethanol and locate the base of the sternum. Insert the needle between the last 2 ribs and slightly to the right of the center. Using a controlled and singular

motion, begin withdrawing the blood from the heart. With practice, this procedure can typically recover 500–800 μL of whole blood. When finished, remove the needle from the syringe prior to transferring the blood to the microcentrifuge tube. Forcing the blood through the needle will induce cell lysis and inhibit serum collection.

11. For improved visualization or certain immunohistochemistry applications, frozen sections can be prepared in lieu of formalin-fixed, paraffin-embedded tissue sections. For frozen sections, place a small amount of OCT compound into a block mold on dry ice. Remove the lung tissue *en bloc* and place in the mold on top of the small amount of frozen OCT. Slowly and steadily fill the remaining block and tissue with OCT. Make sure to minimize air bubbles as this can affect your ability to appropriately section the tissue. Store molds at −80 °C until ready for sectioning.
12. If lungs have been punctured, formalin can be carefully injected into the lungs using a needle and syringe until lungs are inflated.
13. There are multiple protocols for lysis of red blood cells. However, the protocol described here is optimized for downstream assessments of cell morphology and differential counts. For downstream procedures where higher resolution with reduction of background is important, such as for Fluorescence-activated cell sorting (FACS) analysis, red blood cell lysis via ACK lysing buffer may be a good alternative.
14. Differential staining allows for basic assessments of cell morphology. To ensure optimal results, cytospin should be performed on the same day as the harvest. Diff-Quik based protocols allow the differentiation between granulocytes (such as neutrophils, eosinophils, and mast cells) and mononuclear cells (macrophages and lymphocytes). However, depending on the experience of the researcher, confirmation of cell types present in the BALF should be performed by either FACS analysis, immunohistochemistry, or with the assistance of a trained cytopathologist.
15. The PBS used to resuspend the pellet should contain not more than 1% FBS. FBS can be added to the PBS in order to keep cell viable during flow analysis.
16. For this protocol the gates were set for all single cells.
17. The Amnis ImageStream software allows for the calculation of the total number of objects/mL in a given sample and is useful in determining cell counts with the appropriate gate settings.
18. The cells described in this protocol were not counterstained for visualization. Rather, the autofluorescence of the cells (Excitation/Emission: 488/530) was used.

Acknowledgments

Funding for this work was provided by the Virginia Tech Institute for Critical Technology and Applied Science and the Virginia Maryland College of Veterinary Medicine. Nanoparticles utilized in this protocol were provided by Prof. Richey M. Davis from the Virginia Tech Department of Chemical Engineering.

References

1. Djupesland PG (2013) Nasal drug delivery devices: characteristics and performance in a clinical perspective-a review. Drug Deliv Transl Res 3(1):42–62. https://doi.org/10.1007/s13346-012-0108-9
2. Turker S, Onur E, Ozer Y (2004) Nasal route and drug delivery systems. Pharm World Sci 26(3):137–142
3. Fortuna A, Alves G, Serralheiro A et al (2014) Intranasal delivery of systemic-acting drugs: small-molecules and biomacromolecules. Eur J Pharm Biopharm 88(1):8–27. https://doi.org/10.1016/j.ejpb.2014.03.004
4. Engelhardt L, Rohm M, Mavoungou C et al (2016) First steps to develop and validate a CFPD model in order to support the Design of Nose-to-Brain Delivered Biopharmaceuticals. Pharm Res. https://doi.org/10.1007/s11095-016-1875-7
5. Muralidharan P, Malapit M, Mallory E et al (2015) Inhalable nanoparticulate powders for respiratory delivery. Nanomedicine 11(5):1189–1199. https://doi.org/10.1016/j.nano.2015.01.007
6. Grassin-Delyle S, Buenestado A, Naline E et al (2012) Intranasal drug delivery: an efficient and non-invasive route for systemic administration: focus on opioids. Pharmacol Ther 134(3):366–379. https://doi.org/10.1016/j.pharmthera.2012.03.003
7. Fromen CA, Rahhal TB, Robbins GR et al (2016) Nanoparticle surface charge impacts distribution, uptake and lymph node trafficking by pulmonary antigen-presenting cells. Nanomedicine 12(3):677–687. https://doi.org/10.1016/j.nano.2015.11.002
8. Ramishetti S, Huang L (2012) Intelligent design of multifunctional lipid-coated nanoparticle platforms for cancer therapy. Ther Deliv 3(12):1429–1445. https://doi.org/10.4155/tde.12.127
9. Suk JS, Kim AJ, Trehan K et al (2014) Lung gene therapy with highly compacted DNA nanoparticles that overcome the mucus barrier. J Control Release 178:8–17. https://doi.org/10.1016/j.jconrel.2014.01.007
10. Mastorakos P, da Silva AL, Chisholm J et al (2015) Highly compacted biodegradable DNA nanoparticles capable of overcoming the mucus barrier for inhaled lung gene therapy. Proc Natl Acad Sci U S A 112(28):8720–8725. https://doi.org/10.1073/pnas.1502281112
11. Roberts RA, Shen T, Allen IC et al (2013) Analysis of the murine immune response to pulmonary delivery of precisely fabricated nano- and microscale particles. PLoS One 8(4):e62115. https://doi.org/10.1371/journal.pone.0062115

Chapter 14

Non-Enzymatic Tissue Homogenization for Biodistribution Analysis

Danielle M. DiPerna, Alesia V. Prakapenka, Eugene P. Chung, and Rachael W. Sirianni

Abstract

Biodistribution is a valuable technique used to determine payload delivery from nanocarrier to organs of interest in preclinical models. Fluorescent probes can be used as drug surrogates, providing indirect but relevant measurement of tissue exposure to the carrier. This may be useful, for example, to perform a first-pass evaluation of how targeting affects delivery of encapsulated compounds to target organs. This protocol is designed for non-enzymatic tissue homogenization of a variety of organ types allowing tracking of small molecule fluorophores injected freely or encapsulated in nanoparticles.

Key words Biodistribution, Tissue homogenization, Mechanical homogenization, Nanoparticles, Drug delivery, Small molecule fluorophores

1 Introduction

Preclinical evaluation of drug carriers often involves analysis of the biodistribution of their delivery to various tissue sites. Measurement of either payload or carrier concentration in target tissue is an important aspect of evaluating whether targeting was achieved; this initial evaluation can be an essential step toward more detailed pharmacokinetic analysis of specific drug payloads [1]. Biodistribution assessment can be performed in a variety of ways, including in intact tissues (for example, with magnetic resonance imaging, positron emission tomography, or fluorescent imaging [2–4]). Here, we will focus on extraction of drug or label from tissue homogenates, which is a simple and easily implemented technique requiring enzymatic or mechanical homogenization of tissue. Enzymatic methods of homogenization are often time-intensive due to long incubations and introduce chemical variables into the samples. The use of detergents, lytic enzymes, and choatropes can alter fluorescence signal by denaturing proteins and altering the

Rachael W. Sirianni and Bahareh Behkam (eds.), *Targeted Drug Delivery: Methods and Protocols*, Methods in Molecular Biology, vol. 1831, https://doi.org/10.1007/978-1-4939-8661-3_14, © Springer Science+Business Media, LLC, part of Springer Nature 2018

fluorophore-tissue environment. While there are several methods of non-enzymatic homogenization available, we have observed significant variation in the degree of homogenization achieved in different organs, which complicates comparison of extraction from different organs. Here, we demonstrate a non-enzymatic method for mechanically homogenizing a variety of organs (brain, heart, lung, liver, spleen, blood, uterine horn, spinal cord, kidney, and muscle) using a single protocol. We provide an example of utilizing this approach to detect fluorescence in mouse organs.

2 Materials

2.1 Tissue Collection

1. Peristaltic pump.
2. GP tubing 1.6 mm.
3. Leur lock syringe needles (25G × 1 ½).
4. 1 mL insulin syringes with needle (29 G × 1/2 in) attached.
5. 2 mL microcentrifuge tubes.
6. Tubes for blood collection (K2 ethylenediaminetetraacetic acid [EDTA] for whole blood or sodium heparin coated for plasma).
7. Heparinized Saline: 10 units of heparin to 1 mL of 1× saline (*see* **Note 1**).
8. Ketamine/Xylazine: A standard solution contains 16/1.6 mg katamine/xylazine per mL sterile saline (0.9% sodium chloride), which is equivalent to 100/10 mg/kg when administering 100 μL to a 16 g mouse (*see* **Note 2**).
9. Alcohol Prep pads.

2.2 Tissue Mincing, Homogenization, and Probe Sonication

1. Probe sonicator.
2. Bead homogenizer.
3. Small diameter (e.g., 0.156″) stainless steel homogenization beads.
4. Polystyrene weighing dishes.
5. Razor blade.
6. Surgical tweezers, forceps, and fine scissors for dissection.
7. Large magnet, suitable for sliding along the outside of tubes to retrieve beads.
8. Microcentrifuge tubes (2 mL) with locking lid.
9. 15 mL sterile conical tubes.

2.3 Fluorophore Detection

1. 96-well bottom plates (black, flat bottom).
2. Dimethyl sulfoxide (DMSO).

3 Methods

Personal protective equipment should be worn according to institutional policies and MSDS guidelines (*see* **Note 3**). Keep samples on ice and protected from light at all times (*see* **Note 4**). The following protocol has been optimized for measuring biodistribution of fluorescent small molecules in mice and assumes the agent has already been administered to the mouse and allowed to distribute for an appropriate amount of time. Typical measurements might be made at 0.5, 2, 6, 12, and 24 h, although the exact time points should be chosen to span the expected kinetics of the agent being tested.

3.1 Tissue Collection

1. Set up the perfusion pump, dissection board, clean surgical instruments, a beaker of diH_2O, and pre-labeled sample tubes on top of an absorbent laboratory pad.
2. Attach a 25G needle to the free end of the perfusion pump tubing.
3. Prime tubing with heparinized saline to ensure no air bubbles are present (*see* **Note 5**).
4. Approximately 10 min prior to the planned collection time point, anesthetize mouse with an overdose of ketamine/xylazine or according to the institution's IACUC protocols (*see* **Note 6**).
5. Once deeply anesthetized and unresponsive to toe pinch, place mouse supine on dissection board and secure limbs with dissection needles. The abdomen should be taut.
6. Firmly wipe the abdomen with an ethanol pad to dampen the fur.
7. Using surgical scissors, make a vertical incision at the level of the hind limbs. Carefully cut toward the diaphragm, using tweezers in the non-dominant hand to pull skin upward, which will help to avoid nicking internal organs.
8. Grasp the sternum with a pair of tweezers and pierce the diaphragm with the scissors (pneumothorax). Once the diaphragm is pierced, the mouse will begin to gasp and dissection must proceed quickly. Rotate the scissors and continue cutting to one side along the bottom of the ribcage. Rotate the scissors a second time to cut up through the rib cage toward the collarbone. Repeat this procedure along the other side to fully release the ribcage.
9. Lift the entire ribcage by grasping the sternum with tweezers. Pin securely in the open position to expose the heart and lungs.
10. A blood sample can be collected by cardiac puncture. Hold a pair of tweezers in the non-dominant hand and use them to grasp the apex of the right ventricle. Use the dominant hand to hold an insulin syringe, resting the back of the thumbnail on

the bottom of the plunger to enable one-handed manipulation. Holding the heart steady with the non-dominant hand, use the dominant hand to insert the syringe needle carefully into the right ventricle, taking care not to pierce through the septum or into the atrium. Slowly withdraw 100–500 μL of blood. This may take anywhere from 3 to 15 s. If the ventricle collapses, pause to allow blood to refill and proceed at a slower rate.

(a) If analysis is to be performed on whole blood, immediately eject the sample into a K2 EDTA coated tube.

(b) If analysis is to be performed on blood plasma, collect a minimum of 500 μL of blood and immediately eject into a sodium heparin coated tube. After collection, place blood vials on ice. Blood samples should be spun down and processed within 1 h of being collected (*see* **Notes 7** and **8**). Tubes should be processed according to the manufacturer's instructions for optimal blood plasma separation. After centrifugation, collect 60 μL of plasma without disturbing the blood pellet. Place the plasma aliquot in a 2 mL microcentrifuge tube (*see* **Note 9**).

11. The right atrium can be identified by its dark color relative to the ventricle. Use scissors to snip the top. Blood should begin flowing freely into the exposed cavity.
12. Use tweezers in the non-dominant hand to again grasp the heart by the apex of the right ventricle. Insert the perfusion needle into the left ventricle, directing the needle along the inferior-superior axis and taking care not to pierce the septum or left atrium.
13. Release the grasp of the heart and maintain needle position in the left ventricle with the dominant hand. Initiate perfusion. Fluid should flow out of the incision previously made in the right atrium; it will first be dark red and should lighten to eventually become clear. The color of peripheral organs should also lighten, which will indicate a successful perfusion (*see* **Note 10**).
14. Collect desired organs. Carefully remove fat and connective tissue to isolate the organ of interest. Rinse tissue thoroughly with diH_2O, ensuring any tissue particulate, blood, and/or fur is removed.
15. Place each sample into individual, pre-labeled, 2 mL microcentrifuge tubes (*see* **Note 11**).
16. Store organs at −80 °C until ready to process.

3.2 Tissue Mincing, Homogenization, and Probe Sonication

1. Prior to tissue processing, 2 mL locking lid tubes should be pre-labeled and pre-weighed. If the locking apparatus of the tube is missing or appears damaged, the tube should be discarded (*see* **Note 12**).

2. Remove organs, including control tissue, from −80 °C and allow to thaw on ice (*see* **Note 13**). For each study, the same organ for all subjects should be processed on the same day. This will allow for a single standard curve for quantification to be generated.
3. Fill a large beaker with ice water and place under the probe tip at a level that allows the sample to remain cold during sonication.
4. Mince tissue using a scalpel and razor blade. Mincing should be done on a hard surface such as a plastic weigh dish (*see* **Note 14**). Tissue must be completely minced with clean cuts, such that no fibrous or connective tissue remains intact. After mincing, the organ should have a viscous or gelatinous consistency.
5. Transfer the organ to the pre-weighed tube. Re-weigh the tube. Determine the amount of diH_2O needed for 10% weight by volume (w/v) of each sample.
6. Add three stainless steel beads to each tube and add the appropriate volume of water (*see* **Notes 15** and **16**). Once the sample, water, and beads are added, the lid may be closed and locked in place.
7. Place tubes in the high-throughput bead homogenizer. Ensure there is a tight fit with no extra space between the tubes and the apparatus. Run the homogenizer at maximum speed for 5–10 min or until tube contents are liquefied.
8. Remove the tubes from the homogenizer and place on ice for at least 20–30 min to allow any froth generated by homogenization to settle.
9. Use a magnet to remove the steel beads from the tubes. If any tissue is removed with the beads, use tweezers to return the tissue to the tubes. It is normal for some tissue to remain after processing certain organs (e.g., liver). These pieces will be disrupted during probe sonication.
10. Transfer the contents of the microfuge tube to a pre-labeled 15 mL conical tube. We suggest only processing tissue volumes under 3 mL. Otherwise, the sonication energy is not effective.
11. Sonicate the sample at an amplitude of 40% for 10 s. Quickly swirl the conical tube in ice water to ensure contents remain cold.
12. Allow the sample to de-froth for 20–30 min. Once defrothed, sample fluid should be relatively clear and can be transferred to the pre-labeled sample homogenate tube (*see* **Notes 17** and **18**).
13. Repeat **steps 11** and **12** for each organ sample.
14. Store samples at −80 °C until ready to analyze.

3.3 Quantification

1. Remove samples from −80 °C.
2. Vortex each sample for 10 s immediately before plating.
3. Pipette 50 μL of sample or control homogenate into individual wells of a 96-well plate.
4. Add 10 μL of DMSO to each well to reach a final volume of 60 μL.
5. Read fluorescence of all samples on a plate reader using settings appropriate for detecting the signal of interest (*see* **Note 19**).
6. Based on the sample readings, make a serial dilution of the fluorophore in DMSO.
   (a) Adjust the standard curve to as needed to incorporate all the sample points. Ensure all samples lie within the linear portion of the standard curve.
7. If analysis needs to be delayed, plates can be sealed and stored at −80 °C.
8. Arbitrary fluorescent units read from sample homogenates should then be converted to concentration by comparison to the control curve (example data are provided in Fig. 1).

4 Notes

1. Heparinized saline can be made in advanced if stored at 4 °C. Allow the solution to reach room temperature prior to performing perfusion.

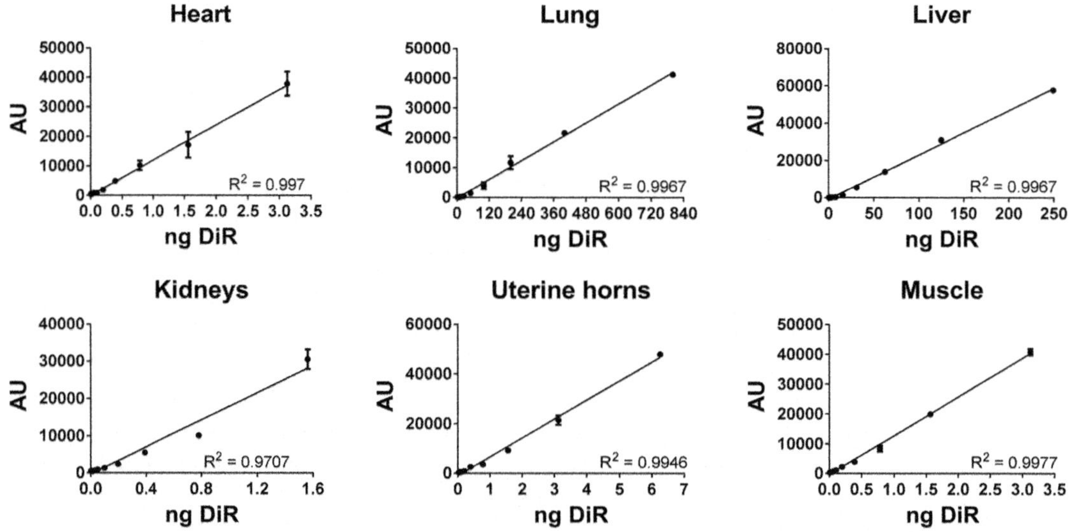

Fig. 1 Example control curves demonstrate a highly reproducible and linear relationship between the quantity of spiked fluorophore in organ homogenate and the fluorescence readout. The fluorophore in this example was DiR, and three replicates are represented per time point

2. Ketamine/xylazine solution should be prepared in a sterile, nonpyrogenic empty vial. The solution can be stored effectively and remain stable up to 2 weeks at 4 °C.
3. We recommend wearing gloves and a laboratory coat for all experiments. A disposable gown, eye protection, and disposable face mask are recommended during perfusion, to protect from splashes.
4. We have observed significant changes to extraction efficiency as a function of temperature. All samples should be held on ice unless otherwise specified. They should also be covered and protected from prolonged exposure to light at all times.
5. Tubing for perfusion can be re-used if it was used with heparin or saline during prior perfusions. Tubing previously used with fixative (e.g., formaldehyde) may still contain traces of the chemical; this tubing should not be re-used, as it may cause the perfusion to fail.
6. The mouse must be deeply anesthetized with the heart still beating for a perfusion to be successful. Too-heavy anesthesia can compromise circulation and should be avoided. Use of inhaled anesthesia may prove difficult, due to the challenge of keeping the mouse's nose in contact with a nose cone while manipulating their body. We have found that injectable anesthesia is both reliable and convenient. Depth of anesthesia should be assessed by performing a toe pinch on both feet prior to beginning perfusion. For the purposes on this procedure, a tail pinch should not be substituted with a touch pinch. The tail is not as sensitive as the feet. Thus a mouse may not respond to a tail pinch but will respond to a toe pinch if it is not yet deeply under anesthesia.
7. Do not freeze blood prior to centrifugation, as the cells will lyse once frozen.
8. A swinging bucket rotor is preferable for centrifugation, because this will place the pellet at the bottom of the tube instead of the sidewall. It is easier to extract plasma this way.
9. After the blood plasma has been collected, the blood pellet can also be processed. The pellet may be frozen in its original tube at −80 °C until the day of processing.
10. Once an efficient perfusion is complete, the liver will have changed from a deep red color to light brown-gray hue. This color change is usually obvious within 10–15 s of perfusion. If the liver does not begin to clear in that time frame, try re-adjusting the needle, or removing and re-inserting the needle into the left ventricle. If the wall dividing the left and right ventricles has been pierced, it may help to clamp between the left and right sides of the heart with tweezers or forceps. We

have found that achieving complete perfusion of the lungs can be difficult, with even very small pockets of inadequately perfused tissue adding high inter-subject variability. To improve perfusion consistency between subjects, we choose to perfuse the lungs separately. After the liver has cleared, re-position the needle toward the pulmonary veins. The lungs will swell with fluid, which will exit via the nostrils. After a count of 3, the needle is removed.

11. Printable tube labels can save a significant amount of time at this stage. We specifically recommend using Cryo-Babies which can withstand storage up to −196 °C (9187–1700, USA Scientific, Ocala, FL, USA).
12. Avoid opening and closing the latch on the lid, which weakens the plastic and can result in breaks. Tubes with broken latches have an increased likelihood of opening during bead homogenization, which may result in sample loss.
13. The number of animals required for a study depends on biological variability in delivery, as well as on the skill and consistency of the perfusion and organ collection. We find that $n = 5–6$ subjects is often sufficient to detect moderate differences in delivery (e.g., comparing a targeted to a non-targeted formulation in a single organ, with an expectation of 50–100% increase in signal in the targeted group). Control tissue should be collected and pooled to construct control curves, which are spiked with known quantities of nanocarrier after being processed to produce homogenates. Some organs (e.g., brain, liver) are relatively large, and $n = 3–4$ subjects will suffice. Other organs (e.g., spinal cord and lungs) are small, and up to 12 subjects will be needed to obtain a sufficient quantity. We routinely collect and store control tissue from non-treated subjects to ensure control organs are available and can be processed in parallel with samples. Control and sample tissues should be subjected to the same number of freeze thaws. i.e., do not generate a single batch of control homogenate and then repeatedly dip into the stock on different days (this will produce signal drift).
14. To minimize waste when mincing samples, the plastic weigh dishes can be re-used. Confirm that the plastic has not been damaged with repeated use, rinse in clean water, dry with a laboratory tissue, and wipe with ethanol. Residual ethanol should be allowed to evaporate prior to next use.
15. The use of three beads was determined to be optimal for all organ types. Adding less than three beads will not provide enough force to homogenize the tissue of more fibrous organs. Adding more than three beads will not provide ample room for the beads to move in the tube, which causes the tissue to

clump. The number of beads may need to be re-optimized if a different diameter is used.

16. All tools, including the probe sonicator and beads, should be cleaned in between subjects. To best clean the homogenization beads, it is important to remove every trace of sample. We clean beads by three washes in distilled water followed by three washes in ethanol. The probe sonicator should be rinsed with clean water, dried with a laboratory tissue, and wiped with ethanol. Residual ethanol should be allowed to evaporate prior to next use.
17. It is important to collect as much of the sample as possible. If, after 30 min, the sample had not de-frothed enough to allow for sufficient pipetting, perform a quick centrifugation to collect the remaining sample before moving forward. Additional diH_2O can be added to the empty tube to collect remaining tissue debris, which can then be disrupted by additional sonication.
18. During probe sonication or vortexing, any fat that was not removed will aggregate and form a layer in the sample that may incorporate with any foam that is present. When pipetting the sample, turn the tube to a 45° angle and pipette below the layer of the foam.
19. We find that readings tend to benefit from a brief shake of the 96-well plate on the plate reader for 10 s. Fluorescent gains should be optimized for each organ (i.e., gains do not need to be matched between organs, and each control curve may have a different gain that should be matched to its own organ). If the experiment requires multiple plates to be read for the same organ, ensure the controls are present on all plates to control for plate to plate variability.

References

1. Schuster BS, Ensign LM, Allan DB et al (2015) Particle tracking in drug and gene delivery research: state-of-the-art applications and methods. Adv Drug Deliv Rev 30(91):70–91
2. Lee PW, Hsu SH, Wang JJ et al (2010) The characteristics, biodistribution, magnetic resonance imaging and biodegradability of superparamagnetic core-shell nanoparticles. Biomaterials 31(6):1316–1324
3. Sirianni RW, Zheng MQ, Patel TR et al (2014) Radiolabeling of poly(lactic-co-glycolic acid) (PLGA) nanoparticles biotinylated F-18 prosthetic groups and imaging of their delivery to the brain with positron emission tomography. Bioconjug Chem 25(12):2157–2165
4. Cook RL, Householder KT, Chung EP et al (2015) A critical evaluation of drug delivery from ligand modified nanoparticles: confounding small molecule distribution and efficacy in the central nervous system. J Control Release 220:89–97

Chapter 15

Methods and Study Designs for Characterizing the Pharmacokinetics and Pharmacodynamics of Carrier-Mediated Agents

Allison N. Schorzman, Andrew T. Lucas, John R. Kagel, and William C. Zamboni

Abstract

Major advances in carrier-mediated agents (CMAs), which include nanoparticles, nanosomes, and conjugates, have revolutionized drug delivery capabilities over the past decade. While providing numerous advantages, such as greater solubility, duration of exposure, and delivery to the site of action over their small molecule counterparts, there is substantial variability in systemic clearance and distribution, tumor delivery, and pharmacologic effects (efficacy and toxicity) of these agents. In this chapter, we focus on the analytical and phenotypic methods required to design a study that characterizes the pharmacokinetics (PK) and pharmacodynamics (PD) of all forms of these nanoparticle-based drug agents. These methods include separation of encapsulated and released drugs, ultrafiltration for measurement of non-protein bound active drug, microdialysis to measure intra-tumor drug concentrations, immunomagnetic separation and flow cytometry for sorting cell types, and evaluation of spatial distribution of drug forms relative to tissue architecture by mass spectrometry imaging and immunohistochemistry.

Key words Nanoparticles, Carrier-mediated agents, Pharmacokinetics, Pharmacodynamics, Immune system, Mononuclear phagocyte system (MPS)

1 Introduction on Carrier-Mediated Agents and Pharmacology

The number of available nanoparticle-based drug systems has seen exponential growth in the past decade. In 2006 alone, nearly 130 nanotechnology-based products were estimated to be undergoing the drug development process worldwide [1]. While the number of agents used clinically is still limited, the plethora that are emerging as potential therapeutic agents warrants the need for detailed studies of their unique pharmacology and mechanisms of action in humans. Caron et al. summarize currently available and late stage development of chemotherapeutic CMAs in supplementary Table S1 [2].

Rachael W. Sirianni and Bahareh Behkam (eds.), *Targeted Drug Delivery: Methods and Protocols*, Methods in Molecular Biology, vol. 1831, https://doi.org/10.1007/978-1-4939-8661-3_15,

The disposition of CMAs is dependent upon the carrier and not the therapeutic entity until the drug gets released [3]. The nomenclature used to describe CMA pharmacokinetics includes: encapsulated (the drug within or bound to the carrier), released (active drug that gets released from the carrier), and sum total (encapsulated drug plus released drug) [4, 5]. After the drug is released from its carrier it is pharmacologically active and subject to the same routes of metabolism and clearance as the non-carrier form of the drug [5]. In theory, the PK disposition of the drug after release from the carrier should be the same as after administration of the small molecule or standard formulations. Thus, the pharmacology and PK of CMAs are complex and comprehensive. Analytical methods must be performed in order to assess the disposition of encapsulated or released forms of the drug in plasma and tumor [6]. Considerable inter-patient variability exists in the PK/PD of CMAs, and while the exact factors are unclear, it is hypothesized that the mononuclear phagocyte system (MPS) (or reticuloendothelial system) plays a key role [7].

The PK of liposomal encapsulated drug and released drug is very different, and compared with conventional small molecule anticancer agents, the PK variability in liposomal formulations is often much greater [5, 8]. Inter-individual variability in drug exposure, represented by area under the concentration versus time curve (AUC), of encapsulated drug can be 20–100-fold. Factors with the potential to affect CMA PK include CMA-associated physical characteristics and host-associated characteristics [9]. Perhaps the greatest influence on the PK variability of CMA, however, is the MPS. Figure 1 illustrates the unique clearance mechanisms associated with CMA as compared with conventional small molecules which include clearance via the MPS in the liver, spleen, and blood, and the enhanced delivery and retention (EPR) effect in tumors [2].

The development of effective chemotherapeutic agents for the treatment of solid tumors depends, in part, on the ability of those agents to achieve cytotoxic drug concentrations or exposure within the tumor [11, 12]. It is currently unclear why within a patient with solid tumors there can be a reduction in the size of some tumors while other tumors can progress during or after treatment, even though the genetic composition of the tumors is similar [13]. Such variable antitumor responses within a single patient may be associated with inherent differences in tumor vascularity, capillary permeability, and/or tumor interstitial pressure that result in variable delivery of anticancer agents to different tumor sites [11, 12]. However, studies evaluating the intratumoral concentration of anticancer agents and factors affecting tumor exposure in preclinical models and patients are rare [12, 14, 15]. Moreover, it is logistically difficult to perform the extensive studies required to evaluate the tumor disposition of anticancer agents and factors that determine the disposition in patients with solid tumors, especially in tumors

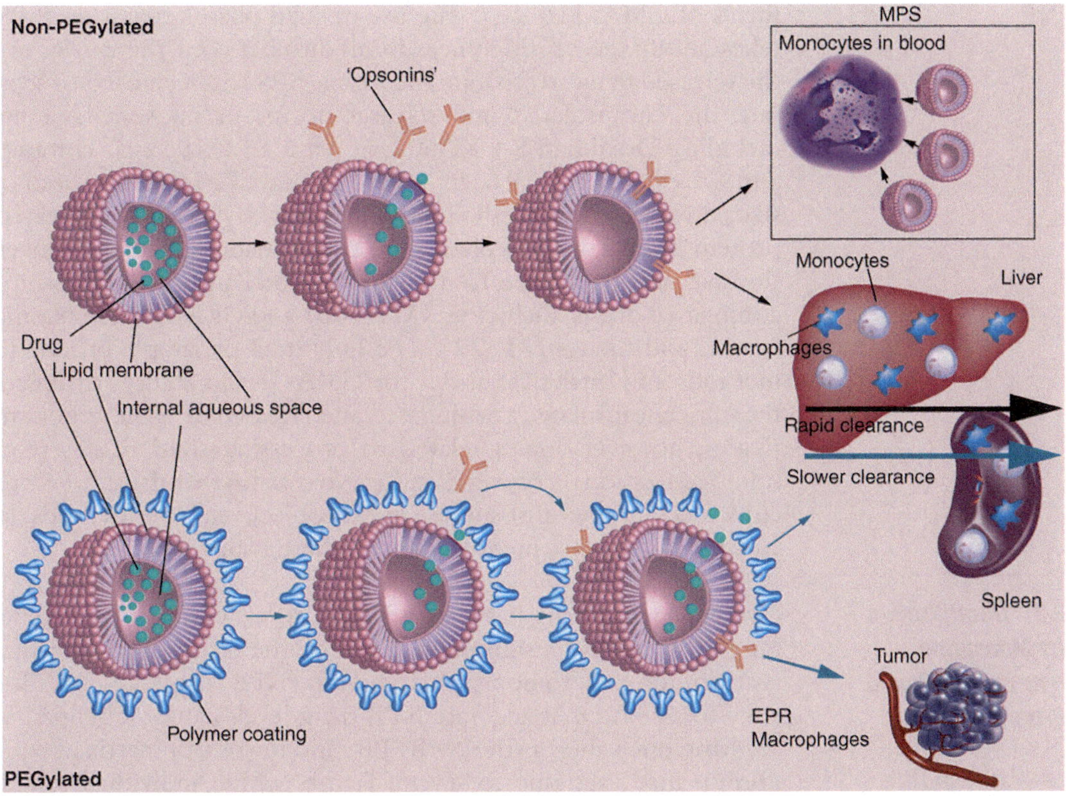

Fig. 1 Clearance of nanoparticles and CMAs via the mononuclear phagocyte system (MPS). When non-stabilized liposomal agents were first tested, they were found to only minimally increase the circulation time of the small molecule agent encapsulated within the carrier (rapid clearance). However, stabilization with polyethylene glycol, (PEG) has helped to reduce uptake and CL of CMA by MPS (slower clearance). While the clearance of pegylated liposomes is slower than non-pegylated liposomes, both are phagocytized by peripheral blood mononuclear cells (PBMC), phagocytes of the liver and spleen. Greater tumor exposure is seen after administration of PEGylated liposomes, which in part due to the enhanced permeability and retention (EPR) effect and possibly, the MPS in tumors [2]. Republished with permission from [10]; permission conveyed through Copyright Clearance Center, Inc.

that are not easily accessible. Thus, there is impending need to develop and implement techniques and methodologies to evaluate the disposition and exposure of anticancer agents within the tumor matrix as well as plasma.

2 Analytical Methods

2.1 Measuring Encapsulated/Conjugated and Released Drug Forms

As CMAs consist of the inactive-encapsulated or inactive-conjugated drug and active-released drug, it is critically important to be able to measure these forms of the agents separately. Different types of methods, including solid phase separation, filtration, size exclusion, chemical conversion, and UV-Vis spectroscopy, have been used to separate the encapsulated/conjugated and released forms of CMAs [16–18]. The use of solid phase separation (SPS) takes advantage of differences in affinity between the carrier and the released drug to separate the forms. SPS has been used to separate the encapsulated and released forms of liposomal agents, including Doxil and S-CKD602, in plasma [2, 19, 20]. Filtration and size exclusion have been used to separate CMA forms based on size; however, nonspecific binding to the device and recovery of protein bound drug in plasma are problematic. Chemical conversion has also been used to measure the total and released form of conjugated drugs, including XMT-1001 and CRLX101, in plasma, tumor, and tissues [21, 22]. The holy grail of sample processing methods and analytical assays for CMAs is the ability to directly measure encapsulated/conjugated and released drug in tumor and tissues; however, issues related to processing solid tissues (e.g., homogenization), recovery, and ex vivo release of drug have precluded achievement of success in this objective. New methods are currently in development to address these issues.

2.2 Ultrafiltration for Measuring Non-protein Bound Drug

Once the active drug has been released from a CMA, protein binding (PB) can have a significant effect on the drug's activity, which is attributed only to non-protein bound (NPB) drug [23, 24]. It is risky to assume that accurate NPB drug levels can be obtained by applying one value, as the NPB/PB ratio in control matrix at equilibrium may vary due to several factors within individual sample conditions. There can be sample-dependent differences in the levels of some proteins that bind drugs, including differences that are affected significantly by certain diseases [25] that may change the NPB/PB ratio at PB equilibrium. Also, samples might be collected before PB equilibrium is reached. Therefore, NPB drug levels should be determined experimentally for optimal data reliability.

NPB drug levels typically are determined by separation of NPB drugs from PB drugs using a molecular weight cutoff membrane in ultrafiltration (UFN) or equilibrium dialysis [26]. We describe here a study to measure NPB concentrations of docetaxel, which is reported to be between ~85% bound to plasma proteins at equilibrium [27]. UFN (using centrifugation to drive smaller molecular weight components of plasma through a membrane, cutoff MW 30,000) was selected for determining the PK profile of NPB docetaxel in human plasma, as the shorter time needed for UFN could minimize PB equilibration after sample collection. The process becomes more complicated if GLP quality data are required because introduction of an internal standard would disrupt the equilibrium between PB and NPB drug.

One challenge of the analysis was due to the water insolubility of docetaxel in aqueous ultrafiltrate (UFT). Isolation of UFT from plasma (200 μL) was not quantitative, as only 100 ± 10 μL of UFT were obtained. Pipette removal of a fixed volume of the UFT was reproducible for the volume, but not for the concentration of docetaxel, even though replicates from the same UFT were pipetted. Reproducible results for docetaxel in UFT obtained from replicates of the same spiked plasma required a quantitative transfer of the UFT followed by a wash of the collection cup with an organic solvent, then extraction of the transferred UFT for LC/MS/MS analysis. The docetaxel result observed upon analysis required adjustment for the UFT volume collected to obtain the final NPB concentration reported for the plasma sample. UFT volumes were determined from the UFT weight collected for each sample (UFT density = 1.0 g/mL). An IS added to plasma could be used to monitor UFN isolation efficiency, but this was not done as this introduction could disrupt the PB-NPB equilibrium. An IS can be used, but it must be added after UFN. The attributed issues observed with pipetting docetaxel in UFT are thought to be due to its poor solubility, producing a non-uniform distribution, perhaps through micelles or due to nonspecific binding of docetaxel to the receiver cup [27].

Another challenge was related to the composition of the calibration standards and quality controls (QCs), where it is risky for these to match that of unknown samples. Generation of NPB levels by adding docetaxel to plasma for standards and QCs was not pursued due to a concern that analytical run acceptance would be based on NPB levels that could not be controlled or known with certainty. As an alternative, UFT spiked with docetaxel to specified concentrations was used for calibration standards and QCs, which required a different processing from that used for docetaxel in plasma of unknown samples. The validation was successful for docetaxel in UFT, including stability in UFT at −80 °C. This information was useful, but was incomplete relative to the complex range of activities of NPB docetaxel in plasma. Additional tests were performed to augment the validated methodology in order to increase its relevance to biological sample analysis. Although NPB accuracy cannot be determined, accuracy relative to an initial reference result allowed a limited evaluation of NPB stability in fresh plasma during short-term storage, freeze thaw cycles, and long-term frozen storage. An additional limitation of using UFT QCs was that they could not be used to confirm that isolation of NPB docetaxel from unknown samples by UFN was operating as expected in the sample analysis runs. This important information was demonstrated by using a reference preparation of docetaxel that was spiked in fresh plasma and was analyzed to afford an initial NPB result before being aliquoted and frozen (−80 °C). Aliquots of this reference plasma preparation were included in all NPB sample analysis runs. Reproduction of the initial NPB results demonstrated that there was a continuity of isolating NPB docetaxel in UFT across all of the sample analysis runs.

2.3 QC Concerns with SPS and Ultrafiltration

QCs are artificial samples, prepared in the laboratory by adding analyte to matrix to produce a specified final concentration. QCs offer the greatest versatility when they are made in a large volume and divided into single use aliquots that can be stored frozen. They are analyzed against an independently prepared calibration curve to establish the observed QC concentration. QC use is required for regulated analysis [28], and although QC use is optional in non-regulated assays, their incorporation can improve confidence in the data quality.

One function of QCs is to test for laboratory calculation and/or preparation error. This is indicated when the difference between the result expected for a QC, based on its preparation, and the result observed upon analysis is greater than the typical experimental error (±15% for regulated bioanalysis). Another function of QCs is to provide accuracy and precision results obtained in three independent runs [28], the foundation of a full validation. Once acceptance criteria have been demonstrated by a QC set, it is advantageous to include the set in subsequent validation and sample analysis runs. These QC sets then also perform a "sentinel" or monitoring function to determine if the method continues to perform as it did during the validation accuracy and precision runs. A final function of QCs uses incorporation of the same QC set in multiple analytical runs to demonstrate analytical continuity. If QC results are comparable in each run, it indicates a reduced risk when making comparisons between data obtained from different analytical runs.

QCs can be used to verify method performance when included as part of an analytical run for unknown samples. Sometimes, it is not possible to create an artificial sample (i.e., a QC) that can be used to duplicate the conditions experienced by unknown samples during the analytical process. The challenge for the laboratory in these situations is to find alternatives that come as close as possible to capturing the information that would be provided if the appropriate QC match could be created. An example of such QC limitations is discussed in the case presented in the above Subheading 2.2.

Another example of QC limitations involves quantitation of encapsulated and released forms of drugs in nanoparticles, where the use of QCs containing the encapsulated drug is limited due to the potential for unacceptable QC results originating from issues not related to analytical performance, such as the release of drug during nanoparticle breakdown or leakage during freeze/thaw cycles or refrigerated storage over relatively short times. Using a common set of encapsulated QCs across all analytical runs introduces risks because low QC results could not be used to differentiate between method performance failure or nanoparticle leakage.

One option is to use separate bulk QC preparations for encapsulated analyte and non-encapsulated analyte, as this might provide adequate stability to characterize validation performance over three consecutive days. However, survival of an encapsulated QC would not be expected during any long-term storage needed for sample analysis involving multiple runs. This is especially difficult in clinical studies where patient enrollment might occur over a long period and sample storage before analysis might be varied. Therefore, a QC preparation containing only released analyte might be the only option for limited reliable monitoring for continuity of assay performance in a lengthy study. The challenge remaining is to demonstrate that the separation of encapsulated and non-encapsulation was performed correctly for each preparation day.

A third QC limitation occurs when the appropriate QC matrix either is not available or its use is restricted by cost or ethical limitations. In these situations, the preparation of QCs in a substitute surrogate matrix can be used if the sample preparation properties of analyte and internal standard can be demonstrated as comparable in the sample matrix and the surrogate matrix. A surrogate matrix can be of biological origin, such as the same species but different age (for pediatrics), strain, or matrix type as the samples, or the same type of matrix but different species. Alternatives to using a surrogate matrix of biological origin are the use of solvents in which the analyte and IS demonstrate properties comparable to the sample matrix. When using a surrogate matrix, there should be awareness that unless demonstrated, analyte stability in the sample matrix might not be matched by analyte stability in the surrogate matrix. In all uses of a surrogate matrix, the more thorough the demonstration of equivalence of the analyte and IS between the sample and surrogate matrix, the greater the confidence in the data generated with its use.

2.4 Use of Microdialysis to Measure Released Drug Forms in Tumors and Tissues

2.4.1 Methods to Measure Drug Disposition in Tumors and Tissue

Until recently, drug uptake into tissues and tumors has been described indirectly based on modeling from plasma pharmacokinetics or measured directly from tissue biopsies. As stated above, modeling of tumor exposure based on plasma exposures without incorporation of factors representing tumor heterogeneity is unreliable [11, 12, 29]. The use of tissue or tumor biopsies is associated with several problems. Obtaining serial biopsies is most often logistically impossible, highly invasive, and associated with patient discomfort [12, 30, 31]. Thus, biopsies are usually only available for a single time point or measurement. Measurements of drug concentrations from biopsies are measured in tissue or tumor homogenates, where it may be difficult to control ex vivo catabolism and differentiate between various forms of the drug. Several new advanced techniques, such as magnetic resonance imaging (MRI), positron emission tomography (PET), and microdialysis, have been developed to quantify the concentrations of anticancer agents in vivo [30–32]. However, the use of MRI and PET is complicated by the lack of ability to differentiate between different forms and metabolites of a drug, availability of imaging equipment, chemical synthesis of effective probes, and cost [31, 32]. The use of microdialysis to evaluate the disposition of anticancer agents in tumors and surrounding tissue, on the other hand, is a methodology that has several advantages over other existing methods [11, 33–35].

2.4.2 Introduction and Advantages of Microdialysis

Microdialysis is an in vivo sampling technique used to study the pharmacokinetics and drug metabolism in the blood and extracellular fluid (ECF) of various tissues [34–36]. The use of microdialysis methodology to evaluate the disposition of anticancer agents in tumors is relatively new [12, 14, 15]. Microdialysis has been used to evaluate the tumor disposition of 5-fluorouracil, capecitabine, and epirubicin in patients with primary breast cancer lesions and carboplatin [14, 15]. Microdialysis has also recently been used to determine intratumoral concentrations of methotrexate in patients with high-grade gliomas and cisplatin in patients with oral cancer [37, 38]. These studies depict the clinical utility of microdialysis in evaluating the tumor disposition of anticancer agents in patients with accessible tumors. Microdialysis is based on the diffusion of NPB drugs from interstitial fluid across the semipermeable membrane of the microdialysis probe [34–36]. A schematic representation of a microdialysis probe in subcutaneous tissue or tumor is depicted in Fig. 2 [39]. Microdialysis provides a means to obtain drug measurements from tumor ECF from which a concentration versus time profile can be determined within a single tumor [12, 14, 15, 35].

Microdialysis provides several advantages over autoradiographic studies of tumor biopsies as a method to evaluate anticancer drug concentrations in tumor tissue. With microdialysis techniques it is possible to obtain serial sampling of anticancer drugs from the ECF of a single tumor with minimal tissue damage or alteration of fluid balance [12, 34, 35]. The microdialysis probe can remain in peripheral or central nervous system (CNS) tissue for up to 72 h without complications, such as increased risk of infection, inflammation, or alteration in probe recovery. Samples can be immediately obtained and analyzed from a single probe that allows for the real-time evaluation of physiologic, pharmacologic, and pharmacokinetic changes [34, 40–42]. In addition, a single microdialysis probe can simultaneously sample several analytes of interest, thus allowing for the measurement of drug concentrations and pharmacologic end points that are required for

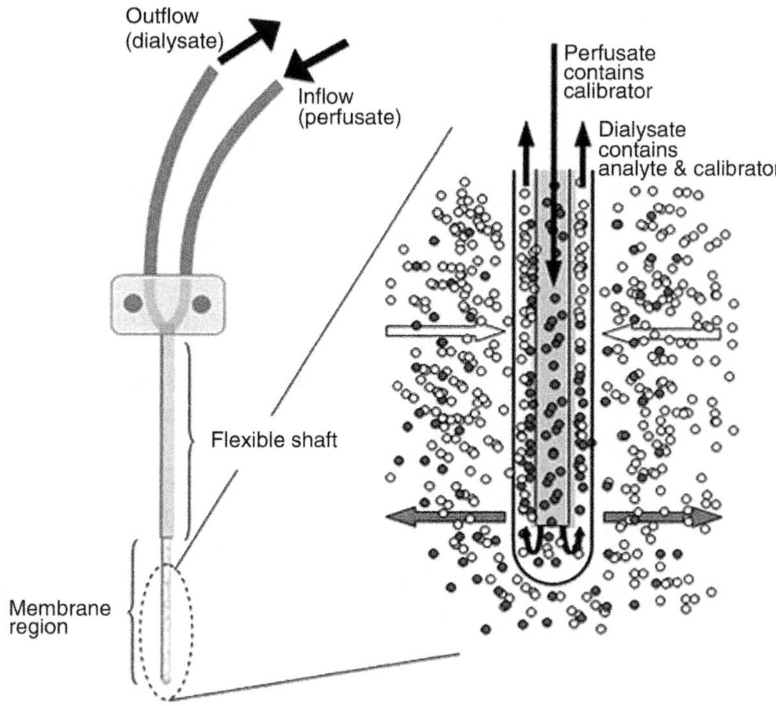

Fig. 2 Schematic of a commercial microdialysis probe with a visual representation of osmosis occurring at equilibrium. Reproduced from *The AAPS Journal*, 2007 with permission from the AAPS [39]

pharmacodynamic studies. Furthermore, the drug concentration can be measured specifically rather than quantitating radioactivity, which may be nonspecific. Because of the pore cut-off size (20 kDa) of the semipermeable membrane, the use of microdialysis allows for the differentiation between liposomally encapsulated, conjugated-drugs, protein-bound drugs, and active-unbound drug in the tumor ECF [33, 43]. Using microdialysis techniques, serial sampling of the non-protein bound, active-form of anticancer agents can be obtained from a single site in a brain tumor, peripheral tumor, or surrounding tissues. In addition, multiple microdialysis probes can be placed in a single tumor to evaluate intratumoral variability of the analyte of interest [6, 12]. Thus, the data obtained with microdialysis techniques may more closely reflect the disposition of the active form of the drug within the tumor ECF [6, 34, 44].

2.4.3 Use of Microdialysis to Evaluate the Tumor Disposition of Nanoparticle Agents

The tumor distribution and pharmacokinetic properties of S-CKD602, a PEGylated liposomal formulation of CKD-602, a camptothecin analogue, were compared to CKD-602 in female SCID mice bearing A375 human melanoma xenografts and are shown in Fig. 3 [19]. Microdialysis was used to determine the released fraction of CKD-602 from S-CKD602 in the tumor ECF as compared with nonliposomal CKD-602. Mice were given S-CKD602 at 1 mg/kg of CKD-602 equivalent, and CKD-602 at 30 mg/kg. Despite the 30-fold lower dose, S-CKD602 plasma AUC of released CKD-602 (36,905 ng/mL•h) was four-fold higher than nonliposomal CKD-602 (9117 ng/mL•h). Eighty-two percent of S-CKD602 remained encapsulated out to 75 hours following administration. Tumor ECF AUC $_{0-75h}$ of CKD-602 was lower (187 ng/mL•h) following S-CKD602 administration than following non-liposomal CKD-602 (AUC $_{0-\infty}$) administration (639 ng/mL•h), but more importantly, the duration of exposure above 1 ng/mL was 3.6-fold longer following S-CKD602. These results are consistent with antitumor response data of S-CKD602 compared with non-liposomal CKD-602 [12, 45].

2.5 Immunomagnetic Cell Sorting: A Powerful Tool for Isolation and Analysis

2.5.1 Conventional Methods in Cell Separation

Having the ability to separate and analyze a heterogeneous cell population based on a specific cellular characteristic provides a significant analytical resource for researchers. Current anti-cancer CMAs in development are becoming more actively targeted in comparison to their earlier counterparts that rely on passive targeting strategies, utilizing the EPR effect to accumulate within tumor tissues. By identifying a specific marker of interest for CMAs to target, researchers can equally use the same marker to improve and focus their analytical studies by quantifying uptake of targeted CMA formulations into the cells of interest (those expressing the marker of interest) compared to surrounding cells.

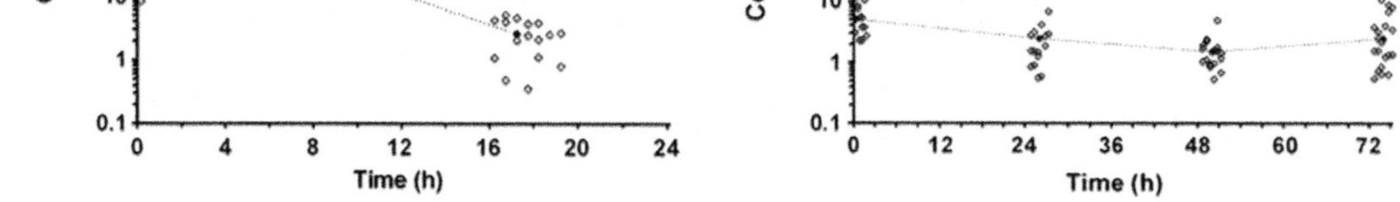

Fig. 3 Concentration versus time profile of CKD-602 in plasma, tumor, and tumor ECF after administration of nonliposomal CKD-602 (**a**) and S-CKD602 (**b**). The plasma and tumor sum total concentrations represent the mean of three mice at each time point. Microdialysis studies (n = 3–4 mice per interval) were obtained every 20 min from 0 to 2 h and every 30 min from 4 to 8 h and 20 to 24 h after administration of either CKD-602 (**a**) or S-CKD602 (**b**), ◇, mean tumor ECF concentration at each time point. - - -◆ - - -, average tumor ECF concentration at each interval. The CV% for the plasma and tumor sum total concentrations at each time point for all samples was <25%. Reproduced from *Clinical Cancer Research*, 2007 with permission from American Association for Cancer Research

Various physical and biochemical cellular separation methods exist, including density gradient centrifugation, erythrocyte lysis, or adherence. In the last four decades, advances in cellular biology and immunology have led to various types of cellular probes that instead are able to differentiate cells based on the presence or absence of specific surface markers. These markers can vary in their individual characteristics, but examples include DNA content, membrane organization, intracellular pH, and surface receptors [46].

Being able to conduct such analysis and separation is based on the ability to identify, or label, a specific property of interest, such as a cellular receptor. In the case of specific cellular separation, the label is further exploited to isolate cells from the rest of the population, especially if the cell type is rare, such as progenitor or stem cells. A number of different labeling technologies exist, but the most specific labels are those that will interact with single cell-associated molecules, commonly employing the use of monoclonal antibodies [47]. These immunological labels can then be coupled with various compounds, such as fluorophores or magnetic beads, which allow for differentiation or separation from a population. Once target-specific cell populations are separated, conventional bioanalytical techniques, such as those reviewed above, can be used to determine drug concentration versus time data within the targeted population of interest.

The most common immunofluorescent technology, where a fluorescent tag is covalently attached to a probe that is used for cell separations, is fluorescence-activated cell scanning/sorting (FACS). FACS systems allow for the added benefit of being used for both phenotypic analysis and sorting and can be utilized in a wide platform of applications, from basic biological practices to clinical determination of disease [46]. This method has several advantages, including utilizing either positive or negative (null) selection, the ability to utilize multiple marker selection, and sorting of cells using intracellular markers (such as green-fluorescent proteins). While this method allows for high purity (>98%) and high specificity of sorting, the method is technically complex and requires specialized equipment that limits its high-throughput appeal. FACS can be considered a more expensive technique due to the need for capital investment and dedication of personnel and facilities once the equipment is available. It is further limited by the time required for complete separation, which can take several hours for a single sample due to the serial sorting nature of the device. This sorting time can be reduced, but at the expense of specificity. While newer instruments that employ a "parallel sorting" technology are in development, none is currently available on the open market. Another issue with using FACS is that when dealing with the large surface areas involved in cell separation (due to the high number of cells in a population), FACS probes can potentially bind to cells nonspecifically in larger cell populations. This can create issues when trying to achieve high enrichment rates, especially when attempting to sort out rarer cells from the total population.

2.5.2 Immunomagnetic Cell Separation Technologies

On the other hand, a number of immunomagnetic technologies are now available on the market, typically where antibodies (or sometimes lectins) are coupled with magnetic beads less than 100 nm in diameter. This magnetic-activated cell separation (MACS) primarily provides cell separation with the most representative products being separators produced by Dynal and Miltenyl Biotec. These MACS-based systems have also provided a similar wide platform of applications to FACS, from basic biology to clinical treatment of disease, since their inception [48–51].

The primary principle behind MACS is that a cell population can be labeled with antibodies conjugated with paramagnetic particles targeted to a certain cell target. This mixture of magnetically labeled and non-labeled cells is applied to a column filled with a ferromagnetic matrix or another separation vessel and placed within a magnetic field. The magnetically labeled cells will be retained in the column/vessel due to the magnetic field, while the remaining non-labeled cells can be washed out. Once removed from the magnetic field, the labeled cells can then be washed and collected. This method can allow for either positive selection, which labels cells to be retained from the eluted cell population, or negative selection, which labels cells to be removed (depleted) from the eluted cell population. There is currently no method for null selection, as in FACS sorting, using MACS.

Overall, MACS allows for the combination of advantages found in conventional cell sorting methods [49, 52]. The small size of these magnetic particles allows for highly specific and quantitative labeling to occur [49, 52, 53]. It is possible to obtain high purities (>90-98%) and specificity using MACS. MACS is also a gentler method to separate cell populations, as there are no added mechanical forces applied via FACS fluidics that could affect cell viability or integrity. Seeing that cell populations are being sorted in parallel simultaneously, between 10^9 and 10^{11} cells can be processed in roughly 30 minutes. Further, the magnetic labels do not interfere with FACS analysis for later analytical studies and do not inhibit regular cellular functions. However, the true advantage of MACS lies in the low technical complexity, and it is able to be performed on the bench in-house for modest financial impact.

The greatest limitation of MACS is its use in multiple marker selection; multi-parameter, high gradient magnetic cell sorting devices are in development, but current multi-step separations require multiple label separation strategies. The principle behind a multi-parameter cell sorting with MACS is using multiple individual separations. For instance, after an initial cell separation, the magnetic particles can be cleaved from the label using enzymatic digestion before labeling again with a second immunomagnetic probe. The cell mixture is then run though a new column in a magnetic field, retaining cells with the secondary trait, while those not labeled for this second trait are eluted. Further, MACS is unable to allow for sorting based on expression, such as high versus low expression, which can be achieved with FACS. Samples can only be sorted into positive or negative fractions.

Depending upon the specific product used, MACS can confer specific advantages and disadvantages as well. Dynabeads® by Dynal use a larger magnetic bead (4.5 μm), created from an iron core surrounded by a thin polymer that can then have other biomolecules (i.e., lectins, antibodies, enzymes, etc.) adsorbed to its surface. Due to the size of the beads, cells can be separated from the remaining population using a relatively small, but still powerful, magnet. However, if the density of these beads becomes too great, they can interfere in downstream applications and cell-cell interactions, and thus it is recommended to typically cleave and remove these beads before use. Of note, Dynabeads® are not suitable for every type of cell separation, as in some cases their usage has been shown to strip the antigen from the cell surface, making the separation unachievable.

The MACS separation system by Miltenyl Biotec differs in from the Dynabeads® system in that the magnetic beads consist of iron oxide and polysaccharides and are much smaller (roughly 50 nm) in comparison. Due to their smaller size, a far stronger magnetic field is required to separate cells from the population. However, the beads do not need to be removed after separation as they will be internalized by viable cells, so there is no interference in the interaction of cell adherence or cell-cell interaction. This system also requires a relative larger investment in equipment (cost of the separation magnet) and supplies (magnetic bead costs) but is still much cheaper compared to FACS.

In the sorting of rare cells, where the frequency of a cell is very low (<1%), such as circulating tumor cells, successful isolation is contingent upon highly specific labeling of a cell population coupled with a short processing time to maintain cell viability and ensure marker shedding has not occurred. MACS separation techniques have been successfully demonstrated in isolating rare cell populations while maintaining cell viability, such as in CD34-expressing haematopoietic stem cell progenitor cells, which make up a total of 0.1% of peripheral mononuclear cells (PBMCs) [54, 55]. There is no other method available to obtain $CD34^+$ cell subsets that can achieve similar enrichment, up to 20,000-fold, and cell recoveries from both tissues and peripheral blood [56–58]. Other successful applications include isolating fetal cells from the peripheral blood of a pregnant woman [59] and isolating allergen-specific B-cells from peripheral blood of a donor [48]. The use of MACS technologies in equipment for the detection of rare cell subsets has even led to FDA-approved clinical diagnostic tests in the detection of circulating tumor cells in patients with metastatic breast, colon, or prostate cancer [60].

2.6 Mass Spectrometry Imaging to Evaluate Spatial Distribution of Drug and Nanocarrier

Liquid chromatography coupled with tandem mass spectrometry (LC-MS/MS) is the gold standard for quantifying anti-cancer drug exposure in plasma, tissues, and tumor in drug development studies. This approach requires the homogenization of tissue followed by extraction of the drug from the matrix (i.e., protein precipitation, liquid-liquid extraction, solid-phase extraction) in order to measure an average drug concentration; however, no information can be gained on the spatial distribution or depth of penetration of the drug within the tissue. Furthermore, when evaluating CMAs in tissue and tumor, there is currently no way to determine by LC-MS/MS if the active drug is encapsulated or released. Knowledge about the relative distribution of the drug in a tissue is desirable in order to obtain a better understanding of how targeted drugs interact with tumor and tissue cells, and to determine if a drug, as well as its relevant entities (i.e., prodrug, metabolite, carrier), is reaching the appropriate target exert its effect.

Recent advances in the field of mass spectrometry imaging (MSI) have utilized the speed, sensitivity, and specificity of mass spectrometry to allow the interrogation of drug distribution and relative amounts in intact tissue. MSI offers a label-free approach to perform simultaneous analysis of the relative amount of drugs and metabolites as well as potential drug targets, which may include endogenous proteins, peptides, lipids, or hormones [61]. It will also address important questions about drug exposure such as the ability of a CMA to pass through the blood-brain barrier or the depth of penetration of a drug into the tumor, which will help to explain pharmacokinetics, efficacy, and toxicity.

In an MSI experiment, a tissue section from a dosed animal is mounted on a glass or metal slide. Analytes in the solid phase within the tissue are transferred to ions in the gas phase and the mass-to-charge ratios (m/z) subsequently analyzed using a mass spectrometer. Individual mass spectra from unique positions across the tissue are processed with sophisticated software to correlate ion abundance with location on the tissue, thus generating a map of the distribution of each analyte of interest. The sample processing, ionization, and mass analyzer used should be tailored to address the questions sought in the experiment. While these topics are addressed below, there are numerous reviews that have been written on the topic of instrument optimization for MSI of drugs in tissues [62–67].

MSI can be applied to tumor, tissues, organs, or even whole body sections [64, 65, 68]. For an MSI experiment, the sample (e.g., organ) is harvested, rinsed, and processed quickly to minimize ex vivo effects, such as drug degradation or diffusion throughout the tissue [63]. Tissue is typically flash frozen in liquid nitrogen or frozen in a container within an isopentane/dry ice bath as not to compromise the shape and integrity of the tissue. Formalin-fixing and paraffin embedding is generally incompatible with mass spectrometry because formalin allows diffusion of the drug whereas paraffin suppresses the analyte signal, although MSI of paraffin-embedded tissue has been demonstrated [63, 69, 70]. The tissue is usually sectioned to a thickness of 5–20 μm [63, 64, 71, 72] and the size of the tissue is limited only by the amount required to secure it for sectioning. MSI data can complement the quantitative data achieved from LC-MS/MS, but studies that require absolute quantitation and spatial distribution should be planned with MS imaging in mind. If a direct comparison of drug distribution will be made between normal tissue and tumor, a section should be prepared that includes both normal tissue and tumor. If immunohistochemistry (IHC) will also be performed, adjacent tissue sections can be collected for MSI and IHC, and the IHC section can be fixed and embedded as desired. Furthermore, if absolute quantitation will be performed by LC-MS/MS, a representative section of the tissue should be reserved for homogenization.

The most common ionization techniques for MSI include secondary ion mass spectrometry (SIMS), desorption electrospray ionization (DESI), and matrix-assisted laser desorption ionization (MALDI) [73, 74]. SIMS, used in the first MSI studies, generates ions by sputtering a surface with a high energy primary ion beam and is capable of high spatial resolution; however, it suffers from limited sensitivity [63]. DESI is a combination of electrospray and desorption ionization where an electrically charged mist is directed toward the sample, desorbing the analytes from the surface and then toward the MS inlet. It is advantageous in that it has good sensitivity and does not require additional sample preparation after sectioning, potentially allowing for IHC after MSI [63]. MALDI is the most widely used ionization technique for MSI and is compatible with a diverse range of analyzers [63]. For MALDI, the tissue section must first be coated with an organic, energy-absorbing compound to promote ionization (e.g., α-cyano-4-hydroxycinnamic acid, sinapinic acid, 2,5-dihydroxybenzoic acid) and this compound can be tuned to preferentially ionize the target analyte [64, 68, 72]. The matrix molecules absorb the energy from a pulsed laser directed at the surface, ablating the tissue surface, along with the drug, resulting in its ionization and detection by mass spectrometry. Infrared laser matrix-assisted laser desorption electrospray ionization (IR-MALDESI) is an alternative technique developed by Muddiman and co-workers [75, 76] that utilizes an IR laser that resonates with water, thus allowing ice to be used a matrix for desorption and subsequent ionization of molecules by ESI. This provides an advantage over MALDI in that no organic matrix is used that could interfere with the analyte signal.

The tissue is interrogated by MSI using a raster technique, where spots of the tissue are sampled at resolutions of typically 20–250 μm in diameter [64, 72, 77], depending on the ion or laser beam. Larger spot sizes collect more material per laser shot, thus improving the signal to noise for the analyte of interest, but sacrifice spatial resolution. Smaller spot sizes are required to obtain high resolution; however, the amount of material per shot is significantly reduced. Furthermore, resolution can be improved by oversampling, where the sample is completely ablated before moving the target by a distance smaller than the laser beam diameter, then ablating the sample in the overlapping spot [78, 79]. A compromise will need to be made to collect enough material to be detected while still obtaining the spatial resolution desired. Matrix effects will affect the sensitivity of an MSI experiment because the tissue matrix of the sample cannot be separated as it is done for absolute quantitation using LC.

Detection of the analytes is achieved by full scan analysis (i.e., measurement of all analytes within a predefined *m/z* range) typically using a quadrupole-time-of-flight (qTOF), Fourier-transform ion cyclotron resonance (FTICR), or Orbitrap mass spectrometer. The physics of how each mass analyzer separates ions by *m/z* differs, but each ultimately achieves high resolution mass spectra. High mass accuracy (low ppm) and resolution, particularly with the Fourier-transform-based ICR and Orbitrap mass spectrometers, is what provides the selectivity required to identify an analyte based solely on intact molecular mass. Full scan analysis provides the opportunity to collect data simultaneously for the active drug and signature ions from the nanocarrier, thus allowing the construction of ion maps to determine the distribution of the encapsulated and released drug forms. In addition, acquisition of full scan spectra allows the investigator to perform a meta-analysis to search for metabolites or other ions of interest if they have been identified after the data has already been collected.

Acquisition of data for an entire tissue section can take hours and generate very large data files. Once the data have been processed, the relative abundance of each ion of interest is correlated with the X-Y position of the tissue [63] thus generating a three-dimensional image of the tissue. If IHC and absolute quantitation were performed with adjacent tissue sections, the IHC data can be overlaid with MSI data to correlate analyte distribution with important features such as vasculature and cell type and the relative amounts can be compared to absolute amounts from LC-MS/MS data. Although imaging data are usually qualitative and measured relative from spot-to-spot and section to section, researchers are developing absolute quantitation techniques for imaging using calibration curves and QCs [71, 80].

We have evaluated the spatial distribution of doxorubicin in tissue after administration of non-liposomal doxorubicin (NL-doxorubicin) or PEGylated liposomal doxorubicin (PLD). Figure 4 shows spleen tissue from tumor-bearing mice that has been imaged using light microscopy (Fig. 4a) and IR-MALDESI coupled with an Orbitrap mass spectrometer where doxorubicin (Fig. 4b) and a signature ion from the PLD (PC 34:1) (Fig. 4c) have been monitored. We can differentially visualize the presence of doxorubicin and the liposomal component in the PLD-treated spleen samples. This demonstrates the ability to achieve spatial distribution maps of drug and the nanoparticle components to complement absolute quantitation by LC-MS/MS. MSI is not yet able to reach detection limits as low as LC-MSMS due to the matrix effects introduced by the tissue. Furthermore, protein therapeutics, such as monoclonal antibodies, are challenging for MSI due to their large size and low copy number.

3 Phenotyping

3.1 Flow Cytometry: A Practical Approach to Immunophenotyping

In general, the immunophenotyping of biological samples describes the use of various tools (e.g., fluorescently conjugated monoclonal or polyclonal antibodies) to detect specific characteristics (i.e. antigens) expressed on or within heterogeneous cell populations [81]. Practically, immunophenotyping using flow cytometry is used to provide information about the expression of specific antigens (e.g., surface receptors) that have been stained

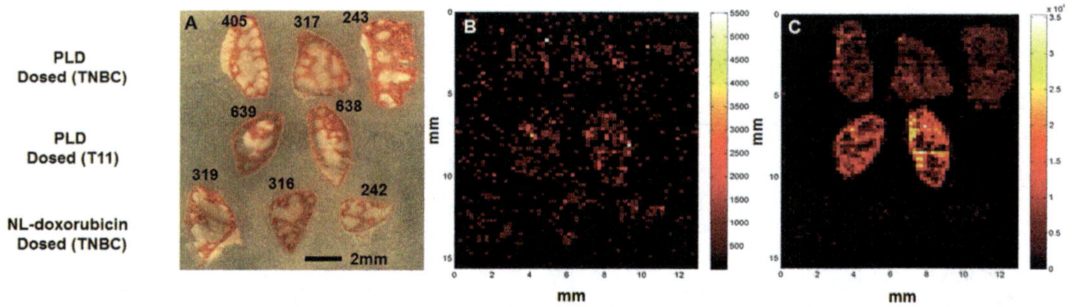

Fig. 4 IR-MALDESI MS imaging of doxorubicin and phosphatidyl choline (32:0) in the spleen of mice bearing an intracranial model of triple-negative breast cancer and genetically engineered mice bearing claudin-low breast cancer tumors (T11) 3 h after administration of 6 mg/kg doxorubicin or PEGylated liposomal doxorubicin (Doxil®) 1 × IV. (**a**) Images of brain tissue by light microscopy; (**b**) Ion map of doxorubicin by IR-MALDESI MSI; (**c**) Ion map of phosphatidyl choline (32:0), which is a liposomal component of PLD, by IR-MALDESI MSI. The color scale in (**b**) and (**c**) refers to relative abundance units

using one or more antibodies. The analysis of these stained cells can non-subjectively confirm the presence, or absence, of the amount of antigen expressed per cell above a certain threshold, and if a pattern can be observed in the expression within the whole cell population of a given sample [81]. The amount of fluorescence emission detected is commonly considered proportional to the number of antibodies bound to the cell provided that the reagent has a stable dye:protein ratio. Flow cytometry can also be used to interrogate other information, such as receptor occupancy and cell function [82–85]. As such, flow cytometry permits any identified phenotypic changes to be put into context with potential changes in function before and after treatment with CMAs or other compounds. These observed changes in phenotype are an important part of the preclinical evaluation process and provide useful information for the further development of CMA formulations.

3.1.1 Flow Cytometry vs. Conventional Microscopy

In the past, cellular phenotypes were studied by microscopy using either enzymatic (immunocytochemistry) or fluorescence (immunofluorescence) approaches. However, flow cytometry has been increasingly used for these immunophenotyping purposes due to several distinct advantages. Compared to microscopy, and other immunophenotyping techniques, flow cytometry is simple and sensitive, allowing for quantitative analysis of multiple antigen targets in a large population of cells, providing high sensitivity/specificity and absolute cell count of a sample within a matter of seconds [86]. Figure 5 shows a standard workflow for the characterization of CMAs in blood by flow cytometry.

The only major disadvantages are the need for single cell dispersed suspensions. Because of this, flow cytometry has been used to great effect in blood and examining rare cell subsets, but its use in cells derived from solid tissue has been limited. Flow cytometry

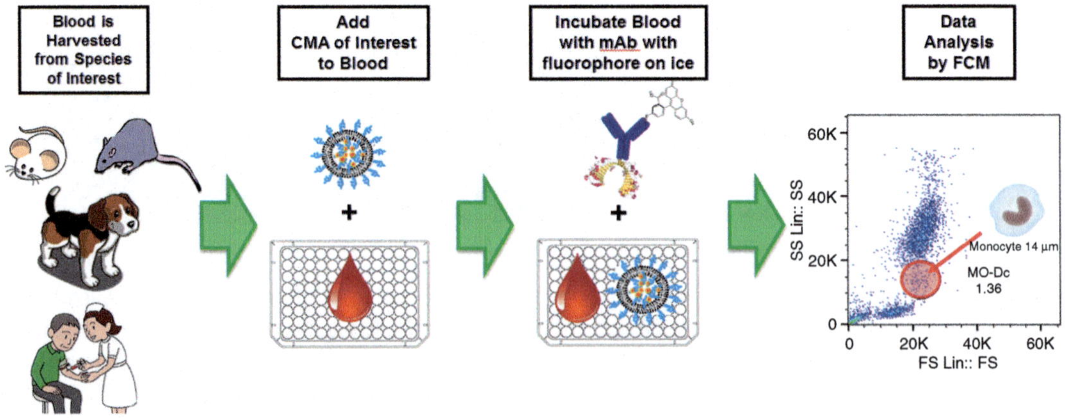

Fig. 5 Workflow for characterization of CMAs in blood by flow cytometry

also lacks clarity in particular morphology and localization of detectable intracellular markers [87, 88]. However, new instruments that combine microscopy and flow cytometry, such as Amnis' ImageStreamX Mark II, begin to bridge the gap of these disadvantages (imaging flow cytometry). In addition to collecting data on the overall stained characteristics of cells, images of individual cells are collected as they are analyzed, generating data on the distribution of antigen markers [89–92].

3.1.2 Variables Affecting the Sensitivity of Phenotypic Detection

The threshold for determining positivity within a sample depends on the sensitivity of the measurement taken. However, this sensitivity relies upon several factors related to the sample preparation, staining reagents, and the instrument used for analysis; these have been extensively reviewed in the literature [46, 93–97]. Most often we focus on manipulation of the staining reagent, commonly a monoclonal antibody conjugated to a fluorescent dye. The affinity of the antibody to the antigen of interest (and thus the concentration of antibody required) and the dye conjugated (using brighter dyes with antigens of less density) are all critical variables in initial panel design and optimization. This use of direct immunofluorescence is preferred for multi-colored antigen reactions due to direct staining of antigens of interest (e.g., anti-CD4-FITC). In comparison, indirect immunofluorescence utilizes a secondary antibody with a fluorescent dye (e.g., antihuman IgG-FITC) to recognize the primary antibody to an antigen, which limits the analysis to a single antigen per sample. Regardless, each new lot of antibody's staining pattern should be confirmed against appropriate controls before use.

Specimens are often whole blood, but may be from other tissues, including cell culture and digests of solid tissues. The types of specimens that can ultimately be processed for flow cytometry can be broadly grouped into three categories: blood containing dispersed cells, red-cell-free single-cell suspension, and solid tissues. While solid tissues will require dissociation into single-cell suspensions (requiring >95% single cells for accurate analysis) prior to staining, antibodies can be applied directly to the other two samples. This will not be the case though if the antigen of interest is also present in extracellular media (such as serum that may contain IgG) or the antigen is expressed in high densities on red blood cells. Other variables to consider within sample preparation include the pH, temperature, and amount of time solutions that are used during cell incubations, as well as those used in any additional steps (i.e., cell washing steps). Certain reagents, including anticoagulants, choice of erythrocyte lysing solution, and fixatives, will also have a direct impact on the sensitivity of the assay. When stained cells cannot be analyzed immediately, samples should utilize a fixative so that the cells are stable for storage. Typically, the optimal sample preparation technique will depend on the type of specimen and the cell population of interest. Preferentially, samples are stained before consecutive red blood cell lysis and washing steps.

Characteristics and configurations of individual optics that define the intrinsic sensitivity of the flow cytometer used are the most important factors that influence the threshold for positivity. Instruments vary widely in their capabilities and format of the data that they generate. The flow cytometer itself should be regularly evaluated for proper function using standardized florescent beads. Further, appropriate controls for using single stains of cells should be performed with each next experiment, as this also will allow for establishing compensation settings needed in the analysis of multiple-color assays. Finally, individual instrument settings will need to be optimized based on the staining protocol used, as identical instruments may not replicate the same results due to the individual variety in their optics (i.e., filters, fluorescence detectors, size/shape of laser spot, and speed of detection).

3.1.3 Quantification of Cellular Phenotypes

Under carefully constructed optimal conditions, the number of molecules bound per cell will depend on the amount of antigen expressed by the cell [98]. Along with the use of internal reference standards added to each sample, a direct relationship between the amount of an emission associated with individual cells and the amount of antigen they express can be made [99]. Several different units have been used to reflect the quantification of antigen expression, including arbitrary fluorescence channel units, standardized units of molecules equivalent of soluble fluorochrome (MESF), and antibody binding capacity (ABC) [93].

Most cell suspensions, even those grown from established cell lines, are heterogeneous in composition. Due to this, characterization of expressed antigen typically requires simultaneous staining with multiple antibodies. By staining for a marker of the cell population of interest as well as the phenotyping antigen, undeniable identification of the cells of interest and their specific expression and/or characterization can be obtained. The level of expression in the cell population of interest can then be reflected as the mean or median fluorescence obtained for those cells (along with coefficient of variation to reflect precision of quantification).

3.2 Immunohistochemical Staining

Carrier-mediated agents are able to exploit the enhanced permeability and retention (EPR) effect to target tumor cells and reduce toxicity to normal cells. The PK of a CMA is defined by the carrier until the small molecule is released and greater inter-patient variability has been demonstrated for the CMA relative to the active small molecule [7]. While numerous factors may play a role in this variability, such as the MPS activity, characteristics of the CMA (size, shape, charge, surface chemistry), and traits of the host (age,

BMI, immune system) [100], it has been suggested that heterogeneity of the tumor microenvironment plays a significant role in the passive targeting of CMAs to solid tumors. This environment includes factors such as tumor-associated macrophages (TAMs), collagen, and abnormal vasculature. TAMS, which are derived from circulating monocytes or reside in the tissue, interact with chemokines, cytokines, and growth factors, which in turn train the macrophage in its function resulting in either promotion or inhibition of tumor growth. Collagen is an abundant, structural protein that makes up the extracellular matrix. Its density may inhibit diffusion of the CMA to its tumor target while having no effect on its small molecule counterpart [101]. The extent of angiogenesis within and among tumors is variable and will also affect heterogeneity of the microenvironment. Profiling the microenvironment of tumors by immunohistochemistry (IHC) will provide a better understanding of which tumor types are conducive to CMA treatment, thus indicating which cancer patients will benefit most from nanotherapy.

IHC is a biochemical technique that takes advantage of the specific interaction between an antibody and its antigen to localize a protein of interest. Harvested tissues are preserved by formalin-fixing and are embedded in paraffin for subsequent sectioning. A general H&E staining protocol can be applied to visualize cellular structures such as nuclei and cytoplasmic and extracellular proteins. For interrogation of a specific target (i.e., protein cell type), additional sample preparation may be required to block nonspecific targets or to make the epitope available for binding (i.e., application of heat or an enzyme). A primary antibody, usually an un-labeled monoclonal or polyclonal antibody raised specifically to the antigen, is applied to the tissue to specifically bind to the antigen of interest. This is followed by the application of a secondary antibody, raised against an immunoglobulin of the primary antibody, which is conjugated to a reporter molecule, typically a fluorescent molecule (e.g., fluorescein, rhodamine). The fluorescent signal can be visualized using a microscope with the appropriate filters for exciting and detection the wavelength of light from the fluorescent probe. Multiple antibodies can be used with different fluorophores to identify the localization of multiple antigens simultaneously.

Several antigens can be interrogated to define the tumor microenvironment. F4/80 is well characterized membrane protein that is used to identify the presence of mouse macrophages. F4/80 staining allows the visualization of TAMS, elucidates the abundance of TAMS, and illustrates any potential change in abundance of time points. Collagen IV is the primary structural component of basement membranes making up the extracellular matrix. A dense network of collagen is thought to inhibit diffusion of a CMA and reduce the exposure of the active drug to the tumor. An antibody to collagen interrogates the density of the collagen in a tumor. CD31 is a protein associated with endothelial cells; thus IHC using an antibody to CD31 demonstrates the presence of endothelial cells and, subsequently, indicates the extent of angiogenesis occurring in a tumor microenvironment.

The role of heterogeneity within the tumor microenvironment on the PK and PD of non-liposomal doxorubicin (NL-doxorubicin) and PEGylated liposomal doxorubicin (PLD) was evaluated for two genetically engineered mouse models of cancer triple-negative breast cancer—C3-TAg (basal-like) and T11 (claudin-low) [20]. PK of doxorubicin and PLD were evaluated in plasma (encapsulated and released for PLD) and tumor (sum total = encapsulated and released). Tumors were treated by IHC staining to evaluate the disposition of TAMS (F4/80), collagen (collagen IV), and vasculature (CD31). Plasma PK was similar between the tumor subtypes for NL-doxorubicin and encapsulated and released doxorubicin from PLD. While tumor PK was similar for NL-doxorubicin, PLD delivery was greater for C3-TAg tumors relative to T11 tumors. As determined by mean tumor volume and survival, efficacy was improved for PLD relative to NL-doxorubicin. Among the PLD-treated mice, the T11 tumors were more responsive while the C3-TAg mice exhibited a prolonged survival, which may be due to the consequence of T11 mice being terminated due to tumor ulceration.

IHC was performed to determine which tumor-associated factors contributed to this observation. F4/80 staining of TAMs showed that baseline levels were the same between the two models and revealed that a nadir occurs at 24 h. This transient decrease indicates that PLD is cytotoxic to TAMS, that they are able to recover from the toxicity, and that a drug-tumor interaction exists. However, the TAM levels present in the tumor microenvironment are not the likely cause for different exposure in the two models. Likewise, collagen IV staining showed that the baseline density of the structural protein was similar in breast tumor subtypes and would not account for differences in exposure between the two tumor subtypes. CD31 staining (coupled with VEG-F quantitation) was applied to evaluate vascularization by blood and lymph vessels. In the T11 model, staining of CD31 illustrated hypervascularization (which is typically observed in claudin-low breast tumors) and ineffective lymph networks, increased interstitial pressure, potentially reducing liposomal transport to tumor. These data indicate that hypervascularization plays the leading role in inhibition of liposomal drug to the tumor target. Each tumor type should be characterized separately to elucidate the optimal treatment formulation.

4 Conclusion

As targeted drug development moves forward, there is evidence that the implementation of the techniques and methodologies described here are contributing to a better understanding of the disposition of targeted drugs. For example, Hu et al. [102] utilized microdialysis to measure methotrexate in rat brains in vivo, and ultimately determined that the type of phosphatidylcholine used in formulation of the liposomal nanocarrier affected exposure and efficacy. Hopkins et al. [103] utilized MACS to isolate CD3+ T lymphocytes, from which they measured teriflunomide, the active metabolite of leflunomide, to probe a correlation between the drug concentration in cells and the high variability in efficacy observed among patients. Often the methodologies and techniques described herein are used in parallel to better correlate drug distribution and efficacy. IHC and flow cytometry are being used to complement each other in all stages of drug development from profiling cell-surface proteins to identify molecular targets for ADCs [104], to predicting how different CMAs will be cleared in vivo using ex vivo tests of MPS activity [105], to correlating the presence of tumor-associated macrophages with the exposure and clearance of various CMAs [106, 107]. Finally, MSI has revolutionized the way that drug distribution is studied in tumor and tissue, and has advanced our knowledge of targeted drug distribution. Several applications include the correlation of intratumoral distribution of receptor tyrosine kinase inhibitors with therapeutic efficacy [108], evaluation of MMAE release in tumor to guide the design of ADCs to target anti-human tissue factor [109], correlation of the heterogeneity or homogeneity of a drug in tumor with efficacy, which cannot be determined with traditional LC-MS/MS measurements [110, 111], and demonstration of the lower tumor exposure of MK-1775 in an intracranial model of GBM compared to flank, underscoring the requirement of therapies to cross the BBB to effectively treat brain cancers [112].

Acknowledgments

We thank Amanda Van Swearingen, Maria Sambade, and Carey Anders (Lineberger Comprehensive Cancer Center, University of North Carolina at Chapel Hill (UNC)) for the TNBC spleen samples; the UNC Mouse Phase 1 Unit (UNC) for the T11 spleen samples; the Animal Studies Core (UNC) for animal handling; Andrew Madden, Gina Song, Allison Schorzman, and William Zamboni (UNC Eshelman School of Pharmacy) for study design and sample processing; and Guillaume Robichaud, Jeremy Barry, and David Muddiman (Department of Chemistry, North Carolina State University) for MALDESI MSI analysis.

References

1. Ge Y, Tiwari A, Li S (2011) Nanomedicine – bridging the gap between nanotechnology and medicine. Adv Mater Lett 2(1):1–2
2. Caron WP, Song G, Kumar P et al (2012) Interpatient pharmacokinetic and pharmacodynamic variability of carrier-mediated anticancer agents. Clin Pharmacol Ther 91(5):802–812
3. Laginha K, Mumbengegwi D, Allen T (2005) Liposomes targeted via two different antibodies: assay, B-cell binding and cytotoxicity. Biochim Biophys Acta 1711(1):25–32
4. Yurkovetskiy AV, Hiller A, Syed S et al (2004) Synthesis of a macromolecular camptothecin conjugate with dual phase drug release. Mol Pharm 1(5):375–382
5. Zamboni WC (2005) Liposomal, nanoparticle, and conjugated formulations of anticancer agents. Clin Cancer Res 11(23):8230–8234
6. Zamboni WC, Gervais AC, Egorin MJ et al (2004) Systemic and tumor disposition of platinum after administration of cisplatin or STEALTH liposomal-cisplatin formulations (SPI-077 and SPI-077 B103) in a preclinical tumor model of melanoma. Cancer Chemother Pharmacol 53(4):329–336
7. Laverman P, Boerman OC, Oyen WJG et al (2001) In vivo applications of PEG liposomes: unexpected observations. Crit Rev Ther Drug Carrier Syst 18(6):551–566
8. Schell RF, Sidone BJ, Caron WP et al (2014) Meta-analysis of inter-patient pharmacokinetic variability of liposomal and non-liposomal anticancer agents. Nanomedicine 10(1):109–117
9. Zamboni WC (2008) Concept and clinical evaluation of carrier-mediated anticancer agents. Oncologist 13(3):248–260
10. Petschauer JS, Madden AJ, Kirschbrown WP et al (2015) The effects of nanoparticle drug loading on the pharmacokinetics of anticancer agents. Nanomedicine (Lond.) 10(3):446–463
11. Jain RK (1996) Delivery of molecular medicine to solid tumors. Science 271:1079
12. Zamboni WC, Houghton PJ, Hulstein JL et al (1999) Relationship between tumor extracellular fluid exposure to topotecan and response in human neuroblastoma xenografts and cell lines. Cancer Chemother Pharmacol 43:269–276
13. Balch CM, Reintgen DS, Kirkwood JM et al (1997) Cutaneous Melanoma. In: DeVita VT, Hellman S, Rosenberg SA (eds) Cancer: principles and practice of oncology, 5th edn. Lippincott-Raven, Philadelphia, p 1947
14. Muller M, Mader RM, Steiner B et al (1997) 5-fluorouracil kinetics in the interstitial tumor space: clinical response in breast cancer patients. Cancer Res 57:2598
15. Blochl-Daum B, Muller M, Meisinger V et al (1996) Measurement of extracellular fluid carboplatin kinetics in melanoma metastases with microdialysis. Br J Cancer 73:920
16. Yuan Q, Hein S, Misra RD (2010) New generation of chitosan-encapsulated ZnO quantum dots loaded with drug: synthesis, characterization and in vitro drug delivery response. Acta Biomater 6(7):2732–2739
17. Dipali SR, Kulkarni SB, Betageri GV (1996) Comparative study of separation of non-encapsulated drug from unilamellar liposomes by various methods. J Pharm Pharmacol 48:1112–1115
18. Mayer LD, St. Onge G (1995) Determination of free and liposome-associated doxorubicin and vincristine levels in plasma under equilibrium conditions employing ultrafiltration techniques. Anal Biochem 232(2):149–157
19. Zamboni WC, Strychor S, Joseph E et al (2007) Plasma, tumor, and tissue disposition of STEALTH liposomal CKD-602 (S-CKD602) and nonliposomal CKD-602 in mice bearing A375 human melanoma xenografts. Clin Cancer Res 13(23):7217
20. Song G, Darr DB, Santos CM et al (2014) Effects of tumor microenvironment heterogeneity on nanoparticle disposition and efficacy in breast cancer tumor models. Clin Cancer Res 20:6083–6095
21. Walsh MD, Hanna SK, Sen J et al (2012) Pharmacokinetics and antitumor efficacy of XMT-1001, a novel, polymeric topoisomerase I inhibitor, in mice bearing HT-29 human colon carcinoma xenografts. Clin Cancer Res 18(9):2591–2602
22. Young C, Schluep T, Hwang J et al (2011) CRLX101 (formerly IT-101)–a novel nanopharmaceutical of camptothecin in clinical development. Curr Bioact Compd 7(1):8–14
23. Musteata FM, Pawliszyn J, Qian MG et al (2006) Determination of drug plasma protein binding by solid phase microextraction. J Pharm Sci 95(8):1712–1722
24. Rowland M (1980) Plasma protein binding and therapeutic drug monitoring. Ther Drug Monitor 2:29–37
25. Tillement JP, Lhoste F, Giudicelli JF (1978) Diseases and drug protein binding. Clin Pharmacokinet 3(2):144–154
26. Taylor S, Harker A (2006) Modification of the ultrafiltration technique to overcome solubility

and non-specific binding challenges associated with the measurement of plasma protein binding corticosteroids. J Pharm Biomedical Analysis 41:299–303

27. Mortier KA, Lambert WE (2006) Determination of unbound docetaxel and paclitaxel in plasma by ultrafiltration and liquid chromatography –tandem mass spectrometry. J Chrom A 1108:195–201
28. U.S. Department of Health and Human Services, Food and Drug Administration Center for Drug Evaluation and Research (CDER), Center for Veterinary Medicine (CVM). Guidance for industry bioanalytical method validation. May 2001
29. Boucher Y, Jain RK (1992) Microvascular pressure is the principal driving force for interstitial hypertension in solid tumors: implication for vascular collapse. Cancer Res 52(5110):1992
30. Presant CA, Wolf W, Waluch V et al (1994) Association of intratumoral pharmacokinetics of fluorouracil with clinical response. Lancet 343:1184–1187
31. Front D, Isreal O, Iosilevsky G et al (1987) Human lung tumors: SPECT quantitation of differences in co-57 bleomycin uptake. Radiology 165:129–133
32. Fishman AJ, Alpert NM, Babich JW et al (1997) The role of positron emission tomography in pharmacokinetic analysis. Drug Metab Rev 29:923–956
33. Brunner M, Muller M (2002) Microdialysis: an in vivo approach for measuring drug delivery in oncology. Eur J Clin Pharmacol 58(4):227–234
34. Muller M, Schmid R, Georgopoulos A et al (1995) Application of microdialysis to clinical pharmacokinetics in humans. Clin Pharmacol Ther 57:371
35. Johansen MJ, Newman RA, Madden T (1997) The use of microdialysis in pharmacokinetics and pharmacodynamics. Pharmacotherapy 17:464
36. Kehr J (1993) A survey on quantitation microdialysis: theoretical models and practical limitations. J Neurosci Methods 48:251
37. Blakeley JO, Olson J, Grossman SA et al (2009) Effect of blood brain barrier permeability in recurrent high grade gliomas on the intratumoral pharmacokinetics of methotrexate: a microdialysis study. J Neuro-Oncol 91:51–58
38. Tegeder I, Brautigam L, Seegal M et al (2003) Cisplatin tumor concentrations after intraarterial cisplatin infusion or embolization in patients with oral cancer. Clin Pharmacol Ther 73:417–426
39. Chaurasia CS, Müller M, Bashaw EW et al (2007) AAPS-FDA workshop white paper: microdialysis principles, application, and regulatory perspectives report from the joint AAPS-FDA workshop, November 4-5, 2005, Nashville, TN. AAPS J 9(1):E48–E59
40. Leggas M, Zhuang Y, Welden J et al (2004) Microbore HPLC method with online microdialysis for measurement of topotecan lactone and carboxylate in murine CSF. J Pharm Sci 93:2284–2295
41. Ettinger SN, Poellmann CC, Wisniewski NA et al (2001) Urea as a recovery marker for quantitative assessment of tumor interstitial solutes with microdialysis. Cancer Res 61(21):7964–7970
42. Ekstrom PO, Andersen A, Saeter G et al (1997) Continuous intratumoral microdialysis during high-dose methotrexate therapy in a patient with malignant fibrous histiocytoma of the femur; a case report. Cancer Chemother Pharmacol 39(3):267–272
43. Thompson JF, Siebert GA, Anissimov YG et al (2001) Microdialysis and response during regional chemotherapy by isolated limb infusion of melphalan for limb malignancies. Br J Cancer 85(2):157–165
44. Conley BA, Ramsland TS, Sentz DL et al (1999) Antitumor activity, distribution, and metabolism of 13-cis-retinoic acid as a single agent or in combination with tamoxifen in established human MCF-7 xenografts in mice. Cancer Chemother Pharmacol 43:183–197
45. Zamboni WC, Gajjar AJ, Mandrell TD et al (1998) A four-hour topotecan infusion achieves cytotoxic exposure throughout the neuroaxis in the nonhuman primate model: implications for treatment of children with metastatic medulloblastoma. Clin Cancer Res 4(10):2537–2544
46. Shapiro H (1995) Practical flow cytometry. Wiley-Lis, New York
47. DePalma A (1997) Developments in biomagnetic separations focus on new affinity mechanisms. Genet Eng News 17:11
48. Busch J, Huber P, Pfluger E et al (1994) Enrichment of fetal cells from maternal blood by high gradient magnetic cell sorting (double MACS) for PCR-based genetic analysis. Prenatal Diagn 14:1129–1140
49. Miltenyi S, Muller W, Weichel W et al (1990) High gradient magnetic cell separation. Cytometry 11:231–238
50. Schmitz B, Radbruch A, Kummel T et al (1994) Magnetic activated cell sorting (MACS) is a new immunomagnetic method for megakaryocytic cell isolation: comparison of different separation techniques. Eur J Hematol 52:267–275

51. Manyonda IT, Soltys AJ, Hay FC (1992) A critical evaluation of the magnetic cell sorter and its use in the positive and negative selection of CD45RO+ cells. J Immunol Methods 149:1–10
52. Molday RS, Molday LL (1984) Separation of cells labeled with immunospecific iron dextran microspheres using high gradient magnetic chromatography. FEBS Lett 170(2):232–238
53. Blanchard D, Gaillard C, Hermann P et al (1994) Role of CD40 antigen and interleukin-2 in T cell-dependent human B lymphocyte growth. Eur J Immunol 4(2):330–335
54. Servida F, Soligo D, Caneva L et al (1996) Functional and morphological characterization of immunomagnetically selected CD34+ hematopoietic progenitor cells. Stem Cells 14(4):430–438
55. de Wynter EA, Coutinho LH, Pei X et al (1995) Comparison of purity and enrichment of CD34+ cells from bone marrow, umbilical cord and peripheral blood (primed for apheresis) using five separation systems. Stem Cells 13(5):524–532
56. Kato K, Radbruch A (1993) Isolation and characterization of CD34+ hematopoietic stem cells from human peripheral blood by high-gradient magnetic cell sorting. Cytometry 14(4):384–392
57. Radbruch A, Mechtold B, Thiel A et al (1997) In: Darzynkiewicz Z, Robinson JP, Crissman HA (eds) Methods cell biology. Academic Press, San Diego, pp 387–402
58. Thiele J, Wickenhauser C, Baldus SE et al (1995) Characterization of CD34+ human hemopoietic progenitor cells from the peripheral blood: enzyme-, carbohydrate- and immunocytochemistry, morphometry, and ultrastructure. Leuk Lymphoma 16(5–6):483–491
59. Irsch J, Hunzelmann N, Tesch H et al (1996) Effects of osteogenic protein-1 (OP-1, BMP-7) on bone matrix protein expression by fetal rat calvarial cells are differentiation stage specific. Immunotechnology 169(1):115–125
60. Miller MC, Doyle GV, Terstappen LW (2010) Significance of circulating tumor cells detected by the CellSearch™ system in patients with metastatic breast colorectal and prostate cancer. J Onco 2010:617421
61. Aichler M, Walch A (2015) MALDI imaging mass spectrometry: current frontiers and perspectives in pathology research and practice. Lab Investig 95(4):422–431
62. Nilsson A, Goodwin RJA, Shariatgorji M et al (2015) Mass spectrometry imaging in drug development. Anal Chem 87:1437–1455
63. Norris JL, Caprioli RM (2013) Analysis of tissue specimens by matrix-assisted laser desorption/ionization imaging mass spectrometry in biological and clinical research. Chem Rev 113(4):2309–2342
64. Prideaux B, Stoeckli M (2012) Mass spectrometry imaging for drug distribution studies. J Proteome 75:4999–5013
65. Solon E, Schweitzer A, Stoeckli A et al (2012) Autoradiography, MALDI-MS, and SIMS-MS imaging in pharmaceutical discovery and development. AAPS J 12:11–26
66. McDonnell LA, Heeren RMA (2007) Imaging mass spectrometry. Mass Spectrom Rev 26:606–643
67. Stoeckli M, Chaurand P, Hallahan DE et al (2001) Imaging mass spectrometry: a new technology for the analysis of protein expression in mammalian tissues. Nat Med 7(4):493–496
68. Christensen J, Litherland K, Faller T et al (2014) Biodistribution and metabolism studies of lipid nanoparticle-formulated internally [^{3}H]-labeled siRNA in mice. Drug Metab Dispos 42:431–440
69. Bruinen AL, van Oevelen C, Eijkel GB et al (2016) Mass spectrometry imaging of drug related crystal-like structures in formalin-fixed frozen and paraffin embedded rabbit kidney tissue sections. J Am Soc Mass Spectrom 24:117–123
70. Casadonte R, Caprioli RM (2011) Proteomic analysis of formalin-fixed paraffin-embedded tissue by MALDI imaging mass spectrometry. Nat Protoc 6(11):1695–1709
71. Vismeh R, Waldon DJ, Teffera Y et al (2012) Localization and quantification of drugs in animal tissues by use of desorption electrospray ionization mass spectrometry imaging. Anal Chem 84:5439–5445
72. Cornett DS, Frappier SL, Caprioli RM (2008) MALDI-FTICR imaging mass spectrometry of drugs and metabolites in tissue. Anal Chem 80:5648–5653
73. Kolarova L, Vanhara P, Pena-Mendez EM et al (2014) Tissue visualization mediated by nanoparticles: from tissue staining to mass spectrometry tissue profiling and imaging. In: Seifalian A, de Mal A, Kalaskar DM (eds) Nanomedicine. One Central Press, Manchester, UK, pp 468–489
74. Greer T, Sturm R, Li L (2011) Mass spectrometry imaging for drugs and metabolites. J Proteome 74:2617–2631
75. Mascini NE, Eijkel GB, ter Brugge P et al (2015) The use of mass spectrometry imaging to predict treatment response of patient-derived xenograft models of triple-negative breast cancer. J Proteomic Res 14:1069–1075

76. Robichaud G, Barry JA, Muddiman DC (2014) IR-MALDESI mass spectrometry imaging of biological tissue sections using ice as a matrix. J Am Soc Mass Spectrom 25:319–328
77. Sampson JS, Hawkridge AM, Muddiman DC (2006) Generation and detection of multiply-charged peptides and proteins by matrix-assisted laser desorption electrospray ionization (MALDESI) Fourier transform ion cyclotron resonance mass spectrometry. J Am Soc Mass Spectrom 17:1712–1716
78. Nazari M, Muddiman DC (2015) Cellular-level mass spectrometry imaging using infrared matrix-assisted laser desorption electrospray ionization (IR-MALDESI) by oversampling. Anal Bioanal Chem 407:2265–2271
79. Jurchen JC, Rubakhin SS, Sweedler JV (2005) MALDI-MS imaging of features snaller than the size of the laser beam. J Am Soc Mass Spectrom 16(10):1654–1659
80. Bokhart MT, Rosen E, Thompson C et al (2015) Quantitative mass spectrometry imaging of emtricitabine in cervical tissue model using infrared matrix-assisted laser desorption electrospray ionization. Anal Bioanal Chem 407(8):2073–2084
81. Pockley AG, Foulds GA, Oughton JA et al (2015) Immune cell phenotyping using flow cytometry. Curr Protoc Toxicol 66:18.8.1–18.834
82. Boland JW, Foulds GA, Ahmedzai SH et al (2014) A preliminary evaluation of the effects of opioids on innate and adaptive human in vitro immune function. BMJ Support Palliat Care 4:357–367
83. Caron WP, Lay JC, Fong AM et al (2013) Translational studies of phenotypic probes for the mononuclear phagocyte system and liposomal pharmacology. J Pharmacol Exp Ther 347:599–606
84. Brahmer JR, Drake CG, Wollner I et al (2010) Phase I study of single-agent anti-programmed death-1 (MDX-1106) in refractory solid tumors: safety, clinical activity, pharmacodynamics, and immunologic correlates. J Clin Oncol 28:3167–3175
85. Latek R, Fleener C, Lamian V et al (2009) Assessment of belatacept-mediated costimulation blockade through evaluation of CD80/86-receptor saturation. Transplantation 87:926–933
86. Dunphy CH (2004) Applications of flow cytometry and immunohistochemistry to diagnostic hematopathology. Arch Pathol Lab Med 128:1004–1022
87. Al-Mawali A, Gillis D, Lewis I (2009) The role of multiparameter flow cytometry for detection of minimal residual disease in acute myeloid leukemia. Am J Clin Pathol 131(1):16–26
88. Muratori M, Forti G, Baldi E (2008) Comparing flow cytometry and fluorescence microscopy for analyzing human sperm DNA fragmentation by TUNEL labeling. Cytometry A 73(9):785–787. https://doi.org/10.1002/cyto.a.20615
89. Knetter SM, Tuggle CK, Wannemuehler MJ et al (2014) Organic barn dust extract exposure impairs porcine macrophage function in vitro: implications for respiratoryhealth. Vet Immunol Immunopathol 157(1–2):20–30
90. Murtas D, Maric D, De Giorgi V (2013) IRF-1 responsiveness to IFN-_ predicts different cancer immune phenotypes. Br J Cancer 109(1):76–82
91. Barteneva NS, Fasler-Kan E, Vorobjev IA (2012) Imaging flow cytometry: coping with heterogeneity in biological systems. J Histochem Cytochem 60(10):723–733
92. Marangon I, Boggetto N, Ménard-Moyon C et al (2012) Intercellular carbon nanotube translocation assessed by flow cytometry imaging. Nano Lett 12(9):4830–4837
93. Wulff S (ed) (2006) Flow cytometry educational guide, 2nd edn. Dako, Fort Collins, CO., Carpinteria
94. Watson JV (1999) The early fluidic and optical physics of cytometry. Cytometry 38:1–14
95. Orfao A, Ruiz-Arguelles A, Lacombe F et al (1995) Flow cytometry: its applications in hematology. Haematologica 80:69–81
96. Mandy FF, Bergeron M, Minkus T (1995) Principles of flow cytometry. Transfus Sci 16:303–314
97. Recktenwald DJ (1993) Introduction to flow cytometry: principles, fluorochromes, instrument set-up, calibration. J Hematother 2:387–394
98. Wittwer CT, Knape WA, Bristow MR et al (1989) The quantitative flow cytometric plasma OKT3 assay. Its potential application in cardiac transplantation. Transplantation 48:533–535
99. Fulton RJ, McDade RL, Smith PL et al (1997) Advanced multiplexed analysis with the FlowMetrix system. Clin Chem 43:1749–1756
100. Lucas A, Madden AJ, Zamboni WC (2015) Formulation and physiologic factors affecting the pharmacology of carrier-mediated anticancer agents. Expert Opin Drug Metab Toxicol 11(9):1419–1433
101. Jain RK, Stylianopoulos T (2010) Delivering nanomedicine to solid tumors. Nat Rev Clin Oncol 7:653–664

102. Hu Y, Rip J, Gaillard PJ et al (2017) The impact of liposomal formulations on the release and brain delivery of methotrexate: an in vivo microdialysis study. J Pharm Sci. https://doi.org/10.1016/j.xphs.2017.03.009
103. Hopkins AM, Moghaddami M, Foster DJ et al (2017) Intracellular CD3+ T lymphocyte teriflunomide concentration is poorly correlated with and has greater variability than unbound plasma teriflunomide concentration. Drug Metab Dispos 45(1):8–16
104. Guo P, Yang J, Bielenberg DR et al (2017) A quantitative method for screening and identifying molecular targets for nanomedicine. J Control Release. https://doi.org/10.1016/j.jconrel.2017.03.030
105. Lucas AT, Herity LB, Kornblum ZA et al (2017) Pharmacokinetic and screening studies of the interaction between mononuclear phagocyte system and nanoparticle formulations and colloid forming drugs. Int J Pharm 526(1-2):443–454
106. Lucas AT, White TF, Deal AM et al (2017) Profiling the relationship between tumor-associated macrophages and pharmacokinetics of liposomal agents in preclinical murine models. Nanomedicine 13(2):471–482
107. Li F, Ulrich M, Jonas M et al (2017) Tumor associated macrophages can contribute to antitumor activity through FcgR-mediated processing of antibody-drug conjugates. Mol Cancer Ther. https://doi.org/10.1158/1535-7163.MCT-17-0019
108. Torok S, Rezeli M, Kelemen O et al (2017) Limited tumor tissue drug penetration contributes to primary resistance against angiogenesis inhibitors. Theranostics 7(2):400–412
109. Fujiwara Y, Masaru F, Manabe S et al (2016) Imaging mass spectrometry for the precise design of antibody-drug conjugates. Sci Rep 6:24954
110. Giordano S, Zucchetti M, Decio A et al (2016) Heterogeneity of paclitaxel distribution in different tumor models assessed by MALDI mass spectrometry imaging. Sci Rep 6:39284
111. Salphati L, Alicke B, Heffron TP et al (2016) Brain distribution and efficacy of the brain penetrant PI3K inhibitor GDC-0084 in orthotopic mouse models of human glioblastoma. Drug Metab Disp 44:1881–1889
112. Pokorny JL, Calligaris D, Gupta SK et al (2015) The efficacy of the Wee1 inhibitor MK-1775 combined with temozolomide is limited by heterogenous distribution across the blood-brain barrier in glioblastoma. Clin Cancer Res 21(8):1916–1924

INDEX

Rachael W. Sirianni and Bahareh Behkam (eds.), *Targeted Drug Delivery: Methods and Protocols*, Methods in Molecular Biology, vol. 1831, https://doi.org/10.1007/978-1-4939-8661-3, © Springer Science+Business Media, LLC, part of Springer Nature 2018

Printed by Printforce, the Netherlands